BLOOD POISON

BLOOD POISON

THE UNTOLD
STORY *of* SEPSIS

PARSA SHAHINPOOR, MD

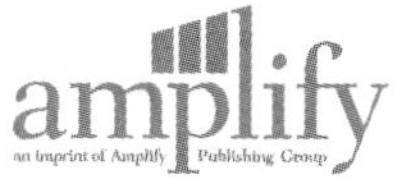

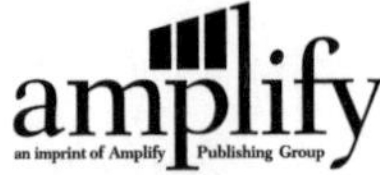

www.amplifypublishinggroup.com

Blood Poison: The Untold Story of Sepsis

This book is not intended as a substitute for the medical advice of physicians. The reader should regularly consult a physician in matters relating to their health and particularly with respect to any symptoms that may require diagnosis or medical attention.

Some names and identifying details have been changed to protect the privacy of individuals.

For more information, please contact:
Amplify Publishing, an imprint of Amplify Publishing Group
620 Herndon Parkway, Suite 220
Herndon, VA 20170
info@amplifypublishing.com

Library of Congress Control Number: 2025925959

CPSIA Code: PRV0226A

ISBN-13: 979-8-89138-716-4

Printed in the United States

The names of the patients whose lives we save can never be known.
Our contribution will be what did not happen to them.
And, though they are unknown, we will know that mothers and fathers
are at graduations and weddings they would have missed,
and that grandchildren will know grandparents they might never have known,
and holidays will be taken, and work completed, and books read,
and symphonies heard, and gardens tended that,
without our work, would never have been.

—DONALD. M. BERWICK, MD, MPP, past president
and CEO, Institute for Healthcare Improvement, 2004[1]

Contents

AUTHOR'S NOTE . . . . *xi*

PROLOGUE . . . . *xiii*
    Rory

INTRODUCTION . . . . *xvii*
    The Silent Killer

Part I

CHAPTER ONE 3
    Bacterial Shock

CHAPTER TWO 19
    Putrefaction

CHAPTER THREE 29
    Germs

CHAPTER FOUR 47
    Magic Bullets and Murphy's Law

CHAPTER FIVE 67
    Changing Patterns of Infection

CHAPTER SIX 83
    "It's Our Response That Makes the Disease"

CHAPTER SEVEN 99
    Trials and Tribulations

CHAPTER EIGHT 117
    SIRS

CHAPTER NINE 135
    The Golden Hour

Part II

CHAPTER TEN 157
The Rips

CHAPTER ELEVEN 173
Bending the World

CHAPTER TWELVE 193
Surviving Sepsis

CHAPTER THIRTEEN 211
Rory's Lessons

CHAPTER FOURTEEN 229
Regulations and Regression

CHAPTER FIFTEEN 251
Mickey

CHAPTER SIXTEEN 271
The Pandemic

CHAPTER SEVENTEEN 283
What Really Matters

CHAPTER EIGHTEEN 297
Getting It Right

CHAPTER NINETEEN 317
Hereafter

EPILOGUE 333
Save a Life, Save the World

ACKNOWLEDGMENTS 339

NOTES 343

INDEX 401

ABOUT THE AUTHOR 415

Author's Note

Since the dawn of medicine, sepsis has been one of its most confounding and dangerous conditions. Its modern understanding first took shape on pre-antibiotic battlefields and hospital wards as "septicemia," or the deleterious effect of microbes and their toxins coursing through the bloodstream. It has more recently been understood as an elusive disorder in which the body's immune response to infection spirals out of control, with immediate and deadly consequences.

Most people associate sepsis with "blood poisoning," but this is a misconception. Though bloodstream infections often cause sepsis, the condition can emerge from virtually *any* infection in the body.

Like cancer, sepsis is not one entity but many. It is not a classical disease with a straightforward cause-and-effect relationship. It is a *syndrome*—a convergence of causes and events happening in sequence. Thus, its fundamental nature makes it difficult to detect and treat.

I wrote this book for anyone interested in sepsis and its history and those who wish to understand how the healthcare system operates today. It is written for both general readers and medical professionals, which was a difficult line to walk at times. There are a few sections where the book may dive deep into science and research. Those who wish to chart a less technical path can gloss over these sections, as they aren't crucial to capturing the overall substance of the story.

There are many footnotes (and even more endnotes). These are mostly for researchers, physicians, experts, or anyone seeking additional details. The book's formidable length will likely be more manageable for those who wish to skip the notes.

This book belongs to generations of dedicated people who have contributed to the field of sepsis, countless individuals whom I've spoken to and interviewed, as well as those who have reviewed the book's content. It encompasses not just my thoughts but those of many others, whom I have gone to great lengths to reference and credit.

Moreover, to paraphrase the physician-author Siddhartha Mukherjee, I stand on the shoulders of giants in writing this book. Its intention, style, and tone are meant to contribute to a long tradition of physician-written narrative nonfiction.

I write *Blood Poison* with great humility. I once thought I understood sepsis; now I see it as a subject so vast that it would take not one lifetime but many generations to fully comprehend. So I offer this book not as an end, but as a beginning.

Above all, this endeavor would not have been possible without the patients and families whose stories have touched my life and shaped me as a physician. I am deeply grateful to these courageous individuals and give my greatest acknowledgment to them as my teachers and inspiration. I share their stories with deep reverence while recognizing the importance of maintaining their confidentiality.

Many of the stories in this book involve real individuals—drawn either from published accounts in newspapers and medical journals or told with the express permission of the patients or their families. In those instances, I have used real names and dates. Other stories are fictionalized accounts based on actual clinical experiences, in which names, dates, medical details, and identifying characteristics have been altered to protect privacy while preserving the essential truths of the encounters. The names and identifying details of some of the other people mentioned in the book have also been changed to protect their privacy.

Rory

NEW YORK CITY, NEW YORK

ON THE EVENING OF FRIDAY, March 30, 2012, Rory Staunton arrived at NYU Langone's pediatric emergency room in critical condition. The ER staff rushed to stabilize his vital signs while a chorus of alarms blared in the background. Amid it all, a doctor pulled his mother, Orlaith, aside.

"Your son is very ill," he said.

The words barely registered.

Rory was a strong, towering twelve-year-old boy. He'd grown up with his sister, Kathleen, in Sunnyside Gardens, a charming village in Queens with family homes made of Hudson brick. Its summers brought backyard barbeques, ball games, and packs of children running from house to house playing tag.

A foot taller than all the other kids, Rory looked after them. It was no surprise that he was the president of Kidadelphia, the Garden Kids' self-declared republic, whose motto was "In God and Fun We Trust."

Now, as his parents stood frozen in the emergency room, nothing made sense. Just hours earlier, Rory had been laughing and talking about his future. And yet here he was, at the brink of death.

Two days before that, Rory had scraped his elbow while lunging for a basketball during gym class. He'd shown it to his gym teacher, who had applied a Band-Aid.

"Go ahead and finish the game," he'd said.

That evening, Rory mentioned it to Orlaith, who thought little of it. Afterward, he finished his homework, ate pizza, and went to bed.

Orlaith awoke in the middle of the night to the sound of retching. She rushed to the bathroom and found Rory hunched over the toilet. He winced as she placed her hand on his back.

"My leg hurts," he cried out.

She tried to comfort him, helping him back to bed and gently rubbing his leg until he fell asleep.

The next morning, he developed a fever of 104°F. Concerned, Orlaith and her husband, Ciaran, called the family pediatrician, who scheduled an appointment for later that evening. At the doctor's office, Rory sat pale and feverish, his heart beating fast at 140 beats per minute, his breathing rapid. A strep test came back negative. Orlaith described his worsening symptoms: the vomiting, the leg pain, and a strange mottled rash developing on his skin.

The pediatrician suggested the leg pain was related to his fall.

"It wasn't a fall. It was a skid," Rory interjected.

The doctor examined his elbow. No redness, no swelling, nothing outwardly concerning. As for the rash on his leg, she said she wasn't concerned about it.

She suspected a stomach virus. One had been spreading in the community. Her recommendation: take Rory to the pediatric emergency room for intravenous fluids.

They arrived at the emergency room at 7:14 p.m. During triage, Rory's pulse was racing, but his temperature had fallen to 100°F—just shy of a fever. After checking him in, a nurse drew his blood and started an IV. An hour later, his white blood cell count came back high—over 14,000, a potential sign of a bacterial infection.

The emergency medicine physician diagnosed him with viral gastroenteritis—a stomach flu. It was nothing to worry about. She signed the discharge papers at 9:14 p.m., writing "patient improved" in the chart.

A few minutes later, Rory's fever spiked to 102°F. The ER staff reassured the Stauntons that they had seen similar patients in the community. Convinced that rest and fluids were all he needed, they took their son home.

That night, Rory burned with fever. He groaned in his sleep, tossing and turning. Orlaith and Ciaran watched over him, taking comfort, believing this was a good sign: his body fighting the infection.

But by morning, something had changed. Rory was a shell of himself. The Stauntons called his pediatrician. She encouraged them to give him fluids and wait it out.

As the day passed, Rory grew weaker by the hour. He could hardly sit up straight, had no appetite, and grew more silent as the day progressed. CNN was playing on the television—one of Rory's favorite channels—but he simply turned away and kept sleeping.

Ciaran contacted the pediatrician again. She said to give more fluids.

"I'm not sure you're getting the picture," Ciaran snapped. "I can't even get him to sit up; I don't know how you expect me to get fluids into him."

It was a tense exchange. The Stauntons were panicked.

The pediatrician finally yielded.

"Take him back to the hospital," she said.

The Stauntons ran Rory back to NYU Langone, rushing through the ER doors at 7:00 p.m. on Friday. By then, his blood pressure was nearly undetectable, his body practically limp.

This time, there was no mistaking the urgency of the situation. The medical staff rushed in from every direction. He was admitted to the ICU in less than an hour.

After that, Rory's condition worsened quickly. A decision was made to initiate life support. As the medical staff hurried around him, the Stauntons remained at his bedside, disguising their concern with small talk. Meanwhile, Rory fixed his gaze on Orlaith.

"Mom, my toes are cold. My toes are cold."

Orlaith held Rory's hand. Before sedating him, a physician assessed his mental status by asking him to name the president.

"Barack Obama," Rory answered.

Orlaith smiled.

"Ah, but Rory, who is going to be the next one?" she asked.

Rory grinned weakly. "Barack Obama."

Even in a weakened state, he held on to the things that mattered most. Politics. Justice. When he was eleven, he'd written a letter to the president of North Korea, asking why he had so many luxuries while his people suffered. In seventh grade, he'd been elected to the student council and led a campaign called Spread the Word to End the Word to stop children from using the word "retarded" as an insult. Orlaith had known Rory was becoming a leader—someone who could shape the world.

By Sunday, a dire truth had emerged. Blood cultures tested positive for

Streptococcus pyogenes, a skin bacterium. It had likely invaded his bloodstream from his elbow wound, festering for days unnoticed until it ignited a full-blown system failure.

With each hour, Rory's organs began shutting down one by one. His kidneys stopped making urine. His fingers, toes, and nose turned black from poor circulation. His blood stopped clotting. Two back-to-back cardiac arrests signaled that his heart was giving out.

The ICU team fought desperately to bring him back, but with each blow, he drifted further out of reach. Family and friends gathered in a vigil around his room. His doctors and nurses struggled to stop the onslaught, remaining at his bedside for most of the day. But by the third arrest, there was nothing left. On the night of April 1, 2012—just four days after scraping his elbow—Rory Staunton's heart beat for the last time.[1]

The Silent Killer

We have the technology and resources today to treat most conditions and injuries, yet infection, which has been killing people since history began, still defeats us.

—PROFESSOR GRAHAM RAMSAY, past president,
European Society of Intensive Care Medicine, October 2, 2002[1]

ON APRIL 1, 2012, A vibrant community in Queens, New York, was shaken by the unexpected death of twelve-year-old Rory Staunton. His cause of death was sepsis, resulting from a minor scrape of the skin. It was a tragedy at the hands of humanity's most enigmatic malady, and it revealed deep fault lines beneath the surface of the world's most advanced healthcare system.

At the time of Rory's death, sepsis remained a vague and misunderstood entity.[2] Most doctors recognized it as the body's extreme reaction to infection, yet its defining characteristics were still a matter of debate. Unlike a heart attack or stroke, sepsis lacked a single defining event. Instead, it emerged as a murky constellation of signs and symptoms—a *syndrome* rather than a straightforward disease with a clear cause-and-effect relationship. This meant that even the most seasoned physicians often struggled to decipher its warning signs before it was too late.

Rory's is one of history's most impactful sepsis accounts, but not the first. Many before him had fallen to this syndrome, their stories etched in the archives of medicine. Even today, millions of patients—many young, previously healthy—slip through the cracks as victims of this silent killer that medicine has yet to fully grasp.

To understand these tragedies, we must first understand sepsis itself: how it hijacks the body's defense system, why it defies easy classification, and how its chameleonic nature challenges even the most advanced healthcare institutions. We must also examine the underlying flaws in the medical system, how doctors think, how hospitals function, and why lifesaving knowledge sometimes takes years to reach the front lines.

The most recent scientific definition of sepsis is "a life-threatening state of organ dysfunction caused by a dysregulated host response to infection."[3] At its core, sepsis is the body's own rebellion.[4] It begins as an appropriate response to infection but spirals into chaos, attacking vital organs like the brain and kidneys.

Once, at sixteen, I landed awkwardly on a friend's foot during a basketball game. I heard a loud snap as my foot twisted outward. My ankle swelled like a balloon, and an intense throbbing pain followed. The doctor diagnosed a severe ankle sprain. The swelling and pain were my body's inflammatory response—an essential mechanism for healing. The injury triggered the response, but the response itself wasn't the injury. It was the body's way of mobilizing resources to repair the damage, but in this case, it was exaggerated.

The body mounts a similar response to infection, which we will discuss in later chapters. For now, the best way to understand sepsis is that it occurs when this response becomes erratic and harms the body itself.

In the words of leading sepsis expert Dr. Mitchell Levy, "Your body liberates inflammatory mediators, and sometimes those mediators help you fight infection, and sometimes they begin to attack organ systems."[5]

The difference between healing and destruction lies in a delicate balance—one that sepsis shatters.

The incidence of sepsis remains muddy as medical experts still disagree about its clinical definition. Current estimates suggest that around fifty million cases occur worldwide each year. In the United States, figures vary widely, ranging from 900,000 to 3.1 million cases annually. A 2017 epidemiologic study placed the incidence at 1.7 million cases, though some experts believe this may be an underestimate.[6]

Sepsis is by far one of the deadliest conditions faced by doctors today, with a mortality rate of approximately 20 percent.* In the US, this translates to 350,000 deaths yearly.[7] Its effects are even more staggering on the global stage, resulting in an estimated eleven million deaths annually, accounting for one in every five fatalities from all causes. It is also the leading cause of death among children worldwide, claiming eight thousand young lives every day.[8]

Even those who survive sepsis often endure lifelong physical and cognitive impairments.[9] Nearly a quarter of survivors are readmitted within months, and almost half die within five years—making sepsis an even grimmer diagnosis than many forms of cancer.[10]

The burden of sepsis falls heavily on society's most vulnerable—children, seniors, pregnant women, and those in low-income communities with limited access to clean water, vaccinations, and medical care.[11] In wealthier nations, it exploits the weaknesses of overburdened healthcare systems, disproportionately affecting patients with chronic conditions, hospital-acquired infections, and preventable diseases such as influenza, COVID-19, and bacterial pneumonia.

Sepsis is also the costliest reason for hospital care, and these expenditures keep rising. A study of American hospitals published in 2020 estimated the total cost of sepsis care to be around sixty-two billion dollars.[12] Globally, the figures vary significantly. A recent review of twenty-six studies shows an average cost of about thirty-nine thousand dollars per sepsis case.[13] Applying this to nearly fifty million cases each year results in an estimated global cost of about two trillion dollars annually, roughly equivalent to the GDP of Italy.†

————

My journey to unravel the mysteries of sepsis began in 2000 as a medical student, confronting its cryptic presence in hospital wards. It continued through my internal medicine residency, where I regularly found myself caring for patients in septic shock—the condition's late and most perilous stage.

At the turn of the twenty-first century, sepsis was recognized in academic medical circles but rarely on the average clinician's radar. It often lacked the urgency given to other emergency conditions like heart attacks, strokes, and

---

* A mortality rate of 20 percent means that, on average, 20 percent (one in five) of affected patients die.

† The cost of sepsis care varies considerably from country to country, but this is a reasonable estimate.

trauma. There were no streamlined protocols, no sepsis alerts. Patients deteriorated gradually, unnoticed, until they'd crossed an invisible threshold into disaster. Meanwhile, outside medicine, the term "sepsis" was virtually unknown. Patients and families stared back in confusion whenever I mentioned it at the bedside. This lack of visibility captures the central struggle of sepsis: a fight for recognition within medicine and in the public eye.

In 2002, an alliance between the sepsis research community and the medical industry launched the Surviving Sepsis Campaign (SSC), one of the largest public health initiatives in history. Its mission was to elevate awareness and standardize best practices for sepsis treatment worldwide. At the same time, stories like that of Rory Staunton began reaching the public, forcing both families and clinicians to pay attention. As the SSC worked to unify clinical care, these personal tragedies galvanized advocacy, spurred hospitals to adopt protocols, and gradually brought sepsis into the mainstream consciousness.

I was part of this movement. Beginning in 2009, as a hospitalist at Kaiser Permanente in Portland, Oregon, I helped lead a sepsis quality improvement program across two major hospitals serving more than one hundred thousand patients yearly.

At first, "quality improvement" appeared to be a lackluster version of the heroism I had always admired. Officially defined as "the framework used to systematically enhance care," it involved tediously understanding workflows, statistics, and human behavior and then using this knowledge to implement incremental changes in frontline operations.

In other words, it was the most unglamorous way to make a difference in the world. It was the monotonous part of a movie squeezed into the montage scene.

I was skeptical. I had gone into medicine to treat patients, not sift through spreadsheets and protocols.

But my mentor, Dr. David Schmidt, put it simply: "You're making a difference not just in the lives of individual patients but in the population as a whole."[14]

Over time, these incremental changes could move mountains.

The first step was as fundamental as awareness. Simply getting frontline professionals to ask, "Could it be sepsis?" often meant the difference between life and death. Half the battle was recognizing there *was* a battle. This insight had eluded too many healthcare professionals for too long. We needed to foster a culture of vigilance, ensuring that doctors and nurses understood sepsis and remained attuned to its earliest, most subtle signs.

Then came complexity. Medicine is a flickering tapestry of a thousand intricate details. Physician-writers like Atul Gawande have drawn attention to this: a system teeming with highly trained professionals, cutting-edge technology, and powerful medications yet still befuddled by conditions like sepsis.[15] Despite our advancements, tragedies like Rory's continue to occur, exposing the limits of even the most sophisticated medical systems.

Awareness was crucial, but it was only the beginning. Real change required orchestrating a complex network—integrating frontline emergency room protocols, computerized early warning systems, and laboratory diagnostics. Beyond technology, we had to master the science, shift ingrained behaviors, and refine the mechanics of how the healthcare system functioned.

———

Today, doctors remain divided on the best approach to sepsis detection and treatment. Since 1991, there have been three major efforts to establish a universal definition of sepsis, yet experts still disagree, leaving frontline clinicians uncertain about who is affected. Others question the evidence base that underpins treatment protocols.

Even when new knowledge emerges, the gears of medicine turn slowly. It can take years, sometimes decades, for scientific discoveries to reach the bedside. The reasons are many: inertia, reluctance to change, and the weight of broader systemic forces. The Surviving Sepsis Campaign offered a case in point. Hailed as a landmark initiative in global sepsis care, it was also shadowed by skepticism and controversy from the start—a reminder of how progress in medicine rarely comes without resistance.

Under mounting pressure from patient advocacy groups and the ongoing tragedy of preventable sepsis deaths, government health agencies have begun enforcing regulations requiring hospitals to adopt standardized sepsis protocols. Many see this as necessary. Others view the regulations as rigid, intrusive, and not firmly grounded in evidence. As we will explore in this book, several medical societies now openly challenge these regulations, highlighting the ongoing pull between policy and clinical autonomy.

In this way, the struggle against sepsis mirrors larger tensions within modern medicine: progress versus resistance, cutting-edge research versus outdated systems, and individual patient care versus large-scale initiatives.

Meanwhile, the healthcare front line has been buckling under the growing burden of chronic disease, deepening socioeconomic disparities, and widespread gaps in access to care. The COVID-19 pandemic only intensified these issues, pushing healthcare systems to the brink as they struggle to uphold even basic standards of care. Adding to this is rising burnout among physicians and nurses and an erosion of public trust in medical and scientific institutions.

———

This book explores the history and science of sepsis, its elusive nature, and the human stories behind the statistics. Through patient experiences and frontline accounts, it will take readers into the heart of the crisis—where doctors and nurses race against time, innovation collides with inertia, and lives are lost and saved.

Above all, I want readers to walk away with a clear answer to a crucial question: what is sepsis? Beyond that, I hope to deepen their understanding of the challenges surrounding its diagnosis and treatment, as well as the vulnerabilities in our healthcare system that are fueling the rising toll of sepsis-related deaths.

At its core, this book is about two simple but profound truths: prevention and early intervention.[16] Hippocrates once wrote, "Prophylaxis is much better than therapy."[17] Medicine has long emphasized treating disease over preventing it. With sepsis, this has left a trail of avoidable death and tragedy, and it is steering us toward an unsustainable future. The bottom line is that many, if not most, sepsis-causing infections are preventable through measures such as hygiene, infection control, and vaccination, to name a few. And once sepsis *does* occur, extensive data show that the sooner we treat it, the more likely patients will survive.

We stand at a crossroads—an increasingly isolated, divided, and uncertain society that faces existential threats. Public trust in medical and scientific institutions is waning. Meanwhile, healthcare workers and public servants face long hours and under-resourced systems. The wounds of the COVID-19 pandemic still linger individually and collectively.

In this light, this story is also one of progress and hope—of what is possible when families, doctors, and advocates refuse to accept the status quo. Rory Staunton's death was a tragedy, but it ignited a movement—a movement that has already saved thousands of lives and holds the promise to save millions more.

Part I

Bacterial Shock

I know it when I see it.

—US SUPREME COURT JUSTICE
POTTER STEWART, in *Jacobellis v. Ohio*, 1964[1]

WHEN I WAS IN MEDICAL SCHOOL in the early 2000s, I learned that sepsis was the body's severe response to infection. Common wisdom confined it to hospital wards and intensive care units—a crisis that unfolded late in the course of illness. By the time patients were diagnosed, they were often very sick, their odds of survival no better than a coin toss.

As students, we discovered that most diseases, like heart attacks and strokes, followed a well-mapped trajectory. For example, in a stroke, an errant blood clot would lodge in a cerebral artery, cutting off blood flow and causing death or necrosis of brain tissue. The effects were immediate and precise, and symptoms correlated with the region of the brain affected.

Sepsis defied such logic. Like a storm, its emergence was gradual, complex, and difficult to define in its earliest stages—an obscure cascade of events rather than a clear, singular occurrence. In other words, a syndrome.

In those days, the word "sepsis" was used interchangeably with "septicemia" or "blood poisoning"—a condition defined by the presence of microbes or their toxins in the bloodstream. "Septicemia" was an antiquated term, having emerged nearly two centuries earlier in the grim hospital wards and blood-soaked battlefields of the pre-antibiotic era, when unchecked bacterial infections decimated entire populations.

During that time, sepsis was typically recognized only after bacteria had already overrun the body, coursing through the bloodstream, resulting in disastrous illness. These dreadful accounts left the medical community with a lasting misconception that sepsis was almost always the result of bloodborne bacterial infections and existed primarily in its most severe state: deadly shock.

As a term, "shock" has its origins in the writings of eighteenth-century French surgeon Henri François Le Dran, who described the *saisissement*—sudden "shock" or astonishment—he observed in gunshot victims.[2] For nearly two centuries, it remained a disorder of the nervous system, believed to be triggered by severe physical trauma.[3] It wasn't until the work of others, notably American surgeon Alfred Blalock in the 1930s, that it became a disorder of blood circulation—the result of inadequate blood flow or perfusion to vital organs.[4]

We now define shock as a condition of persistently low blood pressure in the arteries combined with evidence of low perfusion to organs. Low blood pressure is defined as a systolic pressure of less than 90 or a mean arterial pressure (MAP) of less than 65 millimeters of mercury (mmHg).[*]

By the time I was in training, the standard case study for sepsis was a bacterium known as *Escherichia coli* (*E. coli*). Throughout the second half of the twentieth century, it was notorious for causing severe bloodstream infections (bacteremia) and septic shock.

E. coli is referred to as a "gram-negative" bacterium because its outer membrane fails to retain an aniline dye called gentian violet—the first step in a laboratory procedure known as the "Gram stain." The technique, developed in 1884 by the talented Danish microbiologist Hans Christian Gram, transformed microbiology by allowing scientists to visualize bacteria better under the microscope.[†][5]

---

[*] The term "millimeters of mercury (mmHg)" refers to the fluid pressure required to raise a column of liquid mercury one millimeter up a glass tube. Blood pressure is indicated by two numbers representing the two components of the cardiac cycle: systole (when the heart contracts) and diastole (when the heart relaxes). A normal blood pressure of 110/60 represents a systolic pressure of 110 and a diastolic pressure of 60. The mean arterial pressure (MAP) is the average pressure throughout the arteries during the cardiac cycle (systole and diastole). It is a better indicator of the blood pressure affecting the blood supply or perfusion to vital organs. It's calculated using the following equation: MAP = diastolic pressure + 1/3 (systolic pressure – diastolic pressure).

[†] During Gram staining, gentian violet dye combines with iodine to form a complex that binds tightly to a key polymer in the bacterial cell wall, called peptidoglycan, fixing the stain on the bacterial cell wall, even after an alcohol rinse. Gram-*positive* bacteria have a

Like most bacteria, *E. coli* is usually harmless.[6] One of its natural habitats is the human gut, where it resides as a relatively amicable colonizer or symbiont, peacefully coexisting with other bacteria that make up the normal intestinal flora.[7] Yet certain conditions can make *E. coli* problematic and even lethal, and these conditions have become more common in the modern age.

In the 1950s, doctors began to see a steady rise in infections by *E. coli* and other gram-negative bacteria.[8] By the time I was in medical school, they were one of the most common causes of severe bloodstream infections and sepsis. After infecting a site in the human body, the bacteria multiplied and spread to surrounding areas. In the medical wards, we commonly saw this in bladder and kidney infections, plus infections of the uterus, gallbladder, bile ducts, intestines, and even the lungs and skin.[9] On the surgical wards, we saw gram-negative infections with severe penetrating abdominal injuries like gunshot wounds and stabbings and with spontaneous injuries like perforated stomach ulcers and intestinal ruptures.

Regardless of the source, infections were usually triggered by disruptions in the normal boundaries and conditions where bacteria existed. This allowed bacterial colonists, like *E. coli*, to escape their confines, finding new places to proliferate. It was the definition of *infection*: the unwanted presence and multiplication of germs in the body. In the case of *E. coli*, it also represented a transformation from symbiont to pathogen.*[10]

By the early 2000s, infections of the bladder and kidneys—urinary tract infections (UTIs)—had become some of the most common gram-negative bacterial infections. By the time I was on my hospital rotations, they were also one of the most frequent causes of sepsis.

---

single, thick peptidoglycan cell wall, thus staining brightly violet during the procedure. The gram-*negative* cell wall consists of only a thin layer of peptidoglycan, surrounded by a second outer membrane. Thus, it fails to retain enough violet stain after an alcohol rinse procedure, leaving the bacteria unstained or *negative*. In the final step, a red counterstain called safranin is added, coloring the gram-negative bacteria pink.

*   There are over 700 *E. coli* strains, most of which are harmless. Uropathogenic *E. coli* (UPEC) strains cause about 70 percent of all UTIs. On the other hand, *enteric* strains of *E. coli*, such as enteropathogenic and enterohemorrhagic *E. coli*, cause intestinal infections.

I cared for one of my first sepsis patients as a medical student during my third-year internal medicine clerkship. The patient was a forty-two-year-old diabetic woman named Rosaria, who came in reporting two days of fevers, chills, and back pain.

Rosaria was married with three young children and had grown up in Juarez, Mexico. She had been diabetic for over ten years and had suffered from frequent UTIs. After losing her health insurance, she had run out of insulin, contributing to a worsening of her blood sugar control, among other problems.

"It looks like you have another kidney infection," I said.

"That's what I was worried about," she responded.

UTIs had become increasingly common in the decades leading up to my clerkship, owing to risk factors like diabetes.

I conducted a history and physical examination, carefully evaluating each of Rosaria's vital systems, under the watchful eye of my supervising intern, Jo. A perceptive young physician, Jo was guiding me through the nuances of patient care.

"What's your assessment? Is she sick or not sick?" she asked discreetly.

Sick or not sick? This is the essence of "clinical gestalt." As part of their training, doctors cultivate this cognitive skill—an ability to recognize disease patterns amid a blizzard of data, distinguish critical findings from the insignificant, and gauge the severity of a patient's condition. It's a sophisticated form of reasoning that blends deep medical knowledge with years of hands-on experience.[11]

"A good clinician sees the forest for the trees," as one of my favorite cardiology attendings, Mark Sheldon, used to say.[12]

Most of our clinical training in the hospital involves developing and refining the ability to quickly synthesize a patient's history, physical findings, and diagnostic data into a coherent picture—using experience and knowledge as a template.

Doctors also learn how to think scientifically through a method known as Bayesian inference. It involves forming a general hypothesis about the likelihood of a particular diagnosis based on preexisting knowledge and intuition, then continuously updating that probability as new information emerges. For example, if a patient with cardiovascular risk factors reports chest pain, a doctor's instinct is to consider a heart attack as the most likely possibility. Given the urgency, they might immediately order an electrocardiogram (EKG) and a set of cardiac enzymes. If these tests return positive, the diagnosis of heart attack becomes much more probable. However, if the results are negative, the doctor must recalibrate their working diagnosis, lowering the likelihood of a heart attack while also expanding the list of possibilities to consider causes of chest pain other than the heart.*

This is to say that doctors are highly trained professionals with advanced critical thinking skills. Combined with thousands of years of accumulated medical knowledge and cutting-edge technology, this expertise has propelled modern medicine to remarkable success in diagnosing and treating a wide array of illnesses.

Yet even the most adept clinicians are not immune to bias, ingrained beliefs, or blind spots. This is especially true when their fundamental understanding of a syndrome like sepsis is shaped by outdated knowledge.

When I was in training, sepsis was still a nebulous entity—no test or procedure could definitively diagnose it—forcing us to rely heavily on our clinical gestalt.[13] We were taught to recognize a certain look—something ineffable yet unmistakable—that signaled a patient was septic or "toxic." Most of us deduced that the diagnosis required a convergence of signs and symptoms: dangerously low blood pressure, rapid breathing, and a near-comatose stupor. Sometimes, it was enough if the senior resident thought a patient looked "like crap."

———

Rosaria didn't appear that sick to me, and she certainly didn't look "toxic." She was sitting up in her bed and talking to us. She had some abnormal findings, but I figured they were related to her UTI. We learned that bacterial infections typically cause a constellation of signs and symptoms as the body mounts a response to the infection: inflammation.

Derived from the fourteenth-century Latin word *inflammatio*, meaning "to

---

* Doctors also learn how to practice evidence-based medicine, which involves critically reviewing the medical literature on a particular subject, interpreting the validity of the results, and then using the data to guide medical treatment decisions for individual patients.

set on fire," the term "inflammation" captures the body's instinctive response to infection or injury. It is a complex biological process aimed at eliminating harmful agents and repairing damaged tissue. This response involves the release of specialized proteins and signaling molecules that activate the white blood cells in the immune system.[14] Inflammation ramps up the body's metabolism, helps isolate and destroy invading microbes, and initiates tissue repair. What begins as a localized reaction to a confined infection can, when necessary, quickly amplify into a coordinated system-wide immune response.

The body's response to infection involves a finely tuned balance between multiple overlapping systems, orchestrated by signaling molecules that both promote inflammation (*pro*-inflammatory cytokines) and suppress it (*anti*-inflammatory cytokines). In a healthy response, this creates a targeted attack on invading pathogens with minimal collateral damage to surrounding tissues.

The cardinal signs of local inflammation were first described nearly two thousand years ago by the Roman medical encyclopedist Aulus Cornelius Celsus in *De Medicina*. In his classic formulation, *Notae vero inflammationis sunt quatuor: rubor et tumor cum calore et dolore*—"The signs of inflammation are four: redness, swelling, heat, and pain." It's a phrase every medical student learns in their first year.[15] Wherever inflammation occurs in the body, some or all of these signs typically appear. If you sprain your ankle, it becomes warm, swollen, and painful. If you have an infected splinter, the skin around it becomes red, hot, and sore to the touch.*[16]

A more generalized or systemic inflammatory response can occur in the case of a severe infection, like bacteremia, or a widespread viral illness. This response often resembles a typical flu-like syndrome: fever, elevated heart rate, rapid breathing, and a vague, uncomfortable sense of illness known as malaise. It activates the immune system, mobilizes white blood cells into circulation, and places the body on high alert. Yet in most cases, the response remains tightly regulated and self-limited. We were taught that while inflammation can produce physical findings, such as fever and abnormal vital signs, it represents a normal and *expected* physiologic reaction to infection.

---

* A fifth cardinal sign—*functio laesa* ("loss of function")—was later added, likely by Greek physician Galen but often attributed to German physician Rudolf Virchow, to capture the functional impairment that may result from inflammation.

Rosaria had a fever and an elevated heart rate.*[17] While these were abnormal findings, we considered their presence a predictable response to her infection. Her blood pressure remained normal, which made sepsis less likely in our minds. Her labs showed an elevated white blood cell count, or leukocytosis, another expected sign of infection. It also revealed an elevated blood creatinine level, a marker of kidney dysfunction. Jo suspected this was due to dehydration. Rosaria had been ill with a fever for several days, and patients with infections often become dehydrated from a combination of increased fluid loss through sweating and elevated metabolism, as well as reduced oral intake related to malaise and fatigue.

Sick or not sick? All told, Rosaria had some abnormal findings, but we had a reasonable explanation. After completing our assessment, Jo and I determined that she was stable and wrote a set of admission orders, including prescriptions for antibiotic therapy, intravenous fluids, and urine and blood cultures.

———

When it came to infections in those days, we often waited for alarm bells before a sense of urgency set in. In this case, one came midafternoon when Rosaria's nurse, Sarah, notified us that Rosaria's blood pressure was dropping suddenly, while her heart rate was increasing.

We left our afternoon rounds, darted through the ER, and arrived a few minutes later at Rosaria's room, where it was obvious that something was terribly wrong. Rosaria lay limp, pale, lifeless. Her heart raced on the monitor, and her systolic blood pressure was perilously low in the 70s, almost 20 points below the normal limit.

"Why do you think her blood pressure's dropping?" Jo asked briskly as we began assessing Rosaria's condition.

"Is she getting septic?" I replied.

"Yeah, this looks like septicemia."

"Bacterial endotoxin?" I responded.

"Correct."

---

*   Our concept of "normal temperature" traces back to German researcher Carl Reinhold August Wunderlich, whose 1868 study of Caucasian patients established 98.6°F (37°C) as the average body temperature. Follow-up studies suggest this number is probably too high—the modern average is closer to 97.9°F (36.6°C). Clinically, fever is defined as a temperature of 100.4°F (38°C) or higher.

Toxins are biological poisons produced by living organisms.* They range in harmfulness from the mild venom of an ant sting to the lethal tetrodotoxin of the puffer fish. They are also part and parcel of our earliest conceptions of bacterial sepsis.

The pioneers of modern microbiology first learned of bacterial toxicity when they began injecting putrid pus from rotting wounds into healthy animals during the 1800s. With almost pharmaceutical precision, this injected putrefaction could reproduce sepsis; almost without exception, it would also kill the unfortunate animal. Piece by piece, scientists atomized pus into smaller parts, helping dispel the ancient belief that rot, infection, and sepsis came from anything other than tiny microbes. But one mystery remained: what exactly gave bacteria their deadly, toxin-like properties?

An early and remarkable insight came from Justinus Kerner, a German physician and poet, who published a series of groundbreaking case reports between 1817 and 1822, describing outbreaks of sausage poisoning that had occurred in the village of Wildbad beginning in 1793. Kerner's meticulous observations detailed patients suffering from what could only be the effects of a poison targeting the nerves and muscles: nausea, vomiting, double vision, muscle weakness, and slurred speech.[18]

After carefully measuring sausage extracts, Kerner administered them to animal subjects, reproducing the same symptoms in a dose-dependent fashion. He even administered the extracts to himself.[19] His conclusion was prescient: the poisoning was caused by a biological toxin that paralyzed the nerves. Today we know it as botulinum toxin, the cause of botulism. It's also used in cosmetic surgery as Botox.

In 1895, following a botulism outbreak in Ellezelles, Belgium, microbiologist Émile Pierre-Marie van Ermengem isolated the bacteria responsible for producing it: *Clostridium botulinum*.[20] He went on to separate the bacterium from the toxin it produced and administered the two separately to animal hosts. His findings were striking: the bacteria themselves were virtually harmless. It was the toxin alone that caused the full spectrum of illness. It was one of the earliest demonstrations in medical history of a

---

* Bacterial toxins do not behave exclusively as "poisons" and may even have beneficial properties in certain contexts.

bacterial exotoxin: a potent, secreted poison capable of producing disease in the absence of live bacteria.[21]

Around the same time, French bacteriologists Émile Roux and Alexandre Yersin, at the Pasteur Institute in Paris, demonstrated an exotoxin responsible for diphtheria—once known as the "children's plague."[22] Its culprit, *Corynebacterium diphtheriae*, unleashes the deadly toxin during infection, triggering severe inflammation in the upper respiratory tract. In the worst cases, a thick, leathery film of dead tissue called a pseudomembrane builds up in the throat, gradually suffocating its young victims.

Meanwhile, by the nineteenth century, cholera had emerged as one of the most severe diarrheal diseases in history, caused by a comma-shaped bacterium: *Vibrio cholerae*. It first spread across the globe after an outbreak struck the Ganges Delta in India in 1817, then proceeded to ravage the world population in six successive pandemics, killing millions.*[23]

The causative bacterium was discovered in 1854 by Italian biologist Filippo Pacini, who described tiny "vibrioni" in the intestines of cholera victims. Unfortunately, his work was overlooked for decades.[24] Nearly thirty years later, in 1883, German physician Robert Koch—the world's most renowned microbiologist—independently isolated the microbe while investigating a cholera epidemic in Egypt. He tasked a talented young microbiologist in his lab, Richard Pfeiffer, with illuminating the mechanism behind the disease.[25]

While *Vibrio cholerae* had many features suggesting it also produced an exotoxin, Pfeiffer discovered something unusual about the bacterium. At the time, exotoxins were generally known to be heat labile, meaning they could be destroyed at high temperatures.† However, even after being cooked, *V. cholerae* cultures remained lethal when injected into animal hosts. This led Pfeiffer to conclude in 1892 that it wasn't generating an exotoxin. Its "toxin" was part of the bacterial structure itself—in other words, an *endo*toxin.[26]‡

A year later, Italian pathologist Eugenio Centanni expanded on Pfeiffer's work by extracting a similar toxic substance from multiple other bacteria,

---

* The current, seventh cholera pandemic began in South Asia in 1961 and continues to affect populations worldwide.

† While most exotoxins are heat labile, some are heat stable.

‡ Interestingly, the cholera bacterium also produces an exotoxin, which is responsible for *most* of its pathogenic effects. However, because of its complex structure, it took researchers until the 1950s to finally isolate and identify it in the laboratory.

including *Salmonella typhi*—responsible for typhoid fever. He named the compound *pirotossina*, or "fever toxin," after observing its ability to induce high fevers in animals. Interestingly, Centanni found that endotoxin was present in a wide range of bacterial species, whether or not the bacteria themselves caused disease. It also had similar fever-producing properties irrespective of its source, suggesting that endotoxin was not a disease-specific product, but rather a shared, biologically active component common to many bacterial species.[27]

Decades of research followed into the behavior of endotoxin in two gram-negative bacteria: *Salmonella typhi* and *E. coli*. By the 1940s, microbiologists had purified extracts of the substance and elucidated its structure: a sugary fatty acid molecule, which they named lipopolysaccharide (LPS).[28]

All gram-negative bacteria contain at least some LPS in their outer membrane. When detected by the body, it triggers some of the observed effects of gram-negative bacterial sepsis. Incredibly, LPS makes up about 75 percent of the surface contents of some bacteria and 5 to 10 percent of their total dry weight.[29]

Despite a growing understanding of bacterial toxins, mid-twentieth-century researchers had more questions than answers: How does lipopolysaccharide cause septic shock? Which systems are involved? Most importantly, how can we stop its effects?

More data were needed, but studying septic shock posed significant challenges. Its rapid progression and need for urgent treatment provided little room for real-time examination. Many patients also suffered from underlying medical conditions, making it difficult to isolate the effects of endotoxin from those of frailty. For instance, in a congestive heart failure patient, was low blood pressure due to the bacterial sepsis or the heart's own weakness? Making matters worse, hospitals often lacked the advanced tools necessary to measure the precise impact of sepsis on organ function.[30]

Researchers turned to the laboratory, the primary source of early experimental insights on septic shock.[31] With an isolated, pure form of LPS now available, they could methodically administer it to animals, let it run its clinical course, and analyze every effect down to the individual organs. This allowed the construction of a living simulation or *model* for bacterial shock—one to test potentially lifesaving therapies.

In the laboratory, LPS provoked a swift and intense inflammatory response: fevers, chills, vomiting, diarrhea, and an elevated heart rate. It often spiraled out of control, causing blood pressure to drop and the heart, brain, and kidneys to shut down. The similarities to human sepsis patients were unsettling. In fact, this reaction to LPS was so consistently observed to result in shock that scientists began recognizing it as a case study for sepsis—the "endotoxic shock model."

In medical school, we learned that endotoxic shock results in the widespread dysfunction of blood vessels, causing them to lose muscle tone and become porous and incapable of conducting blood flow. Fluid leakage across the vessel walls also causes a drop in the intravascular volume—the total amount of blood coursing through the blood vessels. The combined effect is to cause blood pressure to drop too low to supply the organs, resulting in dysfunction and eventual failure.

In severe cases of septic shock, endotoxin depresses heart function. This effect occurs almost immediately in animal subjects. In human patients, scientists initially see an *increase* in cardiac function to compensate for the loss of blood pressure, followed by a depression in function as the endotoxemia progresses to a more advanced stage.

One can see here how our modern understanding of sepsis was shaped by studying bacterial endotoxin, particularly from organisms like *E. coli*. The toxin seemed to encode a simple, brutal message to the body: *poison*. The intensity of the response depended largely on two factors: the dose of endotoxin and the host's susceptibility.* In laboratory animals, researchers observed a clear dose–response relationship: the higher the dose of LPS, the more severe the reaction. In hospitalized patients, however, the picture was more complex. The virulence of the infection and the patient's overall health played a critical role in determining just how unforgiving the endotoxin response would be.

———

"Let's give a liter of normal saline," Jo asserted.

"Will do!" Sarah replied cheerfully.

ER nurses never seem to be fazed by anything . . . other than, perhaps, a rookie medical student getting in their way. Sarah gracefully danced around us and grabbed a one-liter bag of normal saline: a 0.9 percent concentrated saltwater solution, one of the standard intravenous fluids for rescuing a patient

---

* There is significant variability in the host response to endotoxin, and some experts believe it may even behave like an adaptive exohormone.

with low blood pressure.* After hanging the bag, she ran it "wide open," so it was running into Rosaria's veins about as quickly as gravity would allow.

The waiting was the hardest part as I watched the saline drip out of the bag. Jo paced back and forth with a scowl, no doubt trying to determine whether we had missed something. Every few minutes, she pushed a button on the monitor to record another blood pressure measurement.

Twenty minutes later, the fluid bolus was complete, but nothing had changed. Rosaria's heart was still racing, and her breaths were rapid and shallow. Sarah checked another blood pressure.

"Still low at 72/40. Do you want to give more fluid?"

"Yes. Please give another liter of saline with a pressure bag this time."

Jo caught my eye. "Call Mark," she said softly.

Mark was our senior. If he was needed, it meant things were unraveling. Rosaria's body was shutting down. Outwardly, she looked lethargic, but her monitor was screaming panic alarms, telling a different story about her *internal* state. Jo's usual confidence had also slipped into a nervous brood. The fluids infused quickly this time, but there was no change. About five minutes later, Mark arrived.

"What's the story?" he asked calmly.

"Forty-two-year-old diabetic woman with probable bacterial shock. Systolic pressure is still in the 70s after two liters," Jo responded.

Mark stroked his beard as he analyzed the monitor, then turned back to Jo. "What do you want to do?"

"I think we should give her more fluid," Jo replied.

Mark considered her plan, then responded, "Sounds good. I'd also give her a dose of gentamicin now."†

Mark was considering all possibilities, including antibiotic resistance. Bacteria are highly resourceful, able to develop strategies to evade or destroy the antibiotics we use against them. By the time I was in medical school, antibiotic resistance had become a common problem, inspiring new antibiotic strategies

---

* Recent studies suggest that, because of its tendence to increase blood acidity, normal saline may be less desirable in sepsis patients than balanced crystalloid solutions, which more closely approximate the electrolyte composition of plasma.

† Gentamicin is an aminoglycoside antibiotic used to treat severe or complex gram-negative bacterial infections. However, the drug itself can be quite toxic—even a slight excess in dosing could result in permanent kidney or hearing damage. Thus, it is reserved for special circumstances and must be administered carefully.

for treating severe infections and sepsis. One such method was to double up on the initial antibiotics to ensure that at least one of them was effective.

Rosaria was now drawing more attention from the other emergency room staff, and one of the charge nurses, Beth, joined the bedside team.

"What do you need help with, hon?" Beth asked.

"Could you hang some gent?" Sarah replied.

I was mesmerized watching the two in action. Within minutes, they'd placed an extra IV in Rosaria's other arm and started running the gentamicin and a third fluid bolus. Mark and Jo watched with furrowed brows.

I decided it was time to ask an obvious question: "What happens if her pressure doesn't improve?"

"Badness," Jo replied.

After two more liters of fluid, Rosaria's blood pressure began climbing, and her vital signs stabilized. She began waking up and interacting with us. I felt a huge relief—it was the first time I had seen a patient brought back from the brink.

"You won't forget this case!" Jo said as she patted me on the shoulder.

Meanwhile, a nurse at the step-down unit called for report, as Rosaria's hospital bed was finally ready after she had spent nearly ten hours in the emergency room.

A harsh, rhythmic beeping sound. Mark groaned under his breath as he snatched his pager from its holster.

"Looks like we've got another admission. Can you two handle it from here?"

"No problem. We'll get her tucked and give the ICU resident a heads-up," Jo replied.

Rosaria improved throughout the night, and by the next day, her fevers had stopped. She was delighted to see us at morning rounds.

"Thank you for taking such good care of me."

"You're most welcome," Jo replied warmly while patting her shoulder.

"If everything goes well today, we could probably discharge you tomorrow."

We debriefed the case as we made our way to our next patient. Rosaria had grown *E. coli* in her blood again, but it was an antibiotic-resistant strain. This partially explained why she got worse even after receiving the first round of antibiotics. Fortunately, we'd been able to administer the gentamicin relatively quickly.

Mark also pointed out something else: Rosaria's initial blood tests revealed that her kidney function was abnormal. He thought her organ systems were starting to show dangerous signs of injury from sepsis. Jo and I had overlooked this, thinking it was a nonspecific finding related to dehydration and her general state of illness.

"What's the current definition of sepsis?" Mark asked.

Jo rolled her eyes. "Here we go again with the Surviving Sepsis Campaign!"

"We're probably underdiagnosing sepsis by waiting until patients are in shock. By the numbers, Rosaria met sepsis criteria right off the bat, even though it probably didn't seem like she was that sick," Mark replied.

Mark was applying for a critical care fellowship, so he was aware of rumblings of a sea change happening in the sepsis world.

"Some major sepsis guidelines are coming down the pipeline. We're about to see a paradigm shift," he said coolly.

———

"Sick or not sick?" This was a question that shaped my clinical training. Each case was like a high-stakes puzzle, demanding assembly before time ran out. It wasn't just about medical knowledge, but clinical intuition and gestalt, honed through countless hours at the bedside.

Still, when it came to sepsis, how sharp was our intuition? How reliable was our clinical gestalt? Back then, most of us equated sepsis with septicemia and shock—a late-stage calamity rather than an evolving threat. "You'll know it when you see it. That was how it was taught to us," as one colleague recalls dryly.[32] And so, we set our threshold too high: when the body was in full revolt and the patient was critically ill. In that sense, our gestalt was telling us something dangerously false: *if a patient isn't in shock or doesn't look "toxic," they don't have sepsis.*

In *The Laws of Medicine*, Siddhartha Mukherjee writes, "Most of our models of illness are hybrid models; past knowledge is mishmashed with present knowledge."[33]

We are indebted to our ancestral knowledge and practices in almost everything we do. The sepsis we understood during my medical training was largely based on observations of the syndrome dating back to the pre-antibiotic era of rampant "blood poisoning."

Yet by the end of the twentieth century, experts had recognized that sepsis was unimaginably complex, with a wider spectrum of severity and the potential to arise from nearly *any* infection. They realized that the outdated model of sepsis had misled doctors for years, leading to delayed treatment and, in some cases, missed diagnoses. Sepsis needed a broader definition, one that encompassed its diverse presentations and varying degrees of severity.

The challenge now was to bridge the gap between emerging research and frontline medical practice, where many healthcare providers still treated sepsis and septicemia as interchangeable. Despite advances in understanding, clinical practice remained years behind the cutting edge of research.

It was an endeavor bound to challenge the establishment to its core. As one of the most ancient maladies, older conceptions of sepsis were ossified in medical culture. To better understand this deeply rooted bias, we should trace its origin to the earliest medical practitioners and the dawn of history.

CHAPTER TWO

Putrefaction

*If, then, thou findest that man continuing to have fever, while that
wound is inflamed, thou shalt not bind it; thou shalt moor (him)
at his mooring stakes until the period of his injury passes by.*

—CASE FORTY-SEVEN, Edwin Smith Papyrus, c. 2625 BCE[1]

ON AUGUST 3, 2000, I joined a group of eager young medical students
at the Convention Center in downtown Albuquerque for the thirty-third
annual White Coat Ceremony for the University of New Mexico School of
Medicine—our formal initiation into the medical profession. We donned our
pristine white coats for the first time and exchanged a handshake with the dean,
then stood and recited the Declaration of Geneva—a pledge adopted in 1948
by the World Medical Association to uphold the highest ethical standards in
medicine. Widely regarded as a modern successor to the Hippocratic Oath,
the Declaration echoes values first articulated some 2,500 years ago in ancient
Greece. Those ideals emerged alongside the Asclepieia, temples dedicated to
Asclepius, the demigod of healing in Greek mythology.[2]

The medicine we practice today is, in many ways, still influenced by our
past. Practitioners and patients exist on a continuum, from the dawn of
history to the unknowable future. Today's medical knowledge is an amalgam

of old and new—a fusion that can sometimes entrench persistent beliefs and traditions.

Sepsis has remained elusive for thousands of years. It's a "disease" within a disease, always entangled with a primary infection.[3] This has kept it from standing out as an entity of its own, always lurking beneath the infections causing it. Until doctors had a more sophisticated understanding of germs, human physiology, and the immune system, it was nearly impossible to fathom what sepsis was, let alone how to treat it.

Tracing its history, we can begin to see how sepsis has eluded our understanding—how past misconceptions continue to confuse us. We can also appreciate how the objectivity and rationality that characterized the scientific revolution still apply today as we strive to create systems that transcend our clinical abilities.

Across the roughly ten thousand years of human civilization, it's only in the last two *hundred* that we've seen significant progress in medicine. For 98 percent of human history, the profession was guided more by tradition and speculation than by science. Now, we are amid a virtual big bang of knowledge. This may give us the impression—perhaps the illusion—that we stand at its apex. But even today, we have an incomplete understanding of disease and health.[4]

———

The word "sepsis" first entered the human lexicon in the eighth century BCE, not in medical texts but in the ancient poetry of the Greek writer Homer. It comes from the Greek word *sepo* ("I rot") and has since become synonymous with the decay of human tissue and other organic material.[5]

Thousands of years ago, observations of decomposing flesh revealed a mysterious process in the universe, which the ancient Greeks named *sepsis*. As it steadily ate away at life, only the vitality of a healthy, living body or the divine power of the gods could defy its onslaught.[6]

We now know that decomposition is caused by putrefaction and autolysis. During autolysis, cells within the body rupture after death, releasing enzymes that liquify its internal organs and other structures. Putrefaction occurs as bacteria break down biological material, releasing foul-smelling gases like hydrogen sulfide.[7]

Ancient observers knew nothing about microbiology, but they could still witness the spoils of billions of invisible bacteria rotting flesh over time. Within just a few hundred years, the term "sepsis" would become commonplace in the medical writings of Greek physicians.

And while the Greeks may have etched their place in medical history by giving us the name sepsis, they weren't the first to notice it. Observations of putrefaction had begun thousands of years earlier in ancient Egyptian death houses.[8]

The earliest Egyptians were keenly aware of decay as a continuous destructive process, from birth and into the afterlife. They also had to stop it at all costs. For the living, this task fell to physicians, and after death, it rested on the shoulders of embalmers.[9]

During mummification, ancient embalmers observed a strong likeness between the stench of feces and the odor of decomposing bodies.[10] Over time, this led to the idea that these "processes" were related to an invisible substance in the intestines called *wḥdw,* or *ukhedu.*[11]

Ancient Egyptians believed that ukhedu could decay the flesh of the dead and rot the wounds of the living. They also believed that disease, in the general sense, resulted from an imbalance of ukhedu in the intestine, which would then enter the bloodstream and sicken the body like a blood poison. They even contended that the aging process was caused by repeated exposure to ukhedu and its cumulative toxic effect on the body.[12] This concept later evolved into the intestinal autointoxication theory of the late nineteenth and early twentieth centuries, which suggested that illness stemmed from the accumulation of toxins produced by fecal matter lingering in the intestines.*[13] As for what ukhedu was made of, the ancients had no idea. It took over four thousand years to discover that bacteria were responsible for putrefaction.

These early observers intuitively recognized an invisible substance present in the world that could decay wounds, cause sickness, and putrefy dead flesh. They did what they could to clear their bodies of the substance and prevent it from being absorbed into wounds. They also created an early concept of disease as something *caused* by a process. This, along with their deductive reasoning skills, led to early work developing wound care practices and wound

---

* The intestinal autointoxication theory has since been disproven, in a manner of speaking, though it has influenced our modern understanding of the microbiome and its effects on health.

salves made of antiseptic substances such as honey, grease, and lint.*[14] It also encouraged generations of Egyptians to regularly purge their bowels of excess ukhedu and consume probiotic foods like yogurt or fermented milk to promote health and longevity.[15]

But how did ancient medical practitioners understand the body's *systemic* signs and symptoms of infection and sepsis? The answer lies deep in the medical archives, where an eerily recognizable account of the syndrome appears in the oldest known surgical treatise, the *Edwin Smith Papyrus*, named after the nineteenth-century antiquities dealer and collector.[16]

Dating around 1550 BCE, the papyrus is a copy of an older document that originated around 2625 BCE and was possibly authored by the priest, architect, and physician Imhotep.[17] Imhotep was the chief minister to King Djoser during Egypt's third dynasty and was later deified as the Egyptian god of medicine. (He's also the main villain in the popular but sensationalized 1999 film *The Mummy*.) The document gives us a glimpse into the mind of an ancient Egyptian surgeon as he describes his approach to forty-eight surgical cases.[18] It also references fever and wound infections, giving us one of the earliest descriptions of sepsis.

From the treatise, we can gather that its author understood that some wounds could become inflamed and infected, leading to fever and serious illness in severe cases. Wounds were often classified as "sick" or "not sick," with sick wounds being those that were infected and released pus, or *ryt*. For instance, in Case Forty-Seven, we see that the surgeon recognized a fever related to an inflamed wound, as well as the need to treat it.[19] However, as ancient Egyptians had no knowledge of bacteria and only a basic understanding of the circulatory system, the treatment was limited to basic wound care and addressing the patient's nutrition.[20]

The patient in Case Forty-Seven was gravely ill, with persistent fever in the setting of an inflamed wound. But from the writing, we learn that the surgeon could do nothing other than to "moor" the patient—in other words, watch and wait. This stark description gives us another clue about the ancients' understanding of sepsis: once it set in, with few options available, there was not much they could do to stop it.[21]

It's not surprising that the earliest clinical descriptions of sepsis came from

---

*   Honey has been shown in the laboratory to have antimicrobial effects.

infected wounds. Wounds are a flesh-and-blood display of deeper inflammatory processes. Ancient Egyptians used the symbol of the brazier to describe the heat emanating from infected wounds and clearly understood the connection between local wound infections and fevers.[22] Fever has since become intimately associated with infection and established as a cardinal sign of disease.[23]

Case Forty-Seven also highlights a crucial distinction in ancient medicine: the difference between visible ailments like wounds and more nebulous *internal* diseases and processes such as sepsis. Because external injuries could be directly observed, ancient physicians could treat them relatively effectively. These early doctors became skilled in wound care, and evidence suggests they could even perform relatively complex procedures like amputations. However, without a deeper understanding of human physiology, microbiology, and chemistry, the signs and symptoms of many infectious diseases—and the body's septic response—must have remained a mystery.

Though ancient Egyptian doctors also used magical spells and rituals, it's interesting that we have almost no reference to these practices in the *Edwin Smith Papyrus*.[24] Maybe this tells us something about Imhotep, or the nature of ancient Egyptian surgical practice. Perhaps surgeons focused on treating external injuries and mainly dealt with wounds that weren't infected or septic—the *not-sick* wounds. It's possible that more mystical practices were reserved for when wounds became *sick*, as described in a later manuscript, the *Ebers Papyrus*.[25]

As Egyptian civilization matured, particularly in the Middle and New Kingdoms, its medicine came to be lauded as the world's most advanced.[26] Meanwhile, careful attention to infected wounds, particularly to the presence of inflammation and pus in those wounds, became its cornerstone. Surgeons often cleaned and debrided wounds, applying drying and antiseptic agents with antibacterial properties.

By the mid-fourteenth century BCE, just as King Amenhotep IV (later Akhenaten) was ascending the throne and plunging Egypt into political and religious turmoil, Egyptian wound care practice seemed to revolve around controlling the degree of "purulence" or pus formation.[27] It operated under a basic yet flawed assumption: "It is good for a wound to rot a little."[28]

We see this teaching inscribed deep within the *Ebers Papyrus*, along with evidence that doctors treated wounds with antimicrobial agents to suppress pus while also using irritants to *draw out* the excess.[29] In the latter case, it would have been like pouring gasoline on a fire—fueling bacterial growth and significantly increasing the risk of a severe infection.

What logic could have led to such an assumption about purulence? It helps to imagine that, in those days, pus was as constant as wounds themselves.[30] Its regular presence could have easily led to the belief that this was the typical evolution of wounds as they healed.[31] Such wounds might have been considered abnormal or "sick" only when they became persistently or excessively inflamed or purulent, followed by systemic fever. It was a fine line that was undoubtedly crossed quite frequently.

Thus, at the root of medical history, there was confusion about normal versus abnormal when it came to wound healing, pus, and inflammation. Without a complete understanding of germs and bacteria, ancient Egyptian doctors might have unknowingly condemned many of their wounded patients to a speedy death and placed generations of future doctors on the wrong path.

In the centuries after Amenhotep IV's reign, Egypt's fortunes rose and fell, and by the end of the New Kingdom, the empire had entered a long decline just as the Greek Empire began its ascent to power. With that, the torch of medicine and an ancient knowledge of sepsis was passed to a new generation.

———

The Greek island of Kos is often celebrated as the cradle of Western medicine. It was the birthplace of Hippocrates, the "father of Western medicine," whose teachings gave the island enduring fame. The Great Asclepieion of Kos was constructed about a century later, dedicated to Asclepius and closely associated with the Hippocratic tradition.[32] During the Hellenistic period, Greeks living in Egypt associated Asclepius with the deified Egyptian physician Imhotep, blending the healing traditions of both cultures.

Hippocrates urged physicians to seek physical rather than divine causes of disease while maintaining an objective and rational approach to clinical observation.[33] As Hippocratic medicine developed, knowledge expanded and medicine began to emerge as a more rational discipline, while the clinical role of priests and mysticism gradually diminished.[34]

Nevertheless, the healing practices taught and refined throughout ancient Greece continued a legacy of thousands of years. Egyptian medicine was highly regarded: Homer praised Egypt as the land of unrivaled drugs, and Herodotus marveled at its specialized physicians. Hippocrates himself was said to have studied in Egypt, and many features of Greek medicine reflected the influence of these older traditions.[35]

The Greeks believed that health and disease were related to a balance of four vital fluids, called "humors": blood, phlegm, yellow bile, and black bile. Although it lacked a sophisticated understanding of biology and physiology, so-called "humorism" still represented significant progress, as it laid out a physical basis for disease. It also opened the door for various methods and treatments doctors could use to fine-tune the balance of humors.

Hippocrates theorized that two interconnected processes, sepsis and pepsis, occurred in the body. Sepsis was associated with rot and putrefaction, the same decay seen in decomposing bodies and infected wounds.[36] Pepsis, by contrast, was a more benign process linked to digestion and fermentation.[37] He believed pepsis governed digestion in the stomach, while harmful *sepsis* arose when matter in the body underwent putrefaction, especially in the intestines.[38] According to his teachings, these two forces existed in balance with each other, and much of his philosophy focused on maintaining this equilibrium through lifestyle and diet.

Sepsis and the germ theory of disease are intimately intertwined in history. Our earliest notions of sepsis came from observing the visible effects of putrefaction, long before microbes could be seen. A generation after Hippocrates, Greek philosopher Aristotle proposed an interesting explanation: he argued that rotting matter spontaneously gave rise to tiny creatures—a process later known as "spontaneous generation."[39]

It was a compelling idea for its time, especially given that the Greeks had no way of visualizing microbes. But Aristotle had reversed the order of events: bacteria *cause* putrefaction, not the other way around. Still, one can see the logic in his conclusion, since insects such as flies and mosquitoes seemed to materialize spontaneously out of putrefying goo in marshes and swamps.[40]

The ancient Greeks also believed the smell of rot and decay in these wetlands was a harbinger of disease and death—an idea associated with Hippocrates. He developed it into the "miasma theory," which held that it was *miasma* ("bad air") transmitting disease. Miasma was promulgated for centuries as the cause of many of the great epidemics and pandemics of history, including cholera, plague, and smallpox. It even motivated the Romans to drain the Pontine Marshes and "fever swamps" throughout their empire and develop city sewer systems.

Miasma likewise inspired what is possibly the first anticipation of germ theory, credited to the polymath Marcus Terentius Varro, who, during Julius Caesar's reign around 47 BCE, speculated that certain "difficult diseases" were caused by animals too small to see, called *animalia minuta*.[41]

Putting the cause aside for a moment, what did ancient Greeks think of the systemic sepsis response in the body? It is clear from Hippocrates's methodical descriptions of diseases that he was observing this response in action, often describing ardent or "violent" fevers, "fever crises," and fevers accompanied by other systemic body symptoms such as delirium, nausea, vomiting, and convulsions.[42] He and his colleagues were also careful observers of infected wounds, which they described as septic or rotting. Yet it's hard to know how much they understood sepsis as part of the body's *response* to an infection. They likely rather saw it as an imbalance in the body's underlying physical processes.

Hippocrates's writings show that he understood the connection between fever and illness. Fever was often attributed to an excess of yellow bile related to fire. It seemed to be a beneficial sign—something necessary to *cook* out the infection.[43] At the same time, a *persistent* fever was an ominous finding.

In one example from *The Book of Prognostics*, he writes, "Should such an abscess disappear, and expectoration not follow, but the fever continuing, delirium and death are to be looked for."[44]

When it came to treating sepsis, Hippocrates's detailed case descriptions reveal a sobering reality: he had little power to alter its course. One such case involved a man named Criton, who lived on the island of Thasos around 400 BCE. While walking drunkenly along the beach, he felt a sudden, sharp pain in his left foot. He initially believed he had stepped on a broken seashell. That night, he was overcome by violent chills, nausea, and fevers.[45]

The next morning, Hippocrates arrived with a group of students to assess him. Criton's condition had worsened: his fever raged, vomiting and diarrhea had set in, and he was delirious. His whole foot had become swollen, turning red with small black blisters. Tragically, there was nothing Hippocrates or his students could do. Resigned, they carefully observed and documented Criton's decline. He died a few hours later.[46]

In retrospect, Criton's illness may have been a fatal case of sepsis caused by *Vibrio vulnificus*, a marine bacterium common to beaches and known to result in necrotizing fasciitis, a severe soft tissue infection often referred to as a flesh-eating disease.[47] A case like this would surely be fatal without proper surgical debridement and powerful antibiotics. *V. vulnificus* infections are also far more lethal in patients with underlying liver disease—from which Criton may have suffered due to his proclivity for wine.[48]

As a student of ancient Egyptian medicine, Hippocrates developed a theory of wound infections, linking them to his concepts of sepsis and pepsis. Notably, like his Egyptian predecessors, he didn't view pus as entirely harmful.[49]

In fact, to Hippocrates, pus could be bad *or* good, depending on its characteristics. For example, cloudy, foul-smelling pus—what he called the "septic" variety—portended a grave outcome.[50] Conversely, odorless, white "peptic" pus was good or "noble"—a sign the wound was healing.[51]

He even famously wrote, "If the pus is white, and not offensive, health will follow."[52]

We can speculate that the odorless "good" pus that Hippocrates observed likely resulted from what we now call pyogenic bacterial infections of the skin and soft tissue.[53] While these infections can be severe, they rarely lead to sepsis once the wound drains.[54] Interestingly, the white pus seen in such infections consists of debris from dying white blood cells, which sacrifice themselves while destroying invading bacteria. In that sense, pus *does* contain something good and noble![55] By contrast, we can speculate that foul-smelling "bad" pus was due to necrotizing soft tissue infections, which are typically polymicrobial—caused by multiple different bacteria—and can quickly result in severe illness, sepsis, and even death.[56]

Hippocrates's observations hinted at a deeper layer to pus formation. However, without knowledge of the underlying biological processes, he and his successors were unable to decipher what they observed, leading to one of the greatest medical misconceptions in history.

A few centuries passed, and with that, Hippocrates's views on pus slowly transformed into a medical doctrine: *pus bonum et laudabile*. It means that pus is laudable and even *necessary* for a wound to heal. With this, a new generation of doctors not only welcomed its presence but sought to *induce* it, often by irritating wounds with heat and cautery in an attempt to promote healing.

This doctrine was not fully credited to Hippocrates but to his successor, physician and philosopher Galen of Pergamon—likely incorrectly.[57] Galen practiced about four hundred years later, during the Roman Empire, and was considered one of the most outstanding physicians in antiquity, making lasting contributions to modern anatomy, physiology, pathology, and pharmacology. He succeeded Hippocrates as the Western medical authority, remaining so for over a thousand years.[58]

From his writings, we now understand that Galen never explicitly promoted the concept of laudable pus. Rather, he saw pus as beneficial only when draining *from* an abscess. The idea nevertheless became associated with his name, and due to his immense influence, it was eventually codified into medical doctrine, shaping wound treatment for centuries.[59]

After the fall of the Roman Empire, Islamic medicine adopted this practice. Even the renowned eleventh-century physician Ibn Sina (Avicenna), often regarded as the "father of modern medicine," discussed it in his famous *Canon of Medicine,* the principal medical textbook used across the Middle East and Europe until the seventeenth century.[60]

The misconception about pus was one of the most damaging in medical history. Throughout the Middle Ages, doctors commonly let wound infections fester while deliberately rankling them with cautery to provoke further inflammation, believing this would accelerate healing. Little did they realize that, in doing so, they were sealing their patients' fates.

A few courageous physicians attempted to challenge the practice. In 1267 AD, the Italian surgeon Theodoric Borgognoni rejected the doctrine in his *Cyrurgia,* recommending instead that wounds be cleaned, sutured, and dressed with wine-soaked bandages. Half a century later, French surgeon Henri de Mondeville likewise criticized the deliberate induction of pus in his 1312 surgical treatise. Nonetheless, the doctrine of laudable pus remained entrenched until the mid- to late nineteenth century—its vestiges persisting in medical journals until as recently as 1916.[61]

Thus, the great prevailing doctrines—laudable pus, miasma, and spontaneous generation—endured for over a thousand years, upheld as immovable dogmas to which the medical community remained bound. In that time, the profession also evolved into a highbrow, paternalistic institution, often resistant to change. This elitist doctor-knows-best model undoubtedly slowed the pace of medical innovation.[62]

Without a fundamental understanding of the invisible microbes that caused infections, medicine would allow pus to flourish, diseases to run rampant, and patients to languish for centuries. As we have limited records and almost no mention of sepsis during this time, we can only speculate about the devastation it caused as a silent partner during the great plagues of the Middle Ages.

CHAPTER THREE

Germs

Science is a process, not an edifice, and sheds old concepts as it grows.

—TIMOTHY FERRIS, *Coming of Age in the Milky Way*[1]

WHEN I WAS SEVEN, I told my father I wanted a starship to explore the galaxy.

He said, "There's an entire universe under your nose. Why not look through a microscope instead?"

I conceded his point, and we went to the store and picked out a Tasco junior compound microscope. I still remember the thrill of analyzing my first sample: a drop of pond water from the woods behind our backyard. With a freshly etched glass slide secured on the stage, I flipped on the light, adjusted the lenses, and turned the focusing knob. *Voilà!* I was transported into a new realm—a dazzling landscape of geometric patterns, cellular structures, and innumerable tiny organisms tumbling in and out of view.

At the turn of the seventeenth century, humanity's eyes began opening to a vast new reality—the hidden world of the microcosm. As with so many great discoveries, this bold new vision was not the work of a single innovator but of several working in parallel. Among them were Hans and Zacharias Janssen, a father-and-son team of Dutch opticians often credited with building the first functioning compound microscope—a device capable of enlarging an object at the end of a metal tube to roughly twenty times its actual size. Others may have reached the same breakthrough independently: Hans Lippershey and Cornelius Drebbel, their contemporaries and rivals, or even Galileo Galilei, who around 1609 is said to have fashioned one of the earliest such instruments, the occhiolino.[2] The true inventor may never be known, but from their collective efforts the microscopic age was born—and within a hundred years, microscopes were magnifying objects fifty to a hundred times their size.[3]

In 1665, English scientist Robert Hooke made a groundbreaking contribution to microscopy with his illustrated atlas, *Micrographia*. Hooke was highly respected among his peers as the Curator of Experiments at the Royal Society of London. His new book showcased stunning observations of biological specimens like hair, fly wings, and cork under a microscope and included the first published report of a microbe: a fungus he'd found in a white mold spot.[4] With *Micrographia*, Hooke demonstrated the power of the microscope and helped lay the foundations for the new science of microbiology.

Ten years later, a cloth merchant living in Delft, Netherlands, named Antonie van Leeuwenhoek astonished the Royal Society with a letter describing single-celled organisms—later known as "Letter on the Protozoa." Eccentric and ingenious, Leeuwenhoek had mastered the craft of building simple yet effective microscopes to inspect fabric quality.[5] After reading *Micrographia*, he was inspired to turn his new optical instruments toward the natural world, examining pond water, rainwater, and even scrapings from his tongue.[6] To his amazement, he discovered a hidden universe teeming with tiny single-celled organisms, which he called "animalcules." Over the years, he communicated with Hooke, who helped him submit nearly two hundred observations of these new organisms to the Royal Society, ultimately earning Leeuwenhoek a place as a Fellow.[7]

Leeuwenhoek's microscopes, capable of magnifying objects up to 275 times, far outperformed others of his time, allowing him to visualize single-celled microbes such as parasites and bacteria.[8] Yet many struggled to replicate his findings with their inferior microscopes.[9] Without Hooke's endorsement, Leeuwenhoek could have been dismissed as a fraud.[10] Lacking formal education, he kept his techniques secret and refused to disclose his methods in detail, which meant the broader scientific world would fail to grasp the full significance of his discoveries.[11] In fact, it would take about 150 years—until the age of Pasteur and Koch—for Leeuwenhoek's pioneering observations to be fully appreciated.[12]

On a cold winter night about a century later, five hundred kilometers south of Delft, the largest hospital in Paris lay engulfed in flames. Its name was the *Hôtel-Dieu* ("Hostel of God"), and it had been the longest-running hospital in Europe.*[13]

Institutions devoted to healing stretch back to the beginning of civilization. In ancient Egypt, Mesopotamia, and Greece, temples and sanctuaries served as centers where religion, medicine, and community care converged. Over time, these evolved into the first true hospitals, from the Greek asclepieia to the Roman valetudinaria and the Christian and Islamic centers of late antiquity. Across their many forms, hospitals have served as centers of healing, compassion, and medical innovation; they have also grappled with persistent challenges, from the spread of infections and deadly epidemics to severe overcrowding.[14]

The Hôtel-Dieu was founded in the seventh century by the Catholic Church and was a bastion of shelter and healing for those in need from all walks of life.[15] However, due to long deteriorating conditions—overcrowding, poor staffing, and abysmal sanitation—it shared another feature common to urban hospitals in that era: it was a death trap. In fact, if you were a patient admitted there in the late eighteenth century, you had a one in four chance of dying.[16]

In his 1788 *Mémoires sur les Hôpitaux de Paris*, surgeon Jacques Tenon presented a sobering review of the Hôtel-Dieu. He described an overwhelmed institution, with only 1,219 beds for an average of 2,500 patients—sometimes reaching 4,800—where many people shared beds with multiple others.[17] Poor conditions led to rampant epidemics of typhus and smallpox, while surgeons performed frequent surgeries directly on patients' beds.[18] Tenon's report linked the hospital's dysfunction to numerous patient deaths, as well as two major fires in 1737 and 1772, the latter prompting King Louis XV to order its demolition.[19]

The hospital's fate was suspended when Louis XV died in 1774, most likely at the hands of smallpox. His successor, Louis XVI, reversed the order and appointed Baron de Breteuil to rebuild the hospital. The baron tasked the Royal Academy of Sciences to form a commission that included notable doctors and scientists, including Tenon, whose memoir served as a thorough account of the problems the Hôtel-Dieu and other Parisian hospitals faced.[20] Although the

---

* Here, we refer to the Hôtel-Dieu in Paris. Many hospitals in France and other parts of the world have the same name.

commission sought to implement improvements based on Tenon's insights, its reforms were constrained by a weakened monarchy and the looming French Revolution.[21]

Tenon's accounts of the Hôtel-Dieu remind us of the law of unintended consequences. Though run by well-meaning individuals, eighteenth-century French hospitals were frequently overcrowded, underfunded, and poorly managed. Often governed by complex hierarchies, they also housed their own decadent and inflexible institutional cultures.

These early institutions—and those that followed as hospitals expanded across Europe, England, and eventually the United States—became fertile ground for sepsis to flourish.[22] Much of our modern understanding of the syndrome comes from the early chronicles of hospitalized patients who suffered its wrath. What's more, the specters of the Hôtel-Dieu, with its overcrowded wards and high mortality, would haunt hospitals for generations, as patients continued to die of infection within their walls.

———

I can remember one of my first nights of hospital call as an intern like it was yesterday. It was a busy night for the internal medicine service, and I was "capped" by midnight—I had already admitted the maximum number of allowable patients for a single trainee. The hospital was bursting at the seams, and we'd been getting punished all night by "cross cover," the stream of pages nurses send when issues flare on patients you're covering overnight.

At 1:00 a.m., I received a call from an oncology nurse named Darika, concerned about her patient, a forty-year-old woman named Janet, who was in the hospital being treated for an aggressive cancer of her lymphatic system, lymphoma. Darika reported that Janet was experiencing increasing pain in her right abdomen, breathing rapidly, and developing an elevated heart rate, also called tachycardia. I reviewed Janet's chart while talking to Darika and saw that she had a known lymphoma mass affecting her small intestine. Her lab values also looked stable, and she hadn't had any fevers during hospitalization.

The number of pages an on-call physician receives in the hospital any night would surprise most people. Even as a staff physician working for a well-resourced organization, I can receive ten to twenty unique calls in an hour. It's impossible to physically see every patient in person, so physicians must triage calls according to their urgency. This means assessing how risky a situation is over the phone with a nurse who is keeping close tabs on the patient and then managing it accordingly. Under these circumstances, nurses are the crucial link between patient and physician.

In Janet's case, Darika was worried. She'd been caring for her all night and had detected an apparent change in her condition. Something seemed wrong. Maybe it was just inadequate pain relief, but as a seasoned oncology nurse, she also knew that many complications could occur in patients like Janet, including hospital-acquired infections, blood clots, and gastrointestinal bleeding.

On the other hand, I was relying on my clinical gestalt, looking for obvious red flags to calibrate my concern. Pain, elevated respirations, and tachycardia? These are common or "nonspecific" findings in the hospital. In this case, I wasn't worried about Janet because I wasn't seeing a clear signal that something was wrong. *Sick or not sick?* Based on the information, I didn't think Janet was in trouble. So, I increased the dose of her pain medication and asked Darika to call me if her condition changed further.

At 5:00 a.m., Darika called again. Janet was now writhing in pain, and her blood pressure was dropping. It was an ominous sign. Severe pain floods the body with adrenaline, causing the blood vessels to clamp down like a vise, typically *raising* blood pressure. Someone writhing around in severe pain with falling blood pressure? Something dreadful was happening.

When I arrived at the oncology ward, I could hear Janet moaning from across the nursing unit. As I entered her room, she was hyperventilating, and her heart rate was elevated at 130. Meanwhile, her blood pressure had dropped thirty points and was now dangerously low at 90/45. I introduced myself and started examining her abdomen. As soon as I touched her, she immediately flinched, letting out an awful howl. I was so startled that I almost jumped back myself.

"That's an acute abdomen," I muttered.

Surgical emergencies are among the more dreadful conditions doctors face. An acute abdomen involves an infected, ruptured, blocked, or otherwise inflamed abdominal organ. It frequently requires immediate surgery to prevent catastrophic injury, sepsis, or both. I suspected that Janet had suffered a perforated intestine, likely related to her cancer. Even worse, this perforation was now seeping irritating and bacteria-infested intestinal fluid—what we call succus—into her abdominal cavity, causing severe inflammation of her abdomen and abdominal lining, or peritonitis. Her infection was also triggering a severe septic response throughout her body, causing her blood pressure to drop sharply. All this meant that Janet urgently needed antibiotics and stabilization of her blood pressure. She also required emergency surgery to wash out the infected succus, a process known as "source control."*

I ordered a set of labs, an abdominal X-ray, antibiotics, and intravenous fluids. I then contacted the general surgery resident on call, who showed up within minutes. After completing her assessment, the resident immediately called her supervising attending. By then, the abdominal X-ray had confirmed my suspicion. It showed free air in the abdomen, a sign that there was, in fact, a perforated intestine, now seeping intestinal gas and succus into the abdominal cavity. Meanwhile, Janet's blood pressure had dropped to 70/40, and she had become lethargic. This was abdominal sepsis, and it was clear that Janet needed emergency surgery.

Surgeons soon swarmed around Janet's room like bees. An intern was setting up to insert a central line—a sizeable intravenous catheter—into her neck to begin administering vasopressors, powerful medications designed to tighten the blood vessels and improve the blood pressure. The resident was on the phone beside him, updating Janet's husband and reviewing consent for her surgery. Across the bed, Darika was swapping out saline bags while the charge nurse, Laura, was scrambling to collect supplies for the central line.

After placing the central line and confirming its position with an X-ray, the surgeons asked Laura to infuse the vasopressor, norepinephrine, also known as Levophed. Within a few minutes, Janet's blood pressure had improved. Meanwhile, Darika had hung a bag of IV antibiotics.

An hour later, Janet was headed to the operating room. Her surgery revealed a perforation caused by her lymphoma, which had eroded through the wall of her small intestine. She survived the surgery and was transferred to the intensive care unit on life support. A week later, she was transferred out of the ICU and had started walking. She was discharged to a rehab facility a few days later.

In retrospect, it was likely that Janet had already been leaking fluid into

---

* Antibiotics, fluids, and supportive care are often insufficient to cure surgical sepsis patients, who frequently require rapid source control to remove the focus of infection. This may involve emergency surgery to drain abscesses, wash out pus and infected fluid, or debride necrotic or infected tissue.

her abdomen from a slowly worsening perforation when Darika had first noticed a change in her vital signs. Her increased heart and respiratory rate could have been heralding the onset of intra-abdominal sepsis, and by waiting to perform an assessment, I had let her get too close to the edge of the cliff. The hospital floods your senses with so many data points that it's often difficult to distinguish the signal from all the noise. It was hard to discern that she was deteriorating until it was almost too late. It was a blurry line between sick and not sick.

Throughout the 1700s and 1800s, conditions in the Hôtel-Dieu and hospitals like it were ripe for bacteria to proliferate, leading to a spectacular rise in hospital infections. The abysmal conditions in which surgeons operated meant that the very contact of the scalpel was akin to "the touch of death," as Dr. Guido Majno writes in his iconic paper, "The Riddle of Sepsis."[23] Surgical infection rates were so high under these overcrowded conditions that they dwarfed the rates reported thousands of years earlier by ancient surgeons performing the same procedures.[24] Even childbirth became far more hazardous than in previous periods, with mothers regularly developing "childbed" or "puerperal" fever—the result of the womb becoming infected during delivery.

At the same time, the expansion of gunpowder use in warfare meant that surgeons were now dealing with more complicated wounds, which were also more likely to become infected. The bullets used in early muskets were bulky and traveled at slow speeds. As they penetrated the body, they would push in bits and pieces of clothing, gunpowder, and bullet debris, contaminating the wound tract with bacteria. The explosive nature of gunpowder injuries also resulted in severe skin burns, open bone fractures, avulsions, and amputations, which were far more likely to lead to severe infections and sepsis. In fact, sepsis was so common after gunshot wounds that, before bacteria were discovered, surgeons even theorized that it was the gunpowder itself that was poisoning the blood.[25]

By the 1800s, a bane of infected wounds caused by gunpowder injuries, childbed fever, and unhygienic surgeries was hitting hospital wards worldwide. Patients were rotting in droves in their beds from germ-infested wounds. The term "sepsis" had survived the ages—it was what doctors referred to when describing contaminated wounds and putrefaction—yet no one could explain what was causing it. By the Middle Ages, it had even become a common belief that putrefaction was related to sin and morality, sparing the bodies of the pious or saintly.[26]

However, by the nineteenth century, medicine was increasingly defined by reason, objectivity, and experimentation. In France, reformers such as Jacques Tenon had set the stage for hospital restructuring. Parisian hospitals, and soon others across Europe and the United States, became not only centers for patient care but also laboratories for clinical observation and hubs for scientific teaching.*[27]

As microscopes revealed hidden worlds of microbial life and experimental science took root, it became increasingly apparent that some deeper force was responsible for infection and decay. Observers could see that corpses, whether of sinners or saints, decayed in precisely the same way.[28] Debate persisted through much of the century, as many scientists still clung to Aristotle's ancient theory of spontaneous generation, but the balance was tipping toward experimentation and evidence.

Meanwhile, doctors were observing many patients with septic wounds regularly developing fevers and other systemic symptoms, such as chills, rapid breathing, and tachycardia. These findings were invariably linked to a higher risk of death, prompting more researchers to begin studying this enigmatic condition.

Physicians also witnessed something both intriguing and troubling when performing autopsies on some of the most severely afflicted patients: pockets of pus appearing in other locations in the body. The implication was that the putrefaction or sepsis was spreading or metastasizing to those areas, the most likely vehicle being the bloodstream.

By 1837, French physician Pierre Adolphe Piorry, best known for his pioneering work in developing physical examination skills, observed the putrid contents of infected wombs of maternal patients spreading throughout the

---

*   This summary necessarily simplifies a much more complex hospital culture and history. Early modern hospitals were shaped by the interplay of physicians, who often drove medical innovation and argued for moral urgency in patient care; nurses, whose daily labor and authority deeply influenced the ward environment; trustees, who focused on governance and resource stewardship; and broader social tensions of class, gender, and race that permeated both hospital life and the societies they served.

body during puerperal fever.* He called this "septicemia," or the spread of sepsis throughout the blood, introducing the modern concept of "blood poisoning."[29]

Hooke and Leeuwenhoek's work over a hundred years earlier had already revealed the microbial world. As hospital-acquired infections and cases of septic illness multiplied throughout the 1700s and 1800s, scientists and doctors spent more time peering into bigger and better microscopes, directly visualizing bacteria, and contemplating the significance of the tiny organisms they were observing. At the same time, they used deductive reasoning and scientific methods to study the problems of putrefaction and rot.

———

In December 1789, the gray-stoned port city of Aberdeen, Scotland, was hit by an epidemic of puerperal fever. Now often referred to as puerperal sepsis, the condition had rapidly become the leading cause of maternal death in Europe, with maternal mortality in affected hospitals often reaching 10 to 30 percent.[30]

At the time, a young Scottish physician, Alexander Gordon, had just entered his fourth year as a staff obstetrician at the Aberdeen Dispensary, one of the outbreak's epicenters.[31] Gordon was far from an ordinary observer. He had a keen mind and sensed something orderly at work behind the onslaught of illness: infections weren't just accumulating—they were *spreading*, from one patient to the next.[32]

But what enabled this transmission? To answer this, he turned to his notes, which contained tables cataloging the time of disease onset, progression, and, most importantly, the midwife and physician assignments. This led Gordon to an inexorable conclusion: the disease was being passed from patient to patient by the caretakers themselves.[33]

In 1795, Gordon published a treatise on the subject, representing one of the first epidemiologic studies of an epidemic. In it, he also emphatically stated his opinion that "the disease was occasioned by a cause very different from the sensible qualities or constitution of the air." In other words, a contagion of sorts—contradicting centuries of dogma.[34] He also proposed infection

---

* Piorry developed skills such as percussing over the skin to estimate the size of organs such as the liver.

prevention measures, including burning contaminated clothes and bedsheets and improving nurse and physician hygiene.*[35]

Sadly, Gordon died within four years of his report's first publication from complications related to tuberculosis. But the treatise lived on and was reprinted multiple times over the next half century. It inspired future physicians, notably American Oliver Wendell Holmes, who himself published *The Contagiousness of Puerperal Fever* in 1843, further adding traction to the germ theory of puerperal sepsis. Holmes also strongly advocated for better hygiene practices, urging physicians to undergo thorough "ablution" (body scrubbing) and change of clothing before attending new mothers.[36]

Three years later, a Hungarian physician, Ignaz Semmelweis, would forever cement his place in history—both as a pioneering figure in medicine and one of its most tragic heroes. In 1846, Semmelweis had just taken on a new role as the first assistant of the obstetrics service at Vienna General Hospital. Vienna General was a teaching hospital that exchanged free medical care for the opportunity to train medical students and midwives. Its service was divided into a "First Clinic" to train medical students and a "Second Clinic" for nurse midwives, with each clinic alternating admitting days. Semmelweis oversaw both clinics as first assistant, functioning much like a modern chief resident.[37]

Though it was a foregone conclusion that childbearing was dangerous, Semmelweis soon discovered that the First Clinic had a rather atrocious reputation. In fact, maternal patients would go to great lengths to be moved to the Second Clinic—pleading, bribing, or even giving birth in the street rather than face the alternative.[38] When Semmelweis examined the data, he found that the patients' intuition was correct: the First Clinic had a mortality rate significantly higher than the Second, sometimes up to tenfold.[39]

This piqued his curiosity. He began analyzing the two clinics, looking for differences. The fact that they alternated days suggested that the distribution of patients between them was likely random, making a difference between the actual patients unlikely.† Hence, the difference had to be something about the clinics themselves. But after considerable sleuthing, he couldn't find it.[40]

A year later, a colleague of Semmelweis, Jakob Kolletschka, developed

---

* Many others had sporadically suggested the same before Gordon. Physician John Burton is also credited with viewing puerperal fever as contagious in 1751. Others, such as John Leak in 1772 and Joseph Clark in 1790, suggested improving cleanliness in maternity wards.

† This is probably not true, as this was not a truly randomized study.

sepsis and died after cutting himself in the cadaver lab with a scalpel. During Kolletschka's autopsy, Semmelweis noted that the findings looked strikingly similar to the puerperal sepsis seen in maternal patients from the First Clinic.[41] In one of medical history's most famous *aha* moments, he made the connection: whatever affected his colleague must have also been affecting maternal patients. He hypothesized that the medical students—who regularly performed autopsies in the cadaver lab and then went directly to the maternity clinic—must have been transferring some "cadaverous material" to the maternal patients, causing sepsis.[42]

His next step was more of a leap: he proposed that medical students wash their hands with chlorine between the cadaver lab and the maternity ward. It was a stunningly effective strategy. Within just a couple of months of instituting the new practice, the mortality rate in the First Clinic decreased by 90 percent.[*][43]

We now know that bacteria, often *Streptococcus*, named for its characteristic appearance of *streptos* or "chains" of spherical cells, cause puerperal sepsis. And while maternal outcomes have since improved, as we will see later in the book, sepsis remains a leading cause of death in maternal patients.

Semmelweis produced some of the clearest early evidence for what would soon be recognized as the germ theory of disease, and he followed it with a spectacular intervention to prevent infections. This feat could have easily transformed contemporary obstetric practice overnight.

Unfortunately, at the time, there was still significant resistance to the germ theory. Despite groundbreaking work by others like Gordon and Holmes, old dogmas persisted, and doctors remained opposed to the notion that they could harm their patients through contamination and disease.[44] As we will soon see, this stubborn trait still hasn't thoroughly washed out of the modern medical profession.

Semmelweis may have had masterful insight and exquisite research skills, but he lacked intuition when it came to implementation and project management.[†] He faced considerable resistance from his colleagues yet waited over ten years to publish his data. He also took their criticism to heart, continuing to bang his drum louder while dishing out snide quips and intimidating rhetoric

---

[*]   It is unclear if Semmelweis was aware of the work of Gordon or Holmes.

[†]   I owe this interpretation to Danielle Ofri's *When We Do Harm*, which illuminates implementation failure as one of the cruxes of Semmelweis's tragic tale.

to his detractors. Additionally, he failed to make handwashing easy for his colleagues. Not many doctors believed in hygiene at the time, and sinks and handwashing stations weren't regular fixtures in hospitals as they are today. The design of these facilities would have to be modified to accommodate this new and tedious activity. By overlooking this critical step, he missed one of the most basic tenets of quality improvement: *make it easy for people to do the right thing.*[45]

As a result of these shortcomings, Semmelweis's ideas were discredited, and he grew more and more despondent, ultimately experiencing a mental breakdown, which landed him in an insane asylum by 1865. In one last tragic sequence of events, in his final weeks, Semmelweis was beaten, placed in a straitjacket, and left in isolation. According to reports, he developed an infected hand wound during this ordeal and died of sepsis, the very condition he had been trying to stop.[46]

Besides being one of appalling misfortune, Semmelweis's story foreshadowed future challenges facing the hospital safety movement. For one, it already showed that the hospital was made up of a complicated system of variables that could easily create its own problems. It also revealed that professionals operating within that system could sometimes be stubborn—and, at times, outright obstinate.

It wasn't enough to have a good idea. To effect change, future quality improvement leaders would have to learn how to inspire their colleagues by winning their hearts and minds. But even then, they would still have to command the more rote mechanisms of human behavior and learn how to cajole their colleagues into doing the right thing.

Even today, many hospitals struggle with hand hygiene: in surveys without targeted interventions, average compliance often hovers around 40 percent. In some well-designed programs, compliance reaches 60 to 70 percent, but such success remains far from universal.[47] Is this because doctors and nurses still don't believe in germ theory? Not at all. It's a problem of complexity and implementation. Getting a group of doctors and nurses to *consistently* wash or sanitize their hands before and after every patient visit is actually a monumental logistical task. Meanwhile, as we will see, hospital-acquired infections remain a significant cause of death and disability in patients worldwide.[48] According to the World Health Organization, better hand hygiene alone could prevent up to half of these infections.[49]

Needless to say, the nineteenth-century medical community missed a huge opportunity to create safer hospitals and save countless lives by failing to heed Semmelweis's warnings. It's hard to imagine how many maternal patients died needlessly in the decades following his death. But the tides were slowly turning, and Semmelweis would have his redemption, eventually being named posthumously the "savior of mothers."

———

In 1859, French chemist and microbiologist Louis Pasteur undertook the experiments that would culminate in his now-famous swan-neck flask experiment, a landmark in microbiology. For years, scientists had observed that nutrient-rich liquids, such as meat broth, would eventually become overrun with bacteria and decay when left undisturbed. Even more puzzling, the bacteria themselves seemed to materialize out of nowhere. To some, this supported Aristotle's theory of spontaneous generation. However, Pasteur, who was deeply knowledgeable in scientific history and steadfast in his commitment to reason, rejected the theory. He was convinced that the bacteria originated from an external source, and he was determined to prove it.

Building on the work of notable experimentalists like Italian biologists Francesco Redi and Lazzaro Spallanzani from over a century earlier, Pasteur devised a clever apparatus to test his theory. He placed nutrient broth in glass flasks with long, S-shaped "swan necks" that allowed air to enter but trapped airborne particles in their curves. The result was striking: broth in intact swan-neck flasks remained sterile, while broth in flasks whose necks were broken or tilted so liquid touched the trapped dust quickly teemed with microbes. He concluded that the bacteria responsible for rotting the meat broth traveled through the air and were not spontaneously generated in the meat. Thus, putrefaction was not only caused by bacteria; these bacteria were originating from somewhere else.*[50]

During this time, Pasteur investigated fermentation and the decomposition of beer and wine. In a series of seminal papers, he demonstrated that these processes were driven by living microbes, laying the foundation of modern

---

*   Italian physician Girolamo Fracastoro is often credited as the first to suggest a modern version of the germ theory of disease in 1546, when he proposed that epidemic diseases were caused by *seminaria* ("seeds") spreading from one person to another, building on earlier observations by Ibn Sina (Avicenna) in *Canon of Medicine*, published in 1025.

microbiology. Pasteur extended his findings to milk, showing that bacterial contamination caused its souring, and he even developed a method—gentle heating, later known as pasteurization—to prevent bacteria from growing, thus preserving the milk.

His papers caught the eye of a British surgeon named Joseph Lister, who made the crucial link between surgical wound infections, putrefaction, and bacteria.*[51] Lister then took an impressive next step, devising a system of antiseptic practices to kill bacteria and *prevent* infections in the first place. He thought to use phenol, or carbolic acid—a chemical then used to prevent wood from rotting— to sterilize surgical instruments and wound dressings. In a now-famous 1867 series of *Lancet* articles, beginning with his report on eleven-year-old James Greenlees, who had suffered an open fracture of the leg, Lister described wounds that healed entirely without suppuration or offensive odor.[52]

More strikingly, he showed that inflammation and granulation—the hallmarks of normal healing—could occur in the complete absence of pus. This observation delivered a crushing blow to the age-old laudable pus doctrine, redefining the very meaning of wound healing. By divorcing healing from suppuration, Lister effectively ushered in the modernization of surgical antiseptic practice.[53]

Meanwhile, more doctors were making the connection between bacteria and septicemia by studying the putrid substance of "septic" infections, aka pus, under the microscope. In 1872, a German doctor named Edwin Klebs, who had been an assistant to the renowned Rudolf Virchow at the Pathological Institute in Berlin, published a treatise demonstrating the presence of bacteria in septic abscesses. The paper stated Klebs's opinion that putrefaction, sepsis, and infection were all interrelated processes caused by bacteria.[54]

Almost simultaneously, other doctors, most notably French physician Casimir-Joseph Davaine, began successfully inducing a septic process by injecting pus from one infected animal into the bloodstream of another healthy animal.[55] With this, doctors began seeing sepsis as related to *infection* . . . not simply as the inevitable process of rot and decay.[56]

In 1882, Alexander Ogston, a Scottish surgeon and early adopter of Lister's antiseptic practices, cut open an abscess on one of his patients and analyzed it under the microscope. He theorized that surgical infections were related

---

* The Listerine brand of antiseptic mouthwash was named after Joseph Lister.

to "some special germ" and set out to identify the microbes in question. To his delight, upon peering into the microscope, he found "beautiful tangles, tufts, and chains of round organisms in great numbers, which stood out clear and distinct among the pus cells and debris." Recognizing these as bacterial "micrococci"—small *kokkos*, or "clusters of grapes"—first described in 1878 by Robert Koch, Ogston concluded that they were the cause of pus and abscesses. He named them "staphylococci," from the Greek word *staphyle*, or "bunch of grapes." Two years later, German surgeon Anton J. Rosenbach isolated and grew two different strains of *Staphylococci* in the laboratory: one with golden-colored colonies (*Staphylococcus aureus*, from the Latin *aurum* or "gold"), and another with white colonies (*Staphylococcus albus*, from *albus* or "white").*[57]

Most of these pioneers were overshadowed by Robert Koch, who is most often credited for proving the connection between bacteria and infections in 1876 through his work with the bacterium that causes anthrax. Koch's success was in his methods, which were elegant, meticulous, and easily reproducible. In 1884, he formally presented the principles that came to be known as "Koch's postulates," a systematic roadmap for linking microbes to specific diseases. The postulates—something every first-year medical student now learns in microbiology class—state that to prove a microbe causes a disease, you must verify cause and effect; to do that, (1) the microbe must be found in the diseased patient, (2) it must be isolated and grown outside of the diseased patient, (3) it must, when inoculated into a healthy patient, cause the same disease, and (4) it must be isolated again from the newly infected patient.[58] By using this systematic method, Koch proved beyond any reasonable doubt the crucial link between certain germs and the diseases they caused.

———

On March 24, 1882, doctors and researchers convened for what should have been a routine monthly meeting of the Berlin Society for Physiology. Yet within minutes of its commencement, the keynote speaker, Robert Koch, stunned his audience with the announcement that he had discovered the cause of tuberculosis.[59]

---

* *Staphylococcus* is a gram-*positive* bacterium.

Also known as the "white plague" or "white death," tuberculosis had besieged civilization and mystified doctors for thousands of years. By the time Koch began studying the disease in the 1800s, it had become responsible for one in four deaths in Europe, affecting people of all ages and earning nicknames like "captain of all these men of death" and "robber of the youth."[60]

Caused by a slow-growing *Mycobacterium*, tuberculosis typically results in a progressive, relentless infection, most often affecting the lungs, but also potentially any other part of the body. Its signature can be seen in skeletal remains dating back 9,000 years to the ancient city of Atlit Yam, off the coast of Israel. Early descriptions of the illness are also found in the accounts of ancient Indian practitioners dating back as early as 3,300 years ago.[61] Doctors had long suspected that tuberculosis was contagious, yet they had no way to prove it. Over the years, its cause and transmission became the subject of wild speculation and fantasy, with theories ranging from a disease of hereditary origin to that of a sickness transmitted by the bite of a vampire.[62]

Even after it was first visualized, the tuberculosis bacterium was a tricky organism for scientists to study, as it was difficult to isolate and grow. (Even to this day, a sample of a patient's sputum must be carefully collected, and it can take weeks to yield any viable bacteria for analysis.) Thus, it was the perfect test for Koch's skills as a master microbiologist and an excellent case study to apply his newly developed postulates.

Koch's fateful evening lecture left little doubt in his audience and is now considered one of the most important presentations in medical history. It included over two hundred carefully prepared microscopic slides demonstrating the *Mycobacterium tuberculosis* organism he had isolated from numerous tissue samples of infected hosts, representing a wide range of the disease forms clinicians were treating at the time.[63]

The discovery of *Mycobacterium tuberculosis* was a turning point in medicine. It provided significant traction to the germ theory of disease by applying it to a prominent scourge. It also prompted immediate public health measures such as the isolation of patients and improved hygiene in hospitals, while later innovations like the use of masks would follow in the early twentieth century. Additionally, as it was becoming clear that microbes caused all infectious diseases, germ theory paved the way for the development of new medical therapies to treat these infections.

This conceptual shift also brought long-standing ideas about sepsis into focus. In 1914, German physician Hugo Schottmüller published a seminal paper titled "Das Problem der Sepsis," in which he wrote, "Sepsis is present if a focus has developed from which pathogenic bacteria, constantly or periodically, invade the bloodstream in such a way that this causes subjective and objective symptoms."[64] This paper provided the first modern definition of sepsis, representing the final synthesis of putrefaction, infection, and bacteria.

———

The twentieth century saw edifices of old medical theories and doctrines begin to crumble, yet this change would take some time to spread throughout the medical establishment. Though there was now clear evidence that bacteria caused infections, putrefaction, and disease, doctors were still slow to accept this reality or to adopt the antiseptic methods proposed by Lister and others.

Lister himself even wrote, "Carrying out this rule implies a conviction of the truth of the germ theory of putrefaction, which, unfortunately, is in this country the subject of doubts such as I confess surprise me, considering the character of the evidence which has been adduced in support of it."[65]

Future researchers would also find sepsis far more complex than Schottmüller's description, and it would be the subject of great debate for decades to come. Nevertheless, now armed with the germ theory of disease, we could begin rooting out the causes of infection, shedding light on countless maladies. Equipped with better antiseptic practices, cleaner surgical techniques, and better wound care, we could also begin to drastically *prevent* more infections and sepsis in hospitals while facilitating a movement toward better patient safety. The stage was now set for a massive counteroffensive against germs.

CHAPTER FOUR

Magic Bullets and Murphy's Law

*I certainly didn't plan to revolutionize all of medicine
by discovering the world's first antibiotic or bacteria
killer. But I suppose that was exactly what I did.*

—ALEXANDER FLEMING[1]

ON MARCH 14, 1942, Anne Miller lay deathly ill in the intensive care unit at New Haven Hospital, Connecticut.[2] One month prior, the thirty-three-year-old had suffered a miscarriage complicated by a streptococcal bloodstream infection, leading to puerperal sepsis. She now had fevers exceeding 106°F, violent chills, and delirium, leaving her barely conscious at times.[3] As she inched closer to death, her obstetrician, Orvan Hess, was gathering his resolve for one final, desperate gambit to rescue her.[4]

A few days earlier, Hess had visited Miller's internist, John Bumstead, at the Graduate Club in New Haven for a second opinion.[5] While seated in the waiting room of Bumstead's office, he'd discovered a *Reader's Digest* article on the use of soil bacteria to combat streptococcal infections in animals.[6] He'd mentioned it to Bumstead, who'd immediately thought of Howard Florey, an Australian pharmacist and pathologist working on an experimental antibacterial medication called penicillin.*[7]

---

*   The article discussed using a bacteria-produced antimicrobial agent called gramicidin.

Discovered fourteen years earlier by Scottish microbiologist Alexander Fleming, it wasn't a synthetic antimicrobial drug but one that occurred naturally—manufactured by another microbe—a *Penicillium* mold. Fleming quickly saw the drug's potential, as it was lethal to certain hardy bacteria, including various species of *Staphylococcus* and *Streptococcus*. Today, we know that penicillin works by blocking the synthesis of peptidoglycan, the key structural component of the bacterial cell wall. Without it, the cell wall weakens and the microbe ruptures in a process known as bacteriolysis.

Fleming was ingenious but lacked the infrastructure or expertise to develop the drug. A decade later, the task was taken up by a team at Oxford led by Howard Florey and German–British biochemist Ernst Chain, with English biochemist Norman Heatley providing crucial methods for extraction and purification. Their work demonstrated penicillin's lifesaving potential but still yielded only tiny amounts of the drug. It was ultimately a collaboration of the Oxford group with the US War Production Board and pharmaceutical companies—including Merck & Co., Pfizer, Squibb, and Eli Lilly—that industrialized penicillin during World War II, making it the first mass-produced antibiotic.[8]

As it happened, one of Bumstead's patients at New Haven Hospital, John Fulton, had been an old classmate and close friend of Florey's at Oxford University.[9] On March 11, Bumstead approached Fulton for help. Fulton reached out through his contacts, and after a flurry of transatlantic coordination involving his Oxford group, the Rockefeller Foundation, and US pharmaceutical partners, five and a half grams of penicillin—nearly half the entire American supply—was delivered to Bumstead's office at noon on Saturday, March 14.[10]

Unsure of the antibiotic's safety, Hess and Bumstead gave Miller a small test dose. There was no adverse reaction. Reassured, they infused the rest of the antibiotic intravenously over the course of the night.[11]

By Sunday morning, Miller's fevers had stopped. A few hours later, she was eating breakfast. She would go on to live to the age of ninety. Never in the history of infection had a drug yielded such a result. Humanity had officially entered the age of antibiotics.[12]

———

Stories like Anne Miller's are immortalized as examples of the windfall that antibiotic therapy and other medical advancements have brought to humanity.[13]

In an era when the dark cloud of infectious diseases cast death and despair over much of the world, medicine turned the tide, launching civilization into a new age—one where infectious diseases could no longer menace our daily lives. During this time, doctors and nurses were elevated to near-superhero status, endowed with seemingly limitless abilities. As Danielle Ofri writes in *When We Do Harm*:

> If the history of medicine over the past two hundred years were a feature film, it would be a swashbuckling adventure epic. Heroes in white coats would brandish stethoscopes and pipettes, decapitating disease in single fell swoops with their medical machetes. Sanitation, antisepsis, and anesthesia would hurl across the screen, flattening 19th-century illnesses. Vaccines and antibiotics would explode like grenades in the early 20th century—rescuing the masses from infectious marauders.[14]

It's a story that's shaped our attitudes about infectious diseases and our impression of what medicine can and can't do.

At the beginning of the twentieth century, infections were the leading cause of death in the world. Diseases like smallpox and cholera were killing millions each year. In the United States, about one in three people perished from bacterial infections like pneumonia, tuberculosis, and diphtheria; a shocking 40 percent of those deaths were children under five.[15] Average life expectancy was a mere forty-six years for men and forty-eight for women.[16]

Staphylococcus aureus bloodstream infections had emerged as the leading cause of hospital and wound infections and were almost invariably fatal, despite treatment, with close to eight out of ten patients succumbing after a long illness of fevers, chills, and metastatic abscesses.[17]

Sepsis, meanwhile, hadn't yet risen in our collective consciousness as a distinct condition. A glimpse into the medical literature in the early 1920s reveals that it was still considered by many doctors to be synonymous with bacterial bloodstream infections, aka bacteremia or septicemia—the most common cause thought to be *S. aureus*.[18] Notwithstanding the ferociousness of bloodstream infections, most experts hadn't yet classified a specific syndrome accompanying them, often describing the clinical picture as "[resembling] that seen in any severe acute infectious disease."[19]

Nevertheless, luminaries like Sir William Osler, one of the founding professors at Johns Hopkins Hospital, began to challenge the common wisdom. After observing a pattern of signs and symptoms associated with septicemia, Osler suspected a mysterious and ominous process at work.

He wrote in 1904, "Except on a few occasions, the patient appears to die from the body's response to infection rather than from it."[20]

When one looks back and traces the natural course of these cases, it's easy to see the disastrous unfolding of what could only be a runaway septic process in action.[21] Furthermore, as we now know that sepsis is the endgame for most severe infections, it undoubtedly had a hand in many deaths during this era, both inside and outside the hospital.

Still, by the turn of the century, the golden age of microbiology was on its way. Scientists were peeling away the layers of a vast new world of microbes and the diseases they caused. Humanity progressed more in just a few decades than it had in the previous ten thousand years. Rotting wounds and decomposition were no longer seen as ungodliness, pus was no longer noble, and the agents of epidemics were now reduced to tiny microbes, as opposed to a shadowy mist of miasma that permeated the air.[22]

These infective agents and the diseases they caused could now be observed, isolated, and cataloged. The germ theory of disease catalyzed a transformation in medicine, as the revelations of Robert Koch, Louis Pasteur, and other researchers exposed the crucial link between germs and infection. A flurry of activity followed toward identifying the cause of infectious diseases. The medical system scrambled to incorporate this new knowledge into its existing schemas, reclassify old concepts, and purge outdated theories—as diseases became linked to their microbial causes, new strategies of defense emerged.

Most of germ theory's early successes came from something absurdly simple: hygiene. We prevented a wide swath of infections by purifying our water, strengthening our sanitation systems, wearing masks, isolating the sick, and cleaning our hands and surgical instruments before operations.*[23]

---

* The practice of quarantining was formalized during the bubonic plague of the fourteenth century, with port officials requiring ships arriving at Venice to sit at anchor and be isolated for forty days before landing—*quaranta giorni*, the origin of the word "quarantine." However, the concepts of contagion and patient isolation had been described centuries earlier by Ibn Sina (Avicenna) in *Canon of Medicine*.

By the late nineteenth century, the explosive growth of urban centers had outstripped their capacity to house and sustain their populations. Overcrowding, insufficient housing, and primitive water and waste-disposal systems were a fact of life and created a perfect setup for germs to thrive. Successive outbreaks of food and waterborne diseases, such as typhoid fever and cholera, hammered cities, killing millions worldwide. As George Rosen writes in *A History of Public Health*, cities like London came to be seen as "devouring Molochs," consuming their inhabitants through disease.[24] In the United States, cumulative cholera outbreaks across the nineteenth century had claimed tens of thousands of American lives, while typhoid fever killed roughly thirty-five thousand in a single year in 1900.[25]

Once public officials understood that germs were causing infectious diseases and that some were transmitted through food and water, they began taking steps to improve sanitation and hygiene in cities and urban centers.[26] By the turn of the century, nearly 90 percent of states had established health departments, and individual counties followed suit within just a few years. Initiatives ranged from overhauling sewage disposal and water treatment systems to bolstering food safety, public education, and handwashing and food handling practices, among other measures.[27]

One of the most important lifesaving interventions was filtering and chlorinating city water supplies. In 1908, Jersey City, New Jersey, became the first city to implement a community water treatment program. Within a decade, thousands of American cities and towns had followed suit. Between 1900 and 1936, this single action cut the number of deaths due to waterborne diseases in half.[28]

The combined effect of hygiene and public health actions was striking. In the early 1900s, typhoid fever and cholera were household names. Louis Pasteur himself lost not one but two daughters to typhoid. Yet by the time I was in medical school a hundred years later, the number of annual cases of typhoid fever had dropped by a thousandfold to only one case per million people; cholera had been reduced even more, to just a few cases per year.[29] Nowadays, in developed countries, most nonmedical people have never known anyone who's suffered from these diseases.

Even more critical were innovations such as antibiotics and vaccinations. Pioneering microbiologist Paul Ehrlich referred to early antimicrobial drugs— precursors to antibiotics—as "magic bullets," having developed the first of their kind, arsphenamine, to treat syphilis. These powerful new drugs could dismantle bacterial cells, defeating bacterial pneumonia, tuberculosis, and numerous postsurgical infections. Within just a few years, deaths from these dreadful illnesses dropped sharply, especially among children and young adults. Meanwhile, vaccines and immunization programs could prevent infections by training the body's immune system to recognize and respond to pathogens more quickly. This eradicated longstanding viral diseases like smallpox and virtually eliminated others such as measles and polio.*[30]

Forward-thinking leaders also saw social and economic factors as just as important in reducing death and disability. With the advent of social programs and public health campaigns, we saw improved nutrition and greater resilience against infections such as bacterial pneumonia and influenza. Expanded access to medical care, combined with sweeping safety reforms in workplaces and on roads, led to astonishing reductions in accident-related deaths by the mid-century.[31]

The results were stunning. A look at long-term mortality data shows that from 1900 to 1937, death rates from infectious disease dropped by about 2 to 3 percent each year. Once antibiotics came onto the scene, they boosted this trend, accelerating the yearly drop to an incredible 8.2 percent per year from 1937 to 1950.[32] By the 1950s, life expectancy for Americans had increased to sixty-seven years for men and seventy-two years for women, roughly amounting to a 45 percent gain. It seemed we were on our way to the most significant period of health and prosperity in history. Technology and innovation were defeating nature, deadly infections were on the run, and life expectancy was on the rise.†[33]

But as you can probably anticipate, the story of infection doesn't have a fairy-tale ending. Despite the advances of germ theory, sanitation, vaccination, and antibiotics, doctors would continue to find themselves in a mortal battle against microbes and sepsis.

---

* Measles was declared eliminated in the US in 2000. However, it has recently resurged due to low vaccination rates.

† These rewards would continue well into the late twentieth century, with life expectancy rising again to close to seventy years for men and seventy-seven years for women by 1980.

During a routine morning in the winter of 2005, I saw a patient, Tom, in the emergency room. I was a first-year intern working alongside my senior resident, Mary, on the inpatient internal medicine service.

Tom was a delightful eighty-five-year-old World War II veteran with a history of congestive heart failure, diabetes, and lymphoma who had been reporting several days of coughing and shortness of breath. His chest X-ray in the emergency room had shown evidence of pneumonia in his right lung.

A cursory look at Tom would not have suggested much of an illness. He was sitting up in bed making jokes. It was his wife, Betty, who had forced him to go to the hospital after she had observed him short of breath walking to the bathroom earlier that morning.

Looks aside, an *objective* assessment of Tom's breathing and respiratory status told a different story. His oxygen levels had been low when he'd first presented in the emergency room, and he now required significant supplemental oxygen therapy to maintain a normal blood oxygen saturation. In addition, his respiratory rate—the number of breaths taken per minute—was troublingly abnormal in the 30s. (A "normal" respiratory rate is around 12 to 18 breaths per minute.)

Tom's other findings weren't very revealing. His heart rate was normal, likely because of a cardiac medication called carvedilol, a beta blocker, which kept it steady at around 60 beats per minute. He also didn't have an elevated temperature, a common phenomenon in older patients whose aging immune systems often fail to generate fevers. His white blood cell count was elevated, but this was a chronic finding related to his lymphoma.

After completing our assessment, we informed the couple that Tom had pneumonia in his right lung as well as an exacerbation of his congestive heart failure. He would have to be admitted to the hospital for antibiotics and close monitoring.

I could see Tom's face grow solemn for a moment, but he immediately smiled and said, "I'm sure you'll take good care of me, Doctor," as he reached out to hold Betty's hand.

Pneumonia is the most common cause of sepsis in the developed world.[34] Its name comes from the Greek word *pneúmōn*, for "lung," and means "disease of the lung." It's transformed over the years in the mainstream to generally refer to a lung infection, but it can also be seen in noninfectious conditions, like autoimmune disorders and drug reactions. It's most often caused by bacteria, followed by viruses like influenza and coronavirus. It can also be caused by fungi, like *Aspergillus* and *Pneumocystis*. In Tom's case, the pattern on his chest X-ray suggested a high likelihood of bacterial pneumonia, prompting us to initiate antibiotics targeting the most likely bacterial agents.

Before the twentieth century, bacterial pneumonia was a dreadful affliction. In the young and healthy, it would often result in a terrible illness lasting up to two weeks, with nightly bouts of fevers, chills, excruciating chest pain, and air hunger. It would drag its victims to the edge of death before settling into an aftermath of exhaustion and debility, sometimes lasting weeks or months.[35] Older patients would have no such luck, often facing a relentless sickness that would gradually smother their life force.

By 1900, pneumonia had become the leading cause of infectious death in developed countries like the United States. Osler even famously wrote in 1901, "Of all acute infectious diseases, pneumonia is now the 'Captain of the Men of Death.'"[36]

For most of history, there was no effective treatment for pneumonia. Osler remarked in 1892 that the disease "has its course uninfluenced in any way by medicine."[37] Yet by the early 1880s, German pathologists were uncovering its microbial basis. In 1882, Carl Friedländer described an encapsulated rod-shaped bacterium (later known as *Klebsiella pneumoniae*), while his contemporary—some might say rival—Albert Fränkel more definitively identified paired spherical bacteria called "diplococci," now *Streptococcus pneumoniae*, as the principal cause of bacterial pneumonia at that time. Hans Christian Gram's newly developed staining technique (1884) helped clearly distinguish the two bacteria, revealing *S. pneumoniae* as gram-positive (staining purple) and *K. pneumoniae* as gram-negative (staining pink).*[38] This understanding presented new avenues for experimental therapies.

---

* Historians describe a three-year debate "of unusual bitterness" between the two pathologists, sparked by an 1883 paper by Carl Friedländer on the bacterial cause of pneumonia.

Within a decade, researchers Emil von Behring and Shibasaburo Kitasato at the Royal Prussian Institute for Infectious Diseases in Berlin had discovered that immunity to bacterial diseases like diphtheria could be *transferred* by injecting serum from a recovered animal into an uninfected host. Shortly after that, Paul Ehrlich fused decades of chemistry and microbiology to propose that whatever was conferring this immunity had to be something tangible, like a protein produced by the body itself. As Siddhartha Mukherjee writes in *Cells*, it was "a *body* produced to defend the body."[39] In other words, an *antibody*, as Ehrlich wrote in an 1891 paper.[40]

We now know that specialized immune cells in the body, called B lymphocytes or B cells, house these antibodies on their cell surface—each B cell with its unique antibody, like a distinct lock-and-key mechanism, waiting to be activated. Once the suitable toxin, germ, or foreign substance binds to the antibody on a B-cell's surface, it triggers a cascade of reactions within the B cell, which, in turn, divides, reproducing into an army of cloned cells, each one capable of mass-producing the same antibody against the inciting agent. The antibody-*generating* microbe or substance thus becomes the antigen.[41] Once activated, the cloned B cells release a barrage of freshly minted antibodies, which scatter throughout the body and bind to their specific antigen, in some cases directly neutralizing its toxicity and in other cases facilitating its destruction by tagging it for immune cells.

Our understanding of antibodies laid the groundwork for modern immunology. It also gave rise to a new form of treatment: antiserum therapy, which entails infusing immunized animal serum and its neutralizing antibodies into infected patients during their illness. In 1894, French physician Émile Roux and a team of doctors used horse antiserum to treat 448 children infected with diphtheria at L'Hôpital des Enfants-Malades in Paris, reducing their death rate by half and saving 117 children in the process.[42]

After presenting his results at the International Congress of Hygiene and Demography in Budapest later that year, Roux received a standing ovation. Antiserum therapy was quickly lauded as a significant feat of medical science.[43] As expected, medical researchers began looking to apply this novel treatment to other diseases, with pneumonia an obvious candidate.

However, fashioning effective antiserum therapy for *Streptococcus pneumoniae* was a complicated endeavor. Research showed that not all *S. pneumoniae* bacteria had the same immunogenic properties, meaning that the antibodies induced by one infection didn't necessarily protect against another. In fact, there were multiple subtypes or "serotypes" of *S. pneumoniae*, each with a unique antibody signature. Thus, to get an antiserum to work, doctors would have to first identify the serotype of *S. pneumoniae* to ensure that it matched the antiserum being used.[44]

In addition to its bacterial cell wall, *S. pneumoniae* is enclosed within a tough outer capsule. Composed of repeating patterns of carbohydrates called polysaccharides, the capsule acts like a layer of chain mail armor, preventing immune cells from destroying it.[45] The type and pattern of polysaccharides in the capsule also serve as a unique identifier or code for each serotype, and over a hundred serotypes have been identified to date.[46]

By 1913, a team led by American physician Rufus Cole at the Hospital of the Rockefeller Institute overcame the challenges of *S. pneumoniae* serotyping and, using the new therapy, cut pneumonia mortality by a stunning 70 percent. Pneumonia serotherapy made its clinical debut in large hospitals throughout the Northeastern United States by the late 1920s.[47]

Antiserum therapy came with many requirements. Treatment had to start early during the illness to be effective, and a patient's serotype needed to be carefully matched to the appropriate antiserum. Serotyping itself was a tedious process, necessitating the rapid and systematic collection of blood and sputum from patients upon hospital admission, incubation of those specimens in the laboratory, and then cross-matching the cultured bacteria against various type-specific diagnostic antisera using techniques such as agglutination and Neufeld's *Quellung* reaction.* The antiserum also had to be infused carefully and patients closely monitored, as antiserum reactions were common.[48]

The establishment of widespread antiserum therapy required considerable infrastructure, coordination between state and federal public health agencies, and a massive educational campaign for both the public and healthcare professionals. This led to significant government guidance and oversight of hospitals and physicians. Serum "typing" stations and depot centers were

---

* Agglutination is a laboratory reaction in which particles—such as red blood cells or bacteria—suspended in a liquid clump together when exposed to a specific antibody that recognizes and binds to them. A related technique, Neufeld's *Quellung* (or "capsule swelling") reaction, introduced in 1902, used type-specific antisera against *S. pneumoniae*. When antibodies bound to the bacterial capsule, the capsule appeared enlarged and more refractile under the microscope, allowing the serotype to be visualized and identified on a slide. (See endnote 48.)

deployed across broad geographic areas. Physicians and patients alike had to unlearn deep-rooted views regarding how and where diseases like pneumonia should be treated.[49]

Medicine was beginning to move away from a *doctor–patient* model to an integrated healthcare *system*, translating cutting-edge research into effective frontline medicine.[50] This also created what US Surgeon General Thomas Parran called a "complicated" relationship between the state and the medical community, as many physicians resisted governmental oversight.*[51]

That said, pneumonia was a terrible scourge. Under Parran's leadership, the US Public Health Service was able to leverage substantial federal funding while coordinating physician outreach to expand antiserum therapy to states nationwide. Consequently, by 1940, two out of three states and territories in the US had established "pneumonia control programs."[52] Meanwhile, public education campaigns had transformed pneumonia into an emergency in the eyes of the public, with one notable educational brochure stating, *"Speed* is the GREAT FACTOR in the DIAGNOSIS and TREATMENT of PNEUMONIA. *Take no chances with this disease!"*[53]

As successful as antiserum therapy was, the arrival of antistreptococcal antibiotics almost entirely overshadowed it. Antibiotics were practical and affordable and didn't require any infrastructure to administer. Starting with sulfapyridine, first reported in 1938, and followed by penicillin a few years later, these drugs shot onto the stage like movie stars, stealing the show.[54]

Beginning in the 1940s, doctors also developed vaccines against the *S. pneumoniae* capsule and influenza, the most common viral cause of pneumonia, marking the start of efforts to prevent these infections altogether.†[55] Meanwhile, advances in intensive care medicine granted healthcare professionals new life-support technologies to maintain patients' vital systems during life-threatening illnesses like septic shock.

Thanks to these new technologies, by the late 1940s, pneumonia had again been relegated to the purview of frontline physicians. During this time, deaths from pneumonia impressively declined, dragging down overall death rates by

---

*   By the 1930s, the medical profession had coalesced into various national medical societies to advocate for physician autonomy and welfare. This gave them a stronger voice, especially when opposing governmental oversight.

†   The first *S. pneumoniae* (*pneumococcal*) polysaccharide vaccine was licensed for public use in 1977, whereas the first influenza vaccine was licensed for public use in 1946.

the 1950s. Not surprisingly, after that, public interest in the disease waned.[56]

Some historians recount a degree of complacency that appeared during this era, with more physicians prescribing antibiotics for all varieties of respiratory infections—often inappropriately—while others began using them to try to *prevent* pneumonia. One 1950s study conducted in South Dakota found that over five years, a startling 92 percent of the population was prescribed antibiotics, with over half of those prescriptions being inappropriate.[57]

———

The evolution of disease rarely follows a straight path. Despite significant advancements in medical care, by the 1980s, pneumonia would once again be a fearsome presence in the corridors of medicine, with resistant strains of *S. pneumoniae* and a fresh ensemble of pneumonia-causing microbes asserting their presence. All the while, patients were becoming older and increasingly vulnerable.

Despite the vaunted successes and magic bullets of the early twentieth century, there was something we hadn't anticipated: *Murphy's Law*. Named after the late United States Air Force engineer Captain Edward A. Murphy, it says that "whatever can go wrong will go wrong."[58] It's a statement about complexity. As things get more complex, more problems appear. Modern medicine was no exception.*

By the 1950s, patients had greater access to medical therapies, such as cancer chemotherapy, open heart surgery, organ transplantation, and immunosuppressive infusions for diseases such as lupus and rheumatoid arthritis. This brought a greater need to implant invasive medical devices like intravenous lines, bladder catheters, and surgical hardware; all the while, more patients were being supported by mechanical ventilators and life-support systems while undergoing advanced surgeries.

Hospitals and large academic medical centers took on a greater role in caring for these complex patients, and the government began supporting an expansion in advanced medical care. In 1946, in response to a considerable demand for hospital services, the United States government passed the Hill–Burton Act, which allocated funding for a substantial increase in community

---

* Not all complexity is disorderly from a physics standpoint. Under the right conditions, entropy can also give rise to orderly complexity.

hospitals across the country. Meanwhile, the growth of the nation's foremost government-funded medical research agency, the National Institutes of Health (NIH), led to significant funding for medical research.

On July 30, 1965, one of the most pivotal pieces of health legislation in history—the Social Security Amendments of 1965—was enacted. It established the behemoth government health insurance programs Medicare and Medicaid, effectively transforming the United States government into the largest payer for advanced medical services in US history.[59]

Additionally, in the 1950s, with the advent of more advanced life-support machines and the improvement of critical care nursing education, hospitals around the country saw a vast expansion in intensive care services. By 1965, more than 90 percent of major hospitals and 30 percent of small hospitals housed intensive care units.[60]

Meanwhile, throughout the second half of the century, doctors saw a sharp rise in diseases of aging and abundance: high blood pressure, heart disease, stroke, cancer, and diabetes. People were living longer, but they were carrying a heavier burden of chronic diseases.

All told, the mid- to late twentieth century saw an impressive rise in advanced medical care and hospital admissions, with the latter peaking at around thirty-nine million per year by 1980.[61] It was a new age in medicine. We had created a world within a world: the American healthcare system, populated by the medicalized patient; with it would come a new collection of problems, complexities, diseases, and patients who were vulnerable on a level we had never seen before.

I entered medical school just as the prevalence of chronic illnesses was rising sharply. By that time, the ninth edition of the World Health Organization's *International Classification of Diseases* manual—the ICD-9—had already recognized over thirteen *thousand* different diseases and disorders.[62] Patient care was getting increasingly complicated, as was the administrative burden of keeping track of all this complexity.

During this time, our technology quickly outpaced our ability to appreciate all its downstream effects, while our past successes left us ill-prepared for the emerging complexities of the future. Before we could understand the full scope of this new world, it was upon us: a large population of highly vulnerable patients, often packed into hospitals, where a new generation of infectious diseases, along with our old adversary, sepsis, was ready to strike.

Mary often remarked that veterans like Tom were "made out of different stuff." He had an incredible demeanor and kept smiling even as he fought for each breath. But his body was frail, and an assortment of medical problems and a weakened immune system stacked the odds against his survival.

I was on call during Tom's second night at the hospital when I received an evening page from his nurse, Mario, informing me that his condition was deteriorating. He was experiencing increased difficulty breathing, and his blood oxygen levels were dropping. I asked Mario to obtain a fresh set of blood cultures, a complete blood count, and another chest X-ray. After hanging up, I quickly grabbed my white coat and headed downstairs.

It's hard to define what it feels like when your patient starts crashing. Perhaps it's best described as your soul being torn from your body. As I raced downstairs to the medical nursing unit, I frantically ran different scenarios through my head.

Maybe it's an MI. Maybe we made the wrong diagnosis.

When I arrived at the step-down unit, Mario was at the bedside with a respiratory therapist, Jill, who had placed Tom on a high-volume oxygen mask. Meanwhile, Tom was still oddly jovial, trying to have a conversation with the two of them as they scurried about organizing the lines and tubes entangling him.

I went through a few rapid-fire questions, trying to rule out any alarming symptoms, like chest pain, which could herald a catastrophic new problem, like a heart attack. Tom sounded a bit confused to me—a concerning sign that he had developed sepsis and an impending system-wide failure. Yet his blood pressure remained normal. Unsure how to proceed, I called Mary, who arrived on the scene a few minutes later.

After what seemed like an eternity, the X-ray was complete. As Mary placed the film over the light board, the image left me speechless. Tom's pneumonia had nearly doubled in size, and he now had widespread inflammatory changes in both lungs.

Sepsis disrupts the delicate web of microscopic blood vessels, called capillaries, which line the lungs' air sacs or alveoli, making their walls leaky. This allows fluid, immune cells, and inflammatory debris to flood the alveoli and surrounding support structures. It can leave the lungs too stiff to expand and impede the vital exchange of oxygen and carbon dioxide in the blood.

In the early stages, a patient suffering from lung injury might feel short of breath, have low oxygen levels, or breathe rapidly. Later, they might require a mechanical ventilator to survive. The most severe form of this lung injury is called acute respiratory distress syndrome (ARDS), and it's a common way patients can die from sepsis.

The combination of Tom's X-ray findings and blood oxygen measurements clearly indicated ARDS. Even more sobering were the blood oxygen levels themselves, which showed that Tom's respiratory system was failing. Mary asked Jill to start therapy with a noninvasive ventilator mask called BiPAP to help him breathe. She then asked me to confirm Tom's DNR status with him while she called Betty.

Sitting beside Tom, I tried my best to hide my trepidation. I held his hand and laid out the situation. Despite his mild confusion, I could tell he understood what I was saying. He even responded, "No, no, no, I don't want that!" while shaking his head when I asked him if he wanted to be on a mechanical ventilator. Ultimately, he agreed to continue the current level of medical care, including adding the BiPAP device. Before getting up, I squeezed his hand one last time, and he gave me a couple of good squeezes back as if to thank me. Jill slid in after that to start fitting him with the BiPAP mask.

I returned to the nurse's station, where Mary was discussing Tom's case with the ICU attending on-call, who recommended changing the antibiotics to cover for more antibiotic-resistant bacteria. We had considered the possibility of resistance when Tom first presented to the emergency room. Still, as Tom hadn't experienced any recent hospitalizations, we figured he had "community-acquired" pneumonia—pneumonia caused by the kinds of bacteria found outside the hospital, usually less likely to harbor resistance. The attending had a different take. He thought Tom's weakened immune system was a strong risk factor for resistant organisms. He felt that this, in combination with Tom's severe illness, had warranted broader antibiotics from the start—antibiotics that could have been pared down once Tom had stabilized. It was a difficult call either way, but the attending's assertion added to my disappointment about the situation.

Antibiotics may be hailed as wonder drugs, but they are hardly a panacea. Among the greatest medical innovations of the modern era, they remain vulnerable to a host of forces that limit their effectiveness.

Antibiotics are tuned to attack specific mechanisms within bacterial cells. Penicillin attacks the bacterial cell wall, swiftly rupturing bacteria, making the drug bactericidal or bacteria *killing*. On the other hand, "sulfa" antibiotics, which emerged about a decade before penicillin, inhibit bacterial synthesis of a vitamin called folic acid, which is essential for bacterial reproduction. This slows bacterial growth, making sulfa antibiotics bacteriostatic or bacteria *slowing*. Moreover, these mechanisms differ between bacteria, making antibiotic selection a critical factor in combatting sepsis.*

Most experts feel that, in severe infections and sepsis, you want to achieve a bactericidal effect with your antibiotic treatment to eliminate the bacteria. An antibiotic's specific mechanism, chemical properties, and ability to be absorbed into one area of the body or another impact its ability to treat a bacterial infection. This becomes especially important when treating bacterial sepsis, often associated with high concentrations of bacteria infecting the body. Selecting the wrong antibiotic, using the wrong dose, or even infusing it incorrectly could have severe and even fatal consequences for patients.

In the early 1900s, *S. pneumoniae* caused most pneumonia cases in the United States. Yet when I was in medical school, the list of causes of pneumonia was seemingly endless. Some of this reflected a greater understanding of the disease and all the possible microbes that can cause it. Another part was a natural shuffling of the order of pathogens, as the frequency of *S. pneumoniae* cases had decreased thanks to antibiotics, vaccination, and smoking cessation programs.[63] Nevertheless, today, doctors must anticipate any number of possible causes, including hospital-acquired pathogens, viruses, fungi, parasites, and multi-drug-resistant bacteria.

---

* The distinction between bactericidal and bacteriostatic is not always clear, as a higher concentration of some bacteriostatic antibiotics can make them effectively bactericidal, and vice versa.

Within an hour, Tom's family members had begun trickling into the intensive care unit. Mary and I convened a meeting at the bedside with Tom, Betty, and their oldest sons, Rick and John. We went through the findings and our assessment and prognosis. The situation was dire. Tom was slowly dying, and despite the recommendations to augment his antibiotics, it was likely too late to change his course. His blood pressure was stable, but his breathing was deteriorating rapidly. At this point, he was unlikely to survive without the BiPAP mask. Mary held Tom's hand and leaned forward.

"Tom, we're having trouble supporting your breathing right now. We think your pneumonia has gotten much worse. We don't think we can keep you going without this breathing mask. Can you give me a thumbs-up if you understand that?"

Tom nodded again and gave a thumbs-up.

"Do you want us to keep going with this mask?"

Tom shook his head emphatically, repeatedly saying, "No, no, no, I don't want it!"

"Are you sure it's what you want, honey?" Betty said.

Tom reached forward to hold her hand, closed his eyes, and nodded. It was all the confirmation Betty needed.

She turned to Mary and whispered, "Okay."

Mary signaled to Jill, who removed the mask and turned off the BiPAP. The machine slowly hissed as it shut down, then became quiet as a sense of calm filled the room. Tom was still breathing rapidly, so Mary asked Mario to administer a small dose of morphine to help with his air hunger. That seemed to help as his breathing slowed down.

We convened one last time with Betty to review the plan. Although she wasn't quite ready to stop the antibiotics, she didn't want to escalate the care any further. She wanted us to keep him as comfortable as possible. I glanced back at Tom one more time before we left. He looked peaceful, surrounded by his family.

———

Mario called me a few hours later with the news that Tom had stopped breathing. I headed to the ICU, where most of the family had now gathered. I took a deep breath as I entered his room. Betty was sitting at Tom's side, along with Rick and John.

They must have known I was in my first year, as John gave a half-smile and said, "I bet you haven't gotten used to this part yet."

I shook my head and said, "No, I haven't."

I offered my condolences and told them I would have to pronounce Tom. Before I left, I conveyed my regrets to Betty one last time, and she thanked me for taking such good care of him.

"I feel terrible. I wish we had done a better job."

She nodded and smiled. "No, you all did a wonderful job. It was just his time."

Her words comforted me, but I wondered if we could have made a difference in his care. It was hard to be sure.

"I hope you all got to spend some quality time with him in the end," I said.

Rick responded, "We did. I even got to lie in bed with him and read him an old bedtime story he used to read me when I was a kid."

Just then, my pager chirped, then vibrated menacingly.

"Sorry, I've got to get this."

"I guess the work never stops." Rick chuckled.

"Take care."

———

Tom's case was one of the more difficult in memory, in part because I was there at every point of his care, including his death. It was hard for me not to feel responsible for his outcome. In addition, back then, treating sepsis related to pneumonia was particularly challenging because we often didn't see it coming. As it didn't present in the same way as the more classic *E. coli* endotoxic shock, we didn't always think of sepsis in pneumonia patients until it was too late. We missed many opportunities to treat it more aggressively and were often caught off guard when patients started deteriorating.

Tom illustrates another valuable lesson: underlying the simple concept of antibiotic therapy is a maddening assortment of complexities, including selecting the right antimicrobial drug or combination of drugs, getting them into the patient urgently, dosing the medication properly, and even knowing when to change course. In the end, it's possible that Tom failed to respond to treatment because he was infected with antibiotic-resistant bacteria, so perhaps broader antibiotics were the missing piece.

Then again, sometimes you can do everything right and still not save a patient. Underneath his warm and generous personality, Tom had a complicated medical makeup and a weakened immune system, making him the perfect target for sepsis. He was a quintessential example of the relentless nature of this syndrome and its ability to seep into every corner of medicine, find the weak points, and attack.

———

Medicine's impressive record of modernization has had a lasting impact on our psyche as both patients and providers, leading to a romanticization of our abilities and, at times, perhaps resistance to a more nuanced approach to healthcare.[64] Until recent decades, we didn't anticipate the need to rethink our paradigm for managing severe infections, sepsis, or hospital care. Perhaps we hoped there would always be another magic bullet around the corner to vaporize the next disease. We still weren't thinking about preventing patients like Rory, Rosaria, and Tom from deteriorating in the first place.

Meanwhile, the twentieth century ushered in a powerful era of medical progress marked by advanced procedures, lifesaving antibiotics, and expanded hospital care. But with these gains came a host of unintended consequences. If one wanted to engineer the perfect conditions for a new wave of severe infections, the blueprint was now in place. And sure enough, by the latter half of the century, rates of severe infections and sepsis were steadily climbing.

CHAPTER FIVE

Changing Patterns of Infection

The hope that antimicrobial drugs would abolish infections as a cause of death has not been adequately realized. Current literature indicates that microbial infections continue to pose life-threatening problems and that antibiotic drugs do not offer susceptible human beings significant protection from certain types of microbial disease.

—DAVID E. ROGERS, MD, October 1, 1959[1]

Antibiotic resistance is rising for many different pathogens that are threats to health. If we don't act now, our medicine cabinet will be empty, and we won't have the antibiotics we need to save lives.

—FORMER CDC DIRECTOR TOM FRIEDEN, September 16, 2013[2]

IN 1959, AMERICAN RESEARCHER David E. Rogers published a report in *The New England Journal of Medicine* titled "The Changing Pattern of Life-Threatening Microbial Disease." It showed that, from the 1930s to the 1950s, antibiotics had transformed the landscape of disease by helping doctors virtually eliminate deaths from tuberculosis and severe streptococcal infections like pneumonia, puerperal sepsis, and scarlet fever.*[3]

Yet deep within the medical wards of American hospitals, severe infections and sepsis were still a serious problem, killing nearly one out of seven patients. More notably, new types of pathogens were replacing old ones. In some cases, such as staphylococcal infections, the microbes were evolving into strains that could evade previously effective antibiotics. In others, they represented an entirely new lineup of infectious organisms scarcely seen in modern times. In addition, as in the historic days of the Hôtel-Dieu, patients were once again getting infected after being admitted to the hospital for other conditions.[4] In fact, by the 1950s, the chance that a patient's severe infection was acquired inside the hospital was about eight times higher than twenty years earlier.[5]

———

In his December 11, 1945, Nobel Lecture, Alexander Fleming issued a prescient warning: "It is not difficult to make microbes resistant to penicillin in the laboratory by exposing them to concentrations not sufficient to kill them."[6]

During many years studying bacteria like *Staphylococcus aureus*, he witnessed their ability to quickly adapt strategies to evade antimicrobial therapies.

Dr. Ian Malcolm puts it best in the iconic film *Jurassic Park*: "Life finds a way."[7]

As evolution unfolds, it constantly shuffles through every genetic possibility, like a spinning raffle drum. With each new challenge the universe doles out, an organism eventually emerges with the ability to prevail.

According to the US Centers for Disease Control and Prevention (CDC), antimicrobial resistance (AMR) "happens when germs like bacteria and fungi develop the ability to defeat the drugs designed to kill them." It's a reality of the biological world that stems from the relentless pressure of natural selection placed against the basic premise of all life: *survive and reproduce*. In short, "it means the germs are not killed and continue to grow," making them "difficult and sometimes impossible to treat."[8]

Early signs of bacterial resistance appeared in eerie lockstep with antibiotics themselves. Clinical strains of *S. aureus* showed resistance to sulfonamide antibiotics within a few years after the drugs were introduced into practice.[9] Additionally, two biochemists from Howard Florey's original penicillin research

---

* Improved hygiene and infection control practices also contributed to the decline in streptococcal infections.

group, Ernst Chain and E.P. Abraham, discovered a penicillin-resistant *E. coli* strain in 1940—years before the antibiotic was ready for clinical use.[10] Sure enough, the same year Anne Miller famously received her first penicillin infusion in New Haven Hospital, researchers Charles H. Rammelkamp and Thelma Maxon of Boston University isolated four strains of penicillin-resistant *S. aureus* (PRSA), while treating patients at two hospitals in Massachusetts.[11]

In 1959, the British pharmaceutical company Beecham Group developed an anti-staphylococcal penicillin called methicillin, which promised to defeat PRSA. However, less than a year after it was introduced into clinical practice, methicillin-resistant *S. aureus* (MRSA) appeared, representing one of the first multi-drug-resistant superbugs.

Along with gram-negative bacteria like *E. coli*, MRSA is now a leading cause of hospital infections, bacteremia, and sepsis. It has also become a frequent cause of skin and soft tissue infections *outside* the hospital. These community-acquired MRSA infections were so common by the time I was in training that it was standard practice to initially treat any suspected *S. aureus* infection with an antibiotic known to kill the superbug.

Antimicrobial resistance has now become one of the most critical problems facing doctors. Resistant pathogens are hazardous because they can keep spreading despite antibiotic therapy, causing disease, sepsis, and even death unless doctors realize what is happening and switch therapy. However, predicting which patients have a resistant infection can be difficult.

Antimicrobial treatment guidelines advise doctors to prescribe broad-spectrum antimicrobial regimens tailored to kill resistant pathogens when the risk of resistance is high. This includes instances when patients acquire their infection while already in the hospital, if they have suffered from prior resistant infections, if they are colonized with resistant bacteria like MRSA, or if they have had a history of multiple antibiotic exposures.*[12]

It is often challenging for doctors to immediately determine whether they are dealing with a resistant microbe. There is also pressure to treat patients urgently. Many sepsis experts believe that when dealing with septic patients, doctors should prescribe antibiotics that cover a broad range of possible pathogens, especially in high-risk situations like septic shock. However, this approach

---

* Other risk factors for resistance include recent antibiotic therapy, history of recurrent skin infections or chronic wounds, presence of invasive devices or catheters, dialysis, or recent hospitalization.

can lead to overtreatment in some cases. As we will discuss later in the book, this issue has created tension in the academic medical community.

Obtaining body fluid cultures, such as blood cultures, is crucial when evaluating and treating sepsis patients. But these tests can take time—sometimes days—to yield results. Additionally, not all cultures demonstrate microbial growth. Only around half of all sepsis patients, and 65 percent of those admitted to the ICU, have a positive body fluid culture result to help guide therapy.[*][13]

Newer metagenomic sequencing and other molecular assays hold the promise of accelerating diagnosis beyond traditional cultures. MALDI-TOF mass spectrometry, a (protein-based) proteomic fingerprinting tool, can identify organisms within minutes once a culture turns positive, dramatically shortening the time from growth to identification. Microarrays, essentially molecular panels with built-in DNA "answer keys," can be applied directly to patient samples—such as blood, urine, and spinal fluid—to rapidly scan for dozens of pathogens and resistance genes at once. Metagenomic sequencing, an open-ended genetic test that looks for all DNA and RNA in a sample, can likewise be used directly on samples to detect virtually any microbe while highlighting resistance markers.[14] Although still limited in availability and imperfect at predicting true drug susceptibility, these technologies point toward a future in which treatment can be tailored far earlier in the course of illness. According to infectious disease expert and past president of the Infectious Diseases Society of America (IDSA) David Gilbert, such advanced tests may eventually increase the likelihood of identifying a specific microbe to as high as 95 percent.[15]

Even when we know we're dealing with antibiotic resistance, treatment often involves second- or third-line drugs—or combination therapies—that can harm the body, particularly the kidneys.[16] This means doctors must consider each case carefully. For instance, in chapter one, the antibiotic gentamicin was effective against Rosaria's resistant *E. coli* sepsis, but it carried a risk of kidney toxicity.[†]

It's now routine for doctors on the front lines to deal with multi-drug-resistant bacteria. The US CDC currently monitors *eighteen* antimicrobial-resistant superbugs that it categorizes as serious or urgent threats to our healthcare system.

---

[*]   A recent review article on sepsis published in *The New England Journal of Medicine* reported that a causative microbe is identified in 60 to 70 percent of sepsis cases. However, this was based on a single 2006 cohort study.

[†]   Most doctors have stopped routinely using gentamicin when treating urosepsis.

Some microbes, such as a group of resistant bacteria known as carbapenem-resistant Enterobacterales, are immune to nearly every antibiotic in our arsenal.[17]

Today, AMR pathogens directly kill around 1.3 million people and are indirectly associated with five million deaths each year worldwide.[18] In the United States alone, there are close to three million AMR infections annually, causing thirty-five thousand deaths.[19]

The forecasts are also dire. A 2019 report by the United Nations Ad Hoc Interagency Coordination Group on Antimicrobial Resistance projected that AMR infections could cause ten million deaths yearly by 2050, lead to twenty-four million people living in extreme poverty, and trigger a global financial crisis.[20] A 2024 study published in *The Lancet* estimated that in the next three decades, resistant infections could directly kill around forty million people worldwide.[21] Thus, prophetic as Alexander Fleming's warning was, as William Rosen states in *Miracle Cure,* it was "an understatement of massive proportions."[22]

What's startling about antimicrobial resistance is how fast it happens. It's an evolution we can watch unfold before our eyes. While, in humans, evolution occurs over thousands to millions of years, in the microbial world, it can occur in just a matter of weeks.[23] This is partly related to how quickly microorganisms can reproduce and transfer genetic information.

In the 1950s, researchers discovered that many genes imparting antibiotic resistance weren't fixed inside the bacteria's core DNA genome. Some were embedded in separate mobile structures of circular DNA called plasmids. Plasmids are self-replicating genetic entities that exist autonomously and encode crafty adaptations like the penicillinase enzyme, which breaks down penicillin.[24] Bacteria regularly pass them from one organism to another using connector tubes named pili during conjugation.[25] In another example of genetic exchange, bacterial resistance genes exist in mobile DNA packets called cassette chromosomes, which can be passed between bacteria and inserted into their native chromosomes.*[26] As a result, bacteria can quickly shuffle and trade plasmids and cassette chromosomes like software upgrades. They can also do this across species, meaning that *Staphylococcus* can pick up a plasmid from *E. coli* and vice versa.[27]

When one considers the prospect of horizontal transmission of mobile genetic elements like plasmids, AMR becomes a tricky problem. The human

---

*   Cassette chromosomes carried by MRSA carry the mecA resistance gene, which imparts resistance to methicillin.

microbiome alone houses around 100 *trillion* microbes, making it an ideal environment for bacteria to exchange resistance genes.[28] Some estimates suggest that, compared to the soil, the rate of horizontal gene transfer in the mammalian gut is about twenty-five times higher. This has led to the idea of the gut resistome: the intestines serving as a reservoir of antibiotic resistance genes. Some scientists even see the gut resistome as continuous with a larger *environmental* resistome, including pools of resistant genes in the greater human population, lakes, sources of drinking water, livestock, the food supply chain, hospitals, plants, and wastewater.[29] Simply existing in this larger ecosystem makes an individual susceptible to acquiring these resistant bugs.

But how did some resistance genes emerge before antibiotics were used? Here, it's crucial to note that many effective antibiotics originate from ancient microbes. For example, penicillin comes from the *Penicillium* mold, and streptomycin is produced by the soil bacterium *Streptomyces griseus*. *Streptomyces* itself is estimated to have existed for around 440 million years.[30] In essence, antibiotics have been part of our ecosystem for much of history.

Evidence also shows that resistance genes have existed as long as antibiotics. They can be isolated from frozen sediments dating back thirty thousand years, and phylogenetic studies trace their origins to over two billion years ago.[31] Thus, bacteria carrying these resistance genes were present long before humans started using antibiotics, waiting for the right conditions to thrive.

There is clear evidence that human behavior significantly contributes to antimicrobial resistance. Reports of antibiotic overprescription began in the 1950s. One North Carolina study at the time found that two-thirds of physicians inappropriately prescribed antibiotics for viral bronchitis.[32] More recently, a 2016 study showed that at least one-third of the 154 million antibiotic prescriptions written annually by emergency and primary care doctors were unnecessary.[33] Meanwhile, antibiotic resistance rates in hospitals have risen from about 15 percent in the 1990s to 60 percent today—a nearly fourfold increase.[34]

Doctors aren't solely to blame for antibiotic overuse. It's a complex issue related to physician time constraints, the desire to satisfy patients, and uncertainty in diagnosing respiratory infections.[35] Public awareness of the risks of antibiotic overuse has grown over recent decades, and fewer patients now demand antibiotics outright, though expectations persist. Physicians nevertheless face ongoing pressure to produce *something* out of their black bag when patients are sick.

Another key factor in antimicrobial resistance is the use of antibiotics in livestock. In 1948, biochemist Thomas Jukes discovered that feeding chickens the antibiotic Aureomycin led to faster growth. This finding spurred feedlots worldwide to start using low doses of antibiotics to promote rapid weight gain.[36] Currently, around 70 to 80 percent of antibiotics produced in the United States are used in livestock, with a global estimate of around 73 percent. Projections only see those numbers rising in the coming decade.[37]

What's more, the antibiotic dosing strategy in feedlots might be perfectly tuned to breed highly virulent strains of pathogens. Antibiotics can serve as hormetic agents—at low doses, they benefit bacteria by stimulating the formation of support structures and other adaptations. For example, antibiotics can induce the creation of a biofilm, a durable coalescence of bacterial cells, which can protect the bacteria from outside attackers. In another instance, low doses of the antibiotic tetracycline can nudge pathogens such as *Salmonella* to form a type III secretion system, a needle-shaped structure that helps the bacteria insert itself into the host's cells. The low doses of antibiotics given in feedlots may induce adaptations in gut bacteria like the *Salmonella* living in animal ruminants, making them more pathogenic to humans.[38]

So why aren't resistant microorganisms dominating the world? The most likely reason is that resistance genes often come with a cost to the bacterium's overall fitness. While these resistance mechanisms provide an advantage in antibiotic-rich environments like hospitals, they can hinder competitiveness outside these settings.[39] For example, some bacteria possess resistance genes for energy-intensive pumps to expel antibiotics, which reduce their overall fitness.[40] However, in patients receiving antibiotics, these resistant bacteria have a decisive advantage over others.

The preponderance of evidence now tells us that antibiotic resistance is inevitable and resistant microbes are everywhere. This suggests that our use of antibiotics is not creating the problem of resistance but rather accelerating it. Anytime additional selection pressure, such as penicillin, is added to a microbial ecosystem, resistant strains will have an advantage over others in that environment.

It also suggests that we can significantly reduce antimicrobial resistance by controlling the spread of resistant organisms and removing their selective advantage by reducing antibiotic overuse. Once we do that, natural selection might do the rest and reshuffle these pathogens back to their original place on the fitness ladder.

———

During the early to mid-twentieth century, hospitals were often considered "the doctor's workshop," with the prevailing attitude that the best hospitals also housed the best doctors. Little attention was paid to a hospital's actual mortality outcomes, and most hospitals didn't track data on hospital-acquired infections and resistant microbes.[41]

This changed in the 1950s, as PRSA began spreading worldwide in a global pandemic, referred to by author Kathryn Hillier as the "Golden Staph Era."[42] This period ushered in the modern infection prevention and control movement, as experts realized one of our most potent tools against resistant bacteria was to identify resistant strains and prevent their spread in hospitals.[43] Notwithstanding these efforts, by the 1960s, 80 percent of *S. aureus* strains had developed penicillin resistance.[44] Today, a staggering 99 percent of *S. aureus* is resistant to the antibiotic.[45]

Despite staphylococcus epidemics in the 1950s and 1960s, hospital infection control programs were uncommon during that time. In the 1960s, the US CDC began integrating infection control research in local hospitals, launching the Comprehensive Hospital Infections Project (CHIP) in 1965, which tested infection control methods in eight community hospitals. As more hospitals adopted these practices, professionals in the field coalesced into dedicated medical societies. By 1972, infection control specialists had formed the Association for Professionals in Infection Control and Epidemiology (APIC). Shortly afterward, hospital epidemiologists established their own society, now known as the Society for Healthcare Epidemiology of America (SHEA).[46]

In the early 1970s, the CDC launched the landmark Study on the Efficacy of Nosocomial Infection Control Project (SENIC), which surveyed over 339,000 patient medical records in 338 randomly selected US hospitals to determine whether infection control practices could prevent hospital-acquired infections. In 1975, data showed that hospitals could effectively reduce their nosocomial infection rates up to 32 percent by implementing core principles of infection control and hiring dedicated infection control professionals and epidemiologists. The projected return on investment associated with these programs was also an astonishing sixteenfold. Not surprisingly, infection control programs had become a requirement for hospital accreditation by 1976. Yet despite these positive developments, many frontline healthcare professionals were slow to adopt infection control principles, and researchers and administrators would continue to debate the cost-effectiveness of hospital infection control programs. Meanwhile, hospital-acquired infections and drug-resistant pathogens would continue to plague the healthcare landscape for decades.[47]

In the late 1990s, the first antibiotic stewardship programs (ASPs) emerged in hospitals—multidisciplinary teams of infectious disease physicians and pharmacists who used existing guidelines and microbiological data to inform the selection, dosing, and duration of antibiotic therapy.[48] This helped maximize the chances of overcoming a specific infection and lower patients' overall antibiotic exposure.

ASPs have since become commonplace in hospitals worldwide. They are essential to reducing antimicrobial resistance and counterbalancing the need to deliver rapid upfront antibiotics in sepsis. In 2019, the Centers for Medicare and Medicaid Services made it a federal requirement for all acute-care hospitals participating in Medicare or Medicaid to implement ASPs.[49]

When it comes to sepsis, there is no question that antimicrobial therapy should be administered rapidly. However, doing this on a massive scale creates the potential for significant collateral damage. As part of a comprehensive strategy to treat today's sepsis while minimizing the toll of *tomorrow's* sepsis, we need to think two steps ahead to limit the further transformation of our bacterial landscape. If we're committed to stopping sepsis, we should not only fight it head-on but also fortify strategies to slow the rise of dangerous resistant organisms. This means pairing urgent upfront antibiotic therapy with downstream antibiotic stewardship to limit the potential negative effects of antibiotic exposure.

The 2000s marked a crucial period when hospitals made greater investments toward infection control and antimicrobial stewardship programs, which paid off almost immediately. Between 2012 and 2017, hospital deaths from resistant organisms decreased by 18 percent, while those from AMR pathogens dropped by 30 percent. Unfortunately, during the COVID-19 pandemic, increased antimicrobial use and a breakdown in prevention systems in overwhelmed hospitals reversed these trends.[50]

Ultimately, history suggests that we can't eliminate antimicrobial resistance, but we can significantly limit its impact, mostly through the unglamorous work of prevention. It begins with the assumption that resistance is out there and that our behavior can significantly impact the problem. Data show that we can make a massive difference in antimicrobial resistance in one way or another. The question is, which way will we sway the results in the coming decades?

———

The 1950s also brought a rise in gram-negative bacterial sepsis, often involving our old adversary, *E. coli*. In addition, clinicians were now recognizing a relatively new category of microbial disease, called opportunistic infections, in which ordinarily *non*pathogenic organisms were transforming into sepsis-causing menaces following a weakening of a patient's immune defenses. During this time, bloodstream infections involving relatively quiescent microbes—like certain gram-negative bacteria, or the yeasts *Candida albicans* and *Cryptococcus neoformans*—were becoming increasingly common.[51]

What David Rogers and others were observing was partly an inevitable result of progress. Dividends from public health programs, vaccination, and other twentieth-century medical advancements were paying off, and people were living longer. At the same time, doctors were able to treat many previously untreatable diseases, like cancer and heart disease. This, combined with the expansion of hospital services and more advanced surgical care in the 1940s and 1950s, meant that hospitals were now housing more complex patients, often burdened by other diseases, while also receiving therapies known to weaken their immune systems.[52]

As infectious disease expert and past IDSA president Martin Blaser explains, "We had more aggressive treatments, like chemotherapies and surgeries, which [were] trying to save lives, which were, at one point, unsavable. One of the consequences of that is that people get prone to infection, and bad infection."[53]

The history of humanity is one of a continuous struggle with microbes. Blaser explains that before the 1900s, humans were killed by so-called high-grade or aggressive pathogens, such as *Streptococcus*.

He says, "As we've been able to control them better, now we get the next line of pathogens, the more opportunistic pathogens, and as we control *those* better, we get the third line of pathogens. When the host is impaired, they are susceptible to infection. We live in a world full of microbes. We can't sterilize the world. We can't sterilize the patient."[*][54]

What normally keeps the body's one-hundred-trillion-microbe ecosystem in check is the integrity of our physical barriers—the skin, respiratory passages, and gut lining—and the complex interplay between our immune system and these resident microorganisms. Even relatively unaggressive microbes that make it into vulnerable areas like the urinary tract and bloodstream can become death-dealing pathogens. As a result, patients suffering from traumatic injuries or undergoing procedures known to disrupt their standard physical barriers are at higher risk for such infections.[55] Patients with chronic ailments or weakened immune systems or those experiencing other acute illnesses in the hospital may be more susceptible to a breakdown in their immune system's ability to control their resident bacteria. Under the right circumstances, these organisms could penetrate the body and cause disease.[†][56]

The composition and health of our microbial ecosystem also serve to keep certain opportunistic microbes in check. One such organism, a spore-producing gram-positive bacterium called *Clostridioides difficile*, has emerged as the leading cause of hospital-acquired infections, with an estimated 224,000 cases and thirteen thousand deaths in US hospitals in 2017.[57] Consequently, many organizations have implemented procedures to prevent the disease and control its spread in the healthcare setting. It's now also spreading outside the hospital in the community. We can estimate that there are nearly a half-million cases in the US each year, causing around twenty-nine thousand deaths.[58]

C. difficile colonizes the colon in up to 60 to 70 percent of healthy newborns and infants.[59] It exists in many children and adults as a harmless commensal inhabitant.[‡][60] Some experts suspect that it might impart some benefit in early

---

[*]   In 1971, an epidemiologist named Abdel Omran proposed the epidemiologic transition theory, which states that as civilizations advance, the burden of infectious disease deaths moves from an "age of pestilence and famine" to an "age of receding pandemics" to an "age of degenerative and man-made diseases." Though some point out flaws in the theory, it nonetheless represents an early representation of the concept of a changing landscape of disease as civilization advances.

[†]   *Staphylococcus epidermidis* is one of our most abundant skin inhabitants and usually exists as a harmless symbiont. It also produces antibacterial proteins called bacteriocins, which are toxic to other more pathogenic bacteria, such as *S. aureus*, thus controlling their ability to invade our skin through colonization resistance. Yet, with the greater frequency of invasive procedures, devices, and catheters breaching the critical skin boundary, *S. epidermidis* has seen increasing misadventures into deeper body regions, leading to serious infections.

[‡]   In 1876, Belgian parasitologist and zoologist Pierre-Joseph van Beneden published *Animal Parasites and Messmates*, an illustrated treatise containing many examples of symbiosis in

life, which is why it's so prevalent in childhood.[61] However, under certain conditions, the bacteria can become pathogenic. Although the factors underlying this transformation are complex, the most direct cause seems to be disruption in a host's microbiome, usually after antibiotic exposure.[62] In other cases, *C. difficile* is acquired through exposure to infectious spores in the environment, such as in a hospital or other healthcare setting.[63]

C. difficile is normally kept in check by other bacteria in our colon, ensuring its concentration is too low to cause significant disease.*[64] Antibiotics disrupt our gut ecosystem, killing off large chunks of bacterial symbionts and making the colon a more hospitable environment for the microbe.[65] Studies show that the diversity of gut bacteria in our colon can decrease within just a few days of antibiotic use. Just like an algae bloom, *C. difficile* can grow uncontrolled in a colon with a disordered ecosystem, leading to infection and sepsis.[66] Additionally, certain antibiotics, particularly broad-spectrum antibiotics, are more likely to put a patient at risk of *C. difficile*. This has led infectious disease experts to sound the alarm when it comes to the risk of excessive broad-spectrum antibiotic use in sepsis.

———

The same factors that can expose patients to opportunistic infections can also put them at risk of developing the dysregulated sepsis response, thus increasing their risk of death. In fact, since the 1960s, research has shown that the most important driver of sepsis mortality risk isn't the specific infection itself but rather the characteristics of the *patient*—what we refer to as host factors.†[67]

---

the animal kingdom. He called one type of symbiosis "commensalism," from the Latin *commensalis,* for "sharing a table." In commensalism, one party benefits while the other is unaffected.

* Researchers are paying greater attention to the myriad factors besides antibiotic exposure that can influence a person's susceptibility to *C. difficile* infections. For example, metabolic products of complex carbohydrates, such as short-chain fatty acids, may protect against *C. difficile* by inhibiting its growth and its ability to produce harmful exotoxins. The standard American diet, which is low in complex carbohydrates and high in fat and simple carbohydrates, may increase a person's risk of getting a C. *difficile* infection.

† Interestingly, the health of the gut microbiome also impacts the likelihood of developing sepsis, with disrupted or unhealthy microbiomes increasing the risk of the dysregulated sepsis response.

Much of our current understanding of the host factors contributing to sepsis comes from the groundbreaking 2020 Global Burden of Sepsis study, led by researchers Kristina Rudd and Mohsen Naghavi.* It showed that of the estimated fifty million sepsis cases seen annually worldwide, about 85 percent occurred in low- to middle-income countries (LMICs), with 40 percent of global cases affecting sub-Saharan Africa. This arguably places socioeconomic status at the top of the list of sepsis risk factors. Age is probably the second most important factor, with most cases occurring in young children or older adults. Over 40 percent of cases, or twenty million, occur in children under five. After this, noncommunicable diseases (aka preexisting conditions) and injuries play a significant role in increasing sepsis risk. Together, they cause about one in three sepsis cases while accounting for almost half of all sepsis deaths. The most common injuries associated with sepsis are motor vehicle accidents, and the most common noncommunicable diseases associated with sepsis are neonatal and maternal disorders.[68] In addition, as we'll discuss later, sepsis remains a leading cause of death in maternal patients.

High-income countries like the United States have a higher burden of chronic disease, which is associated with a higher risk of sepsis. For example, a 2001 study showed that just over half of all adult sepsis patients had at least one chronic disease.[69] In addition, the most recent US CDC estimates suggest that about three in four American adults now have at least one chronic medical condition, and more than half have two or more.[70] We see especially high rates of sepsis in patients with conditions that impair the immune system, such as cancer, AIDS, diabetes, emphysema, and end-stage kidney disease requiring dialysis, as well as those with impaired immune systems related to immunosuppressive med-ications. For example, the risk of sepsis is up to ten times higher than average in a cancer patient and *forty* times higher than average in a dialysis patient.[71] What's more, sepsis *itself* is a risk factor for getting sepsis in the future.

Age and sex also contribute to sepsis risk in high-income countries. In the US, sepsis is more common in infants and older adults. Across all age groups, it's more common in males than females.† In infants, most sepsis cases occur

---

* In this study, researchers analyzed 2017 data from the broader Global Burden of Disease Study (GBD). The GBD is a comprehensive and ongoing international effort by the Institute for Health Metrics and Evaluation to measure health outcomes and systems performance across more than two hundred countries and territories worldwide.

† The reason for lower rates of sepsis in females is still unclear, but researchers feel this is unlikely to be related to sex hormones, as these differences are present across all age groups.

in the neonatal period. In older patients, the higher risk of sepsis is likely associated with a greater burden of chronic diseases and age-related decreases in immune system function.[72]

Race and socioeconomic status also play a prominent role in sepsis risk in high-income countries like the United States. For instance, African-American patients, particularly those aged thirty-five to forty-four, are disproportionately affected by sepsis, which may be related to a higher burden of chronic disease combined with poor healthcare access. Meanwhile, studies consistently show that the syndrome is more common and deadlier in patients of lower socio-economic status.[73]

———

What David Rogers and others were uncovering in the 1950s was a deeper reality underlying infections and sepsis. Infectious disease is not a simple *us versus them* contest against a static lineup of deadly germs. There will never be a day when we will have conquered all disease-causing microbes. Instead, like a rotating kaleidoscope, infection patterns shift, doling out new pathogens and diseases as old ones fade away. In addition, as their host factors change, patients can become more susceptible to insurrections caused by their internal microbial flora. Meanwhile, the new advanced age of medical therapies and the very structures in which we deliver medicine make it easier for specific pathogens to gain a foothold over us. As foreshadowed by historical anecdotes, like that of Semmelweis more than a century ago, we must view sepsis as a problem of complexity while identifying and repairing cracks in our system that allow it to seep into existence.

This brings us back to the pillar of prevention. While these new sepsis-causing infections are largely an expected result of the changing landscape of medicine, as Blaser puts it succinctly, "it doesn't mean we shouldn't try to prevent [them] from happening." As we've been learning since Joseph Lister, we *can* make a huge difference in reducing the risk of infection, even in the most compromising situations, like major surgery.

Today, in the United States, about one in thirty-one patients has a hospital-acquired infection at any given time, with 1.7 million hospital-acquired infections causing around one hundred thousand deaths yearly.[74] According to the World Health Organization (WHO), *hundreds* of millions of patients worldwide are affected annually by healthcare-associated infections, including hospital-acquired pneumonia, catheter-associated urinary tract infections (CAUTIs), catheter-related bloodstream infections (CLABSIs), and surgical site infections, among others.[75] The WHO also estimates that good infection prevention and control programs could prevent up to 70 percent of these infections.

———

The emergence of the modern medical patient, paired with a shift in the type of microbes causing disease, has laid the foundation for much of the sepsis in hospitals and emergency rooms today. These factors also underscore the necessity of stepping outside an older way of treating infections—shifting away from direct confrontations with microbes and toward prevention. We should accept that these pathogens will continue to evade our strategies, making it crucial to be good stewards of existing antimicrobial drugs, continue to develop newer drugs, and explore smarter tactics for eliminating these infections, such as bacterial vaccines and more advanced, precise antimicrobial therapies. Finally, it means we should craft a nuanced approach to germs, understanding that some of them play an integral role in the environment, including our bodies. This means that to combat sepsis, we must also strive to improve our overall health and the health of our microbial ecosystem.

CHAPTER SIX

"It's Our Response That Makes the Disease"

Few critical conditions in medicine are as paradoxical as the events occurring during sepsis. The response of the patient's body to an insult such as infection or severe injury may initially be appropriate, but such defenses can lose their usual balance and destroy the patient.

—DR. ROGER BONE, August 2, 1996[1]

IN THE WINTER OF 2006, a twenty-nine-year-old man named Bobby arrived at the emergency room in severe respiratory distress. Six days earlier, he'd woken up shivering uncontrollably with a dry, hacking cough. Determined to push through, he'd waited it out at home, hoping the illness would pass. But his condition had only worsened. With each day, his strength had faded, and each breath had grown more labored. By the last day, he could barely stand up on his own. Realizing how ill he was, his brother Mike had rushed him straight to the hospital.

By the time they arrived at the emergency room, Bobby was taking nearly forty breaths per minute, his blood oxygen level critically low. His color had turned blue, and he was struggling to keep his eyes open. A chest X-ray revealed widespread inflammation in both lungs—a sign of acute respiratory distress syndrome (ARDS).

The ER team quickly stabilized him with high-flow oxygen therapy, intravenous fluids, and antibiotics, admitting him to the medical ICU. An hour later, a rapid antigen test revealed the culprit: influenza.

As the evening progressed, Bobby's condition worsened, and he needed more oxygen support. By midnight, his respiratory system collapsed, prompting the ICU team to place him on a mechanical ventilator.

I was caring for Bobby the following morning with the daytime ICU team. He had continued to deteriorate overnight and was now on maximum life support. As we discussed his dire condition, I couldn't believe how quickly this invisible virus had dragged a young, healthy man to the verge of death.

Bobby's story illustrates one of the most counterintuitive lessons about sepsis: sometimes the body's response is worse than the disease, and sometimes the response *is* the disease. This erratic behavior of the body's immune system is where our discussion of this syndrome takes a crucial turn.

———

By the second half of the twentieth century, doctors were increasingly observing the ravages of gram-negative bloodstream infections. Careful descriptions from that era detail the first sign of a bacterial intrusion into the bloodstream as a sudden, sharp increase in fever, usually more than 101°F and often as high as 104°F. With infants, it could rise to as high as 106°F. Shock was also observed, frequently occurring within hours of the initial fever. Patients' white blood cell counts were usually elevated, sometimes markedly, and it wasn't uncommon for them to have some degree of kidney dysfunction. Symptoms included chills in the early stages, followed by nausea, vomiting, and, in some cases, diarrhea.[*2]

What the earliest sepsis pioneers had glimpsed a century before—and great minds like William Osler had later underscored—was now becoming undeniable to modern doctors: sepsis was not just an isolated condition but a syndrome, a distinct pattern of signs and symptoms appearing across patients, regardless of the specific bacteria or source of infection.

It also had a remarkably swift onset, with two researchers from the University of Illinois College of Medicine—William McCabe and George Gee

---

* Laboratory studies have shown that within minutes of a bacterial intrusion into the bloodstream, the white blood cell count drops sharply and then rises later. The mechanism behind this is complicated and relates to the innate immune response (which we will discuss shortly). This response leads to the attachment of endotoxin to capillary endothelial cells in the lung. This, in turn, upregulates anchoring receptors that attach to circulating white blood cells in the bloodstream.

Jackson—noting in the early 1960s that "the transition from relatively good health to prostration [could] occur within minutes or a few hours."[*3] This classification scheme matched historical descriptions of sepsis patients showing a "toxic" appearance as the syndrome took hold.

McCabe and Jackson also noted that laboratory animals injected with gram-negative endotoxin rapidly manifested similar findings to those observed in infected hospital patients—a crucial link between the clinical syndrome and experimental endotoxic shock. If you were to open a medical textbook or journal from the 1960s or 1970s, you would probably read all about the endotoxic shock model.[†4]

So here we had "sepsis," a syndrome associated with a set of observable clinical features and, in the case of gram-negative bacterial infection, linked to the physiologic effect of an endotoxic barrage. But what was it about endotoxin that could wreak such internal havoc on the body?

What followed was a succession of discoveries that revealed the complex world of biology's most ancient system of defense: the innate immune system, a built-in first line of protection for detecting and eliminating germs or other foreign agents from the body.[5] It has its evolutionary origins around a billion years ago, first appearing in our most primordial ancestors.[6]

———

In the early 1840s, researchers found that the pus-filled nodules or tubercles in the lungs of tuberculosis patients were filled with white blood cells. Yet the significance of their presence was mysterious. Four decades later, a brilliant, eccentric Russian zoologist named Elie Metchnikoff observed white blood cells called macrophages migrating toward a starfish's injured, inflamed foot. Metchnikoff knew these cells were somehow being beckoned to the site of injury or infection, but it would take researchers nearly another century to

---

[*]   Most modern studies suggest that while molecular signaling begins almost immediately, the measurable systemic host response typically unfolds over a few hours.

[†]   In a 1969 review article published in the *Journal of the American Medical Association*, titled "Bacterial Shock," infectious disease experts Jack A. Barnett and Jay P. Sanford wrote, "The most common offending organisms are gram-negative bacteria, although septic shock may occasionally occur after infection with fungi, rickettsiae, viruses, and gram-positive bacteria."

discover how this happened.*[7]

As bacterial endotoxin, aka LPS, was wreaking havoc in the wards of mid-twentieth-century hospitals, bench researchers were hard at work deconstructing its effects on the body. By the 1940s, some suspected its toxicity resulted from other intermediary chemicals the body fashioned. However, proving it was a difficult task.[8]

In 1943, American pathologist Valy Menkin reported isolating a fever-inducing protein from sterile pus, which he called "pyrexin." When injected into rabbits, this substance produced high fevers, suggesting that inflammation itself could generate a fever-causing mediator. Later analysis, however, revealed that his samples were likely contaminated with bacterial endotoxin. Nevertheless, the idea took hold, and just five years later, American physician Ivan Bennett repeated the experiment under more rigorous conditions, confirming that such a host-derived fever mediator existed—distinct from bacterial endotoxin and produced by white blood cells.[9]

Over the next two decades, evidence increasingly showed that inflammation resulted from chemicals released by the body's provoked or damaged cells. As fevers were one of the most measurable manifestations of inflammation, these substances were aptly called endogenous pyrogens ("internal fever generators").

In 1974, American physician Charles Dinarello successfully isolated and purified two distinct endogenous pyrogens from human white blood cell extracts—proteins that would later be named interleukin-1 alpha (IL-1α) and interleukin-1 beta (IL-1β).[10] Around the same time, researchers began using the term "cytokine"—meaning "that which moves cells"—to describe this new class of intercellular signaling proteins that included the interleukins. These molecules were soon recognized as the body's primary chemical mediators of inflammation and the very substance beckoning Metchnikoff's macrophages.†[11]

As these discoveries circulated in the academic medical world, clinical researchers began refocusing their lenses on the body's response observed in sepsis patients. Conceptually, the previous model of *severe infection causes sepsis* was refined to the more sophisticated *severe infection triggers an inflammatory response in the body—which, in turn, causes sepsis.* Sir William Osler had been

---

* He later observed them attempting to engulf or ingest infectious agents in a process he called phagocytosis.

† Though Dinarello played a significant role, the discovery of cytokines began gradually with the identification of interferons in the 1950s.

right all along in focusing on the reaction over the infection.

As physician-author Lewis Thomas aptly summarized in a 1972 *New England Journal of Medicine* essay titled "Germs," "It's our response that makes the disease."[12]

Inflammatory cytokines were seen provoking swift and dramatic changes in the body. They could quickly induce fever, raise the heart rate, induce rapid breathing, and release white blood cells into circulation. They could also have dramatic effects on the lining of blood vessels—increasing the number of sticky receptors binding white blood cells and opening junctions between the endothelial cells lining blood vessels, making them more permeable. All this intended to ramp up the body's metabolic system while recruiting white blood cells to the site of infection, where they could launch a counteroffensive against invading germs.

Still, by the 1980s, a big question remained: What was the *initial* trigger for the body's immune response? In other words, how were white blood cells first alerted to a pathogen's presence? This vexed American immunologists H. Kim Bottomly and her husband, Charles A. Janeway. (The two often debated the issue.) In 1989, Janeway developed a concept he called the Pattern Recognition Hypothesis, which is now considered foundational to our understanding of innate immunity.[13]

Microbes possess specific groups or patterns of molecules, which are either attached to their surfaces or released during internal metabolic processes. Meanwhile, ordinary cells lining the body are coated with receptors that recognize and attach to these molecules. Once attached, the receptors initiate a cascade of chemical reactions, activating an immune response. In this way, the body and its sentries constantly sweep the environment, looking for danger signals in the form of these aptly named pathogen-associated molecular patterns (PAMPS), using cell surface receptors called pattern-recognizing receptors (PRRs).[14]

By the 1990s, scientists had uncovered entire classes of PAMPs, which enabled them to identify a mechanism by which bacteria (including endotoxin-containing gram-negative bacteria), fungi, parasites, and viruses could trigger an immune response.[15]

A decade later, researchers also identified so-called damage-associated molecular patterns (DAMPs)—molecules released by the *host's* injured cells during infection or injury. First conceptualized in the 1990s and formally named in the early 2000s, DAMPs were shown to trigger the same receptors as microbial

PAMPs, provoking a vicious cycle of immune activation and dysfunction.*[16] Because DAMPs could also be released during trauma, burns, or other noninfectious conditions, it became clear that the body could spiral into a widespread cascade of immune hyperactivation and dysregulation without the slightest presence of pathogens or their toxins in the blood or body.[17]

The innate immune response gets even more intricate, and this can help us appreciate how it can amplify out of control. Coursing throughout the body are tiny specialized proteins that make up the complement system. Normally dormant, they are activated when they encounter PAMPs or DAMPs, with the resulting reactions transforming them into ferocious pro-inflammatory mediators called anaphylatoxins.[18] Others break into fragments and coat microbial surfaces, tagging them for destruction during opsonization. In their most impressive feat, complement proteins can self-assemble into a multiprotein membrane attack complex. This pore-shaped structure inserts itself into a microbe's cell membrane, rupturing the organism.[19]

Our bodies are, in essence, coated and primed with a primordial perimeter defense system—an ancient network designed to recognize and destroy invaders and with enough redundancy to give it the makings of a giant chain reaction.

As Lewis Thomas put it, "Our arsenals for fighting off bacteria are so powerful, and involve so many mechanisms, that we are in more danger from them than from the invaders. We live in the midst of explosive devices; we are mined."[20]

Usually, the innate immune response does quick work on a microbial incursion, and the body goes about its business. However, in some cases, due to an overwhelming infection or any number of pathogen-directed or host-derived factors, this system can wildly overreact, resulting in a domino effect. One can appreciate how uncontrolled activation of even one piece of this response—the complement system—could quickly result in massive collateral damage to surrounding tissues and organs while tripping the body's other defense systems.[21]

———

Bobby's condition was deteriorating rapidly. His lungs' alveolar air sacs had begun to fill with inflammatory fluid and debris, preventing oxygen from

---

* The term "damage-associated molecular patterns" (DAMPs) was coined by researchers Seung-Yong Seong and Polly Matzinger in 2004.

being absorbed into his bloodstream. Meanwhile, his lungs had stiffened from injury, resulting in dangerously high pressures as we ventilated him. Despite maximum support, his blood oxygen levels were too low to supply his body's needs. A decision was made to paralyze his muscles while placing him in a prone or belly-down position to try to open up more of his lungs for gas exchange and make ventilation easier. All the while, a deluge of inflammation spread throughout his body, causing his cardiovascular system to shut down as he tumbled toward septic shock.

Several of Bobby's family members had gathered in the ICU waiting room. Accompanied by my attending physician, I gave them an update. His parents were stunned by what they were hearing.

"How can he be dying? He's so healthy," they said.

Bobby's condition had declined so quickly that there had barely been enough time to get his family up to speed on what was going on, let alone the fact that he was resting on a razor's edge between life and death.

———

Every pathogen has a unique way of tripping the body's immune response, and while almost any pathogen can cause sepsis, there are common offenders. In an extensive 2017 survey looking at infection patterns in ICUs across eighty-eight countries, gram-negative bacteria were isolated in 67 percent of all sepsis cases, gram-positive bacteria in 37 percent, fungi in 16 percent, and viruses in about 4 percent.*[22]

Microbes possess virulence factors, which allow them to evade the immune system while injuring the host in some cases. This includes the formation of protective biofilms, discussed in chapter five, and the production of exotoxins, discussed in chapter one. For instance, *S. aureus* houses an arsenal of about two dozen potent exotoxins, called superantigens, that can short-circuit the immune system, resulting in a surge of pro-inflammatory cytokines. Another familiar bacterium, *Streptococcus pyogenes*, which killed Rory Staunton, carries

---

* The percentages add up to greater than 100 percent because many patients had more than one type of infection in this study. Additionally, these patterns of infection vary significantly based on geographic location.

eleven superantigens.*[23] As we've already learned, in other cases, the simple expression of PAMPs, such as lipopolysaccharide in the case of gram-negative bacteria, can trigger the body's sepsis response.

Influenza is a small, spherical virus, 100 nanometers in diameter—about a twentieth the size of an *E. coli* bacterium and close to a hundredth the size of a red blood cell. It's coated with two proteins, hemagglutinin and neuraminidase, giving it a spiky appearance. Its ability to mutate and shuffle these surface proteins through two processes called antigenic drift and shift leads to different influenza strains, as well as the "H" and "N" designations of these variants. For example, the Spanish flu pandemic involved the H1N1 influenza strain, sometimes called "swine flu." Once it contacts a human respiratory tract cell, the hemagglutinin attaches to sialic acid receptors on the host cell's surface.[24] After it attaches, it's engulfed by the cell through endocytosis. It then releases ribonucleic acid (RNA) as a blueprint or programming code. The RNA seizes control of the host cell's protein manufacturing machinery to mass-produce millions of viral copies. Finally, the new virus particles or virions exit the cell with the help of neuraminidase, which cleaves off the sticky sialic acid receptors, freeing the virus from the cell.

While the virus may enter the cell and engage in its mischief under relative cover, its genetic material can quickly trigger the host cell's defense systems. Once detected, this material activates multiple immune pathways in the cell, unleashing a cascade of inflammatory mediators. It's the balance or *imbalance* of this response that dictates the severity of the reaction. In those like Bobby, who are less fortunate, the response spirals out of control, resulting in an uncontained inflammatory response: a cytokine storm.†

———

Shortly after learning about inflammatory cytokines, researchers discovered a group of cytokines that also suppressed inflammation. The body's inflammatory response was coupled with a compensatory *anti*-inflammatory response.[25]

---

*   *S. aureus* and *S. pyogenes* can inject these toxins into host cells using specialized nanosyringes known as type III secretion systems, which we discussed in chapter five.

†   The damaging effects of a severe influenza infection stem not only from the host's inflammatory cytokine response but also from the virus's direct cytopathic effects on infected cells, as well as secondary bacterial infections.

Some believed that, under normal conditions, these two responses existed in a balance that contained the body's overall immune reaction. Sound familiar? It reminds me of the ancient Greek concepts of sepsis and pepsis existing in equilibrium.

The body's inflammatory cascade was beginning to look like a complex orchestra of chemical mediators, with one part ensuring that the other operated in a controlled fashion. If the inflammatory response intensified out of control, it could overwhelm the compensatory anti-inflammatory response, and you'd get a runaway effect. Instead of the harmonious symphony of a successful immune response, you would have the cacophony of sepsis. On the other hand, an overreactive anti-inflammatory response could clamp down so swiftly and persistently that it might induce an immunocompromised state in the body. This might leave the host susceptible to any number of secondary infections, which could beset the patient just as their response to the initial infection was subsiding.*[26]

———

Bobby remained in critical condition throughout the day, with his system teetering on the brink of collapse. We watched his organ systems slowly fail one by one as the toxic effect of his septic response seethed throughout his body.

By the afternoon, we had initiated extracorporeal membrane oxygenation (ECMO), a form of heart-lung bypass used in the ICU. As Bobby's respiratory system was failing, the ECMO machine would serve as an external set of lungs—a critical lifeline until his sepsis subsided.

But ECMO was no trivial matter. It was a massive undertaking, requiring the surgical insertion of large-caliber catheters while pumping his system with blood thinners to prevent blood clots. Any number of serious complications could occur, including catastrophic bleeding, severe infection, and even stroke. We just needed to buy enough time for Bobby's sepsis to resolve and the inflammation in his lungs to settle down.

---

* While this is a good general framework, as we'll learn in the next chapter, it's still an oversimplification of the complex sepsis response.

———

In addition to the effects of cytokines and complement proteins, researchers have observed something more sinister happening in the blood of sepsis patients. This involves the convergence of the body's separate but interrelated systems of defense and healing.

We can start this discussion with the adage "All bleeding stops, eventually." It's a bit of macabre humor from the old days on surgery rounds, but it refers mainly to the axiom "When there is bleeding, first hold pressure." Imagine you cut your finger and hold pressure for a few minutes. Usually, the bleeding stops. Underlying this simple truth is one of the most intricate systems in the body: the coagulation system.

Most of our understanding of the coagulation system stems from the work of nineteenth-century Italian pathologist Giulio Bizzozero. He observed tiny granular cell fragments in blood samples, which he named *piastrine*, or platelets, for their "plate-like" appearance. In 1881, he observed those same platelets aggregating over a rabbit's recently injured artery to form a patchwork called a *thrombus*, from the Greek word *thrómbos* ("clot").[27]

We now recognize platelets as first responders to blood vessel injury, rapidly aggregating to form an organic plug over the damaged area. Their ability to detect injury comes from receptors embedded on their surface, which react to signal proteins released by damaged blood vessels. The endothelial cells that line blood vessels contain storage granules filled with one of these proteins, von Willebrand factor (vWF), named after the Finnish hematologist who discovered it. When damaged, endothelial cells release vWF, attracting platelets to the injured region and serving as a bridge between platelets and exposed damaged tissue.[28]

The blood circulation also houses a system of specialized proteins, aka clotting factors, which interact with platelets to fine-tune the coagulation process to almost mathematical precision. When injured, damaged blood vessels expose a protein called tissue factor, which activates the first of thirteen clotting factors—factor VII—which triggers a cascade of activity that cleaves a protein named fibrinogen into dense strands called fibrin. Fibrin, in turn, reinforces and crosslinks the platelet plug, forming an organic meshwork that seals the injury and stabilizes the mature clot.[29]

Myriad factors, including mechanical injury, infection, and inflammation, can activate the clotting system. There are also dozens of ways this process can go awry. For instance, the build-up of cholesterol plaque in the inner lining of blood vessels in the heart can lead to increased turbulent blood flow, shearing the surface of the blood vessels, exposing vWF, and leading to thrombus formation in a coronary artery. This blocks the blood supply to the heart muscle, leading to a myocardial infarction or heart attack. The deadliest version of this condition is the ST-elevation myocardial infarction (STEMI), named after the electrical changes seen on the electrocardiogram when a coronary artery is completely blocked. The cornerstone of medical treatment of heart attacks—aspirin—inhibits platelets by irreversibly blocking an enzyme called cyclooxygenase.

In the early twentieth century, bacteriologists started observing the formation of countless little clots or microthrombi inside the blood vessels of patients with endotoxic shock. By the 1930s, it was so common to see overactivation of the clotting system in sepsis that some doctors began treating patients with powerful blood thinners. Unfortunately, many of these patients suffered severe complications, like brain hemorrhages, effectively halting the practice by the mid-century. In the 1970s, it became clear that there was considerable overlap between the inflammatory cascade of sepsis and the clotting system, with cytokines, like IL-1, able to promote clotting by upregulating tissue factor. Decades later, PAMPs, such as endotoxin, were also observed to activate the clotting cascade, as were activated complement proteins.[30]

In sepsis, excessive activation of the clotting cascade can obstruct or disrupt the flow of blood through the microscopic network of tiny blood vessels that supplies the organs. In addition to the large-vessel or macrovascular effects of dilated, leaky, and dysfunctional blood vessels, sepsis inflicts an invisible threat of widespread microvascular disease. While a heart attack is brought on by the occlusion of a single medium-sized coronary artery, sepsis involves the calamitous dysfunction of the *entire* blood circulation—both macroscopic *and* microscopic.*

This unrestrained systemic inflammation and microvascular clotting can have the unfortunate effect of widely impairing blood circulation, which can then disturb and injure internal organs, which rely almost entirely on the blood to supply them with nutrients like oxygen and glucose. Disruptions like this

---

* This is oversimplified, as coronary microvascular disease can sometimes mimic the signs and symptoms of a heart attack, though it rarely causes a true heart attack.

can be measured as changes in specific markers of organ function. In the case of the kidneys, it's reflected in their ability to filter out byproducts of protein metabolism, like creatinine, or by the output of urine produced by the organs' filtration process. What's more, this can all occur under the guise of relatively normal vital signs. Looking back at Rosaria from chapter one, her impaired kidney function was heralding the onset of sepsis before her blood pressure had even begun to drop.*[31]

———

Bobby's first two weeks on ECMO were brutal. Each day brought new complications and collateral damage. In the early stages of his illness, he suffered from a severe lack of blood flow to his extremities, leading to necrosis of his fingers and toes. He was also hit by a succession of secondary bacterial infections (ones that occur during or after treatment for another infection), the worst of which were staphylococcal pneumonia and a lung abscess, which required a surgical chest tube to drain out infected pus. In the mornings, when I wasn't on overnight call, I walked through the ICU doors with trepidation, wondering if he'd still be alive.

By the third week, we started seeing signs of improvement, and we began weaning him off the ECMO machine. At first, when we pulled back support, he would crash and have to go back on. But after a few more days, he was off ECMO and stable on the ventilator alone. It took another week to wean him off all his life support, and by the twenty-first day of his admission, he was awake and breathing on his own. A week later, I visited him on the medical ward before he was discharged. Despite everything, he was in good spirits. By then, he had lost three fingers, severely damaged several others, and suffered significant injury to his kidneys. But he was alive, off oxygen, and walking again. In the end, he had narrowly escaped death.

---

*   It is still unclear to researchers what happens during organ dysfunction in sepsis. Studies have shown that the cells within the organs are not permanently destroyed, so some researchers have theorized that the observed organ dysfunction is an adaptive response to sepsis, almost like hibernation.

As it turned out, Bobby was infected with the H1N1 strain—a direct descendant of the one that caused the Spanish flu. Beginning in March 1918, the virus circled the globe in just a few months. Over the next two years, it infected a third of the world's population and claimed as many as fifty million lives, many of them children and young adults.

Worse than that was how it attacked infected individuals: tearing their lungs apart, flooding their alveolar air sacs with pools of blood and inflammatory fluid, leaving its unfortunate victims drowning in their secretions.[32] The onset of death was often foreshadowed by the appearance of mahogany spots on the cheeks and dusky, dark blue skin, making patients look as "blue as huckleberries."[33]

Even those who survived the first wave of infection often suffered from secondary bacterial pneumonia and sepsis. The virus's proclivity toward damaging the respiratory tract leaves its victims helpless against scavenging bacterial invaders, resulting in a double infection: bacterial pneumonia on top of the flu. Researchers now believe most deaths during the Spanish flu pandemic were related to secondary bacterial pneumonia.[34*]

SARS-CoV-2, the virus that causes COVID-19, can also dysregulate the body's inflammatory response, leading to sepsis. Once it infects a host cell, it uses the cell's machinery to manufacture numerous copies of itself. During peak infection, the number of circulating virion particles can approach 100 billion per host.[35] It evades the innate immune response by hiding its viral PAMPs, possibly within tiny membrane-bound vesicles, while interfering with cytokine production and other host defense proteins. The virus eventually triggers the self-destruction, or pyroptosis, of these hijacked cells, which can result in a significant, and sometimes delayed, inflammatory reaction referred to as cytokine release syndrome.[36] The virus attacks cells throughout the body, including the lungs, heart, brain, blood vessels, liver, and kidney. The most significant organs affected are the lungs, where the surge of inflammation can significantly impair oxygen exchange and, in the most severe cases (as commonly seen in earlier SARS-CoV-2 strains), cause acute respiratory distress syndrome

---

* An essential component of pandemic preparedness involves stockpiling antibiotics and bacterial vaccines in conjunction with viral vaccines and antiviral therapies in order to prepare for secondary bacterial pneumonia.

(ARDS).* In addition to causing the tragic deaths of countless individuals, this virus has the capacity to bring the healthcare system to a halt due to the sheer volume of hospitalized patients during COVID-19 surges. This makes it a critical public health issue.

Viral pandemics add another worrisome dimension to the changing landscape of infection we discussed in chapter five. This is because they are associated with climate change and agricultural and deforestation practices. Many viral diseases, like COVID-19 and influenza, are zoonotic, meaning they are caused by germs that spread between animals and humans.[37] As the climate changes, so does the geographic range of specific animal hosts. This, combined with the disruption of natural habitats and the expansion of farms and human population centers, can increase the commingling risk between species, eventually allowing such diseases to jump to humans—something called zoonotic spillover.

For instance, there's evidence that climate change has altered the global distribution of bats, which are an essential reservoir for deadly viruses, such as SARS-CoV-2, SARS-CoV-1 (which caused the first SARS outbreak in 2002), and are suspected reservoirs of Ebola virus. This has increased their proximity to crossover species, such as pangolins, which, in turn, increases the risk of zoonotic spillover.[38]

In another example, the US CDC is currently tracking H5N1 avian influenza, or bird flu, which we'll discuss more later in the book. Periodic outbreaks of this disease have been linked to the intensification of poultry farming and the globalization of the poultry trade.[39]

Yet the scale of potential risk extends far beyond this handful of pathogens. A 2022 *Nature* study projected around ten *thousand* viruses capable of infecting mammals and birds that could spill over to humans, but only a fraction have been detected or characterized.[40] This tells us that there may be few limits to the number of deadly pandemics that nature can churn out as climate change accelerates.

---

* As the virus has mutated into newer, less virulent variants, and our collective immunity to it has increased, we are seeing fewer episodes of the cytokine storm, with some experts now referring to a cytokine breeze.

By the second half of the twentieth century, sepsis was inching its way into the lexicon of hospital intensive care units, while its enigmatic nature was slowly revealing itself in the laboratory. As a concept, it now encompassed far more than just bacterial blood poisoning or terrible wound infections. Close examination revealed an imbalance of chemical signals underpinning the body's response to various insults, including but not limited to gram-negative bacteremia. Yet there was still ambiguity around this new understanding of sepsis. Although researchers now knew that it involved the host's response to an infection infiltrating the body, it would still take years for this idea to sprout into a mature understanding of sepsis as a process. It would take even longer to translate it into more effective treatment strategies. Moreover, much of the older common wisdom about sepsis remained fossilized in the medical consciousness, leaving many cases undetected well into the twenty-first century.

Trials and Tribulations

More than 100 randomized clinical trials have tested the hypothesis that modulating the septic response to infection can improve survival. With one short-lived exception, none of these has resulted in new treatments. The current challenge for sepsis research lies in a failure of concept and reluctance to abandon a demonstrably ineffectual research model.

—JOHN C. MARSHALL, past chair,
Canadian Clinical Care Trials Group, 2014[1]

FOR MOST OF HUMAN HISTORY, practitioners developed new medical therapies through simple observation and deductive reasoning, passing down their knowledge through anecdotes, personal accounts, and case histories.[*][2] Over time, these reports and insights coalesced into a body of medical knowledge that formed the foundations of pre-modern medicine—shaping practice and guiding future generations of physicians.

Eventually, doctors began to think more scientifically, questioning if a treatment reliably produced the intended effect—what we now call efficacy. In essence, they sought to determine whether the treatment itself was truly responsible for the outcome or if other variables, such as a physician's skills, a patient's constitution, or some other unknown factors, played a role.

---

[*]   Anecdotal evidence can still exist within the scope of the scientific method. For instance, in large medical case studies, data are derived by quasi-experimental methods and is potentially verifiable by others in follow-up studies. However, for most of history, such studies were not systematic and were thus unreliable.

One of the earliest records of such an inquiry appears in the ninth century, in the writings of Persian physician Abu Bakr al-Razi. Among his many travails as medical director of Baghdad's largest hospital, al-Razi faced a succession of diseases and plagues, including a spate of meningitis.[3] By that time, the ancient Egyptian practice of bloodletting—intentionally bleeding patients—had become a widespread treatment for many diseases, famously taught centuries earlier by none other than Galen himself.[4]

Al-Razi had a talent for science and approached many reported therapies with healthy skepticism. In *Kitab al-Hawi*, he described a clever experiment to test the efficacy of bloodletting as a preventive therapy for meningitis.[5] He began by selecting patients who showed an early constellation of signs and symptoms—"dullness and pain in the head and neck [that] continues for three and four and five days or more, and [for whom] the vision shuns light, and watering of the eyes is abundant, yawning and stretching are great, insomnia is severe, and extreme exhaustion occurs." Afterward, he divided them into two groups: one in which he "[proceeded] with bloodletting" and another where he "intentionally [neglected] them."[6] Over time, he observed that those in the bloodletting group were "saved," while all of those in the "neglected" group progressed to meningitis, concluding that bloodletting was indeed an effective preventive measure.[7]

We now recognize this ninth-century experiment as an early example of a controlled clinical trial, in which investigators compare a group of patients undergoing an experimental treatment to an unexposed "control" group. The study was remarkably advanced for its time. However, al-Razi's flawed methods led him to an incorrect conclusion, as we now know that bloodletting is entirely ineffective in treating or preventing meningitis.

Even to the untrained eye, his experimental design reveals several inconsistencies. For example, how did he decide who would receive the bloodletting treatment and who would be left untreated? Could he have otherwise unknowingly treated one group differently? In what ways did he neglect the control group? These uncertainties suggest the possibility that any number of factors besides the experimental intervention may have impacted his patients' survival.

The universe abounds with hidden variables that can easily influence the outcome of any study. It's impossible to manually account for all these invisible confounders when conducting clinical trials. Researchers themselves can also influence results by unknowingly selecting patients who are more or less likely to respond favorably to therapy. Moreover, they can unconsciously change their behavior while caring for one group or the other.[8] In the end, any number of these problems could have skewed al-Razi's results.

In the 1940s, English statistician Bradford Hill continued the work of another Englishman, Ronald Aylmer Fisher, and devised an elegant solution to this problem of hidden variables with a technique called randomization.[9] It involves randomly assigning experimental patients to either treatment or a placebo, thus relying on chance to distribute any potential confounders equally between the two groups and independently of any human influence.

A terrible bout of tuberculosis in 1917 foiled Hill's aspirations for a career in medicine. Hence, he turned his focus to medical statistics, becoming one of the foremost experts in the field by 1937.[10] A few years later, he persuaded the Medical Research Council in Britain to use his method to test the efficacy of the antibiotic streptomycin in treating tuberculosis in what would become the first randomized clinical trial (RCT).[11] In the process, he catapulted the medical profession into a new era of scientific discovery.[12]

RCTs have since become one of the most crucial innovations in medical research and are now the principal means by which researchers test new medical interventions and therapies. As sepsis expert John Marshall explains, "Randomization is the key to understanding causation. Things occur randomly in the universe; if you can control one variable—for example, the treatment delivered—while everything else happens at random, then you can be confident that the nonrandom variable was the cause of any differences seen."[13]

Still, even the most carefully fashioned RCTs, conducted by the most diligent investigators, can be plagued with problems. Did investigators ask the right clinical question? Were patients selected properly? Were the methods sound? Poorly designed trials can sometimes mislead scientists for decades while confusing and frustrating frontline doctors and patients. Like al-Razi, even the best doctors can be fooled by a clinical trial when its methods are flawed.

More importantly, clinical trials don't provide absolute truths. Instead, they are designed to answer specific questions and improve our confidence about certain associations, such as the efficacy of a particular treatment for a group of sepsis patients. As our understanding of the underlying science evolves, so too will the design and results of our clinical trials.[14]

Researchers have repeatedly encountered disappointment when testing advanced sepsis treatments in clinical trials—a challenge I refer to as the "sepsis clinical trials conundrum." While scientific theory has consistently offered promising new therapies, these treatments have often failed to demonstrate consistent efficacy across different trials. This pattern has flummoxed experts and drug developers alike.

Some of the early setbacks resulted from flawed experimental designs, such as the absence of randomization. Others stemmed from patient selection problems, largely driven by the lack of a clear, standardized definition of sepsis.

However, the most important explanation for the sepsis clinical trials conundrum is that it took some time for researchers to realize that sepsis wasn't a single "disease" in the classical sense. "Sepsis," as people were understanding it, was a catchall term representing a staggering *collection* of variations around a common theme. In much the same way that we now understand "cancer" to be a term encapsulating a broad range of diseases stemming from a shared thread, we were beginning to recognize that sepsis is also an assortment of disorders sprouting from a common root.

———

As doctors faced an increasing number of deadly sepsis cases during the second half of the twentieth century, they began to realize that conventional therapies, such as antibiotics and intravenous fluids, were often insufficient to reverse the downward spiral for many patients suffering from septic shock. During this time, researchers began illuminating the underlying processes at play while exploring therapies that could target new pathways. To understand these early experimental treatments, we should first review some basic physiology while taking another historical jaunt.

In 1849, English physician Thomas Addison observed that if a tuberculosis infection were to infiltrate and destroy a patient's adrenal glands, the individual would suffer from a terrible malady of lethargy, depression, and an intense craving for salt.[15] By 1894, two British researchers, George Oliver and Edward Schafer, had found that when they injected an extract of adrenal glands into a laboratory animal, its blood pressure and heart rate abruptly increased. A crystalline chemical from the extract was isolated a few years later, reproducing the same effect. The substance was called epinephrine, also known as adrenaline.*[16]

---

*   The term "epinephrine" is typically used in medical and scientific contexts, while "adrenaline" is more commonly used in everyday language and outside of the United States.

In 1936, Polish–Swiss chemist Tadeusz Reichstein isolated another chemically active compound from adrenal gland extracts, which he named cortisol.*[17]

These researchers were gradually uncovering the body's *endocrine system*, a complex network of glands that regulate various physiological functions and help the body maintain a delicate internal balance, or homeostasis.

The term "homeostasis" was first coined in 1926 by physician Walter Cannon, derived from the Greek for "same" and "standing still." It describes the body's ability to maintain stable internal conditions—such as body temperature, blood pH, and blood pressure—despite an ever-changing environment.[18]

Remarkably, this equilibrium is almost always maintained through a highly coordinated interplay of sensors, chemical messengers, and feedback loops—systems that have evolved over hundreds of millions of years to detect and counteract disruptions in the body's internal state.[19] When we overheat, we sweat, allowing evaporative cooling to regulate body temperature like a built-in air conditioner. When we get too cold, we shiver, generating body heat to restore warmth. It's a perpetual biological dance, constantly resisting the relentless pull of entropy.

The endocrine system releases chemical messengers called hormones, which travel through the bloodstream and interact with distant organs to regulate their function. There are numerous endocrine organs, but the two small, triangle-shaped adrenal glands on top of each kidney are central to our discussion of sepsis.

The inner portion of each adrenal gland, the medulla, produces adrenaline (aka epinephrine), as well as another similar compound, noradrenaline (also called norepinephrine). These two chemicals take part in the well-known fight-or-flight response accompanying a significant stressor or fear, resulting in a rapid increase in heart rate, tightening of the blood vessels, increase in the heart's contractile force, and a burst of glucose released into the blood to prepare the body for the fight or flight of its life. Given their ability to raise blood pressure quickly during shock, doctors began using these substances almost as soon as they learned to isolate and purify them chemically. They have since become the basis for modern vasopressor therapy.

Surrounding the medulla is the adrenal cortex, which forms three zones from

---

* Reichstein and another chemist, American Edward Kendall, discovered a group of corticosteroid compounds from bovine adrenal glands almost simultaneously. According to historians, the two men competed with each other.

outer to inner: the zona glomerulosa, zona fasciculata, and zona reticularis. The outer zona glomerulosa makes a salt-regulating hormone called aldosterone; the zona fasciculata produces cortisol—referred to as a corticosteroid because of its cholesterol-based steroid chemical ring structure—which helps the body regulate blood sugar levels and blood pressure while suppressing inflammation. The innermost zona reticularis makes sex hormones, such as DHEA.

By the late 1940s, studies on rheumatic fever and rheumatoid arthritis indicated that corticosteroids, including cortisol, could reduce inflammation.[20] It was also clear that these hormones could strengthen the body's initial reaction to severe stressors like infections or surgery. Those who developed adrenal gland dysfunction, whether by birth or due to a damaging process later in life, sometimes faced a total collapse of their cardiovascular system and even sudden death during an acute illness—what is now referred to as an adrenal crisis.[21]

The youngest sepsis trials of the 1950s and 1960s focused on harnessing the powerful effects of corticosteroids to dampen the impact of severe inflammation while also supporting the body's stress response.[22] Though conceptually sound for their time, they reflected an incomplete understanding of sepsis, the body's innate immune system, and that system's mediators.[23] These early sepsis trials also demonstrated shortcomings in accepted scientific methodology, which was common in that era, as clinical trial science had just begun evolving toward higher standards.

In a 1974 paper published in the *Annals of Internal Medicine*, Stephen Weitzman and Stephen Berger of the Albert Einstein College of Medicine reviewed thirty-two sepsis corticosteroid trials. Their analysis showed that just under two-thirds of the trials used standardized criteria to select patients, only a quarter employed randomization, and a mere 16 percent blinded both investigators and patients. They concluded, "The historical perspective gained from our review may well incriminate inadequately designed studies for perpetuating confusion and uncertainty."[*][24]

For most of the twentieth century, "sepsis" was a diagnosis made by an experienced clinician utilizing clinical gestalt, often using bacteremia and shock as the most apparent indicators of the disease.[25] However, this approach was problematic when selecting patients for clinical trials. Inconsistencies in the patients recruited for the studies showed that clinical expertise was too subjective

---

[*]   Many 1950s studies also used non-standardized steroid doses, creating a completely different comparison problem.

to select similar patients across different studies reliably.[26] This created an apples-to-oranges comparison problem when experts tried to relate different studies with one another or when frontline doctors tried to generalize the studies to their sepsis patients.

In addition, preclinical animal studies showed that rapid sepsis treatment was associated with significantly better survival in the laboratory.[27] These early trials hinged on the time-sensitive delivery of experimental therapies. Yet this approach was challenging when applied to human patients studied in real-world hospitals. Identifying sepsis patients involved waiting for a frontline doctor's gestalt, which could take hours, or confirming positive blood culture results, which could take days. This led to significant delays in initiating treatment in human clinical trials, potentially reducing any benefit.[28] Furthermore, as we'll discuss shortly, preclinical animal studies had limited applicability to human trials, given the differences in physiology between humans and animals.

This is not to mention that the existing sepsis definition failed to capture its true nature as the body's *reaction* to infection. It was not so much a direct harmful effect of microbes, but rather pieces of these microbes, as well as damaged tissue, tripping the body's innate or nonspecific defense system, that led to the sepsis response. As researchers like McCabe and Jackson were describing as early as the 1960s, this reaction could be seen as a *pattern* of clinical findings known as a syndrome, with many of the findings present long before bacteremia was clinically apparent from laboratory blood cultures or a doctor's recognition of septic shock. All this meant that clinical trial investigators needed a better system to identify sepsis patients early while selecting those with similar manifestations of the disease.[29]

———

The decades leading up to the 1980s saw conflicting results from corticosteroid trials and a growing realization that conventional antimicrobial and supportive therapies were failing to reduce sepsis mortality. This left experts eager to develop a better understanding of sepsis physiology as well as more precise and effective treatments.

By then, bacterial endotoxin was widely understood as a direct and potent trigger of cytokine release, often sending the body's white blood cells into apparent rage, bursting with pro-inflammatory cytokines. Researchers theorized that by blocking endotoxin's interaction with white blood cells, they could stop it from activating the inflammatory response in the first place.[30] It so happens that nature had already devised a clever solution to block toxins—antibodies—so they thought to administer anti-endotoxin antibodies to block endotoxin before it could hijack the body's immune system.

A number of clinical trials explored donor antiserum therapy against endotoxin. While this technique showed promising results in early studies, it was too expensive and impractical to produce a standardized, reliable supply of the serum for clinical use. The 1980s also brought increased fears of HIV infection, adding to the challenge of using donor serum.[31]

Immunoglobulin therapy overcame some of these challenges by isolating and purifying specific antibodies called IgG and IgM from volunteers exposed to *E. coli* infections and then infusing those antibodies into patients. Unfortunately, these trials were mired in design problems, such as a lack of standardization of immunoglobulins and the use of vastly different treatment protocols across different studies. Additionally, investigators didn't always know whether patients recruited to these trials even had high levels of endotoxin in their bloodstream.[32]

By the mid-1980s, a new technology had emerged: monoclonal antibodies, which were produced by cloning entire lines of B lymphocytes exposed to one specific antigen (such as LPS) and then harvesting the resulting clones to produce highly targeted antibodies. With this technology, whole lines of anti-endotoxin monoclonal antibodies could be manufactured in the laboratory and then injected into patients to block endotoxin's effects. Again, though preclinical trials were promising, human trials using this advanced therapy struggled to achieve reliable results that could be validated across multiple patient groups.

In the end, when analyzing the data, there were too many differences in study designs, the definitions of shock used, and how specific types of sepsis patients were identified.[33] Moreover, like prior immunoglobulin studies, many of these trials failed to demonstrate that recruited patients had significant endotoxemia or that the anti-endotoxin antibodies were actually neutralizing the endotoxin. As a result, they failed to show significant benefits in large clinical trials and were ultimately abandoned.[34*]

With the intricate world of cytokines also coming into resolution in the

---

* According to John Marshall, the response to endotoxin is sufficiently complex and conserved, or unchanged, across species, that it could be considered an exohormone, meaning that, in

1980s, therapy shifted away from endotoxin and toward blocking inflammatory cytokines directly. This strategy could effectively widen the net to treat other *non*-endotoxin-mediated infections and noninfectious causes of severe inflammation. With sepsis now deconstructed into a complex series of chemical pathways and signaling molecules stemming from the body's response to infection, it seemed only natural to develop drugs that could block or otherwise halt the *mediators* of that response.

During this period, numerous clinical trials investigated a promising group of anti-inflammatory therapies, including monoclonal antibodies targeting cytokines such as interleukin-1, first identified by Charles Dinarello (chapter six), and another key inflammatory cytokine, tumor necrosis factor-alpha (TNF-α). Physicians hoped that neutralizing these chemical mediators would sufficiently dampen the body's inflammatory response, thus improving sepsis survival. However, despite initial optimism, randomized clinical trials repeatedly failed to show significant benefit when these therapies were applied to average sepsis patients at the time.[*][35]

Indeed, the post-1950s era revealed sepsis to be a vexing disease. Frontline doctors sought more advanced medicines to halt the runaway inflammatory cascade, yet ostensibly beneficial experimental therapies targeting endotoxin and cytokines were falling short in real-world settings. A considerable disconnect was emerging between theory and practice and between preclinical animal and human patient trials.[36] Something just wasn't adding up, leaving the sepsis research community in a dysphoric state. The question "Why have clinical trials in sepsis failed?" became a subject of regular discussion and debate in academic circles.[37]

Public health officials and policymakers were also beginning to take notice. This culminated in the 1974 US Senate-commissioned Special Study Group on Gram-Negative Bacteremia, which examined the issue of gram-negative sepsis.[38] The committee analyzed troves of clinical trial data, noting that many supportive therapies for sepsis used at the time were developed using animal models, which usually involved injecting dogs with massive doses of endotoxin—far

---

some contexts, it may support a healthy response in the body. In fact, trials have shown that mortality increases when endotoxin is targeted in patients with gram-positive infections.

[*]   Cytokine-blocking drugs ultimately transformed into modern-day biologic therapy for autoimmune diseases, such as rheumatoid arthritis and Crohn's disease, and now make up a significant share of global pharmaceutical industry revenue.

in excess of what might be experienced by a human sepsis patient.[39] They also pointed out that a canine's physiologic response to endotoxin differed substantially from that of humans. This meant that any methods of treating septic shock honed in canine laboratories were based on conditions scarcely seen in human patients on the healthcare front line.[40]

In fact, the case study for sepsis in those days was still gram-negative bacterial shock. Moreover, many of the early sepsis preclinical trials used disease models in the laboratory involving extremely sick animals with baseline mortality rates that were much higher than what was being seen in hospitals. Some now argue that, for that reason alone, preclinical trials were more likely to show benefits for new therapies than subsequent human trials.[41] Additionally, while the *model* for sepsis back then was gram-negative bacteremia, many sepsis patients in the hospital had sepsis resulting from other microbes. Even a nonexpert can look at that and say, "How are these the same thing?"

This led some researchers to question the fundamental theory behind sepsis, while others began reexamining the methodology of clinical trials themselves. By momentarily hanging up their lab coats, they conducted an analysis of the *analysis* in the hope of constructing better trials that could more accurately translate the basic science into clinical practice. In the process, they also began reexamining the precise definition of sepsis, realizing that the studied patients might not have represented what doctors saw on the front lines.

They gradually came to realize that sepsis wasn't a single disease with a distinct cause and footprint. Patients weren't experiencing a monolithic or homogeneous process. Instead, sepsis was revealing itself as one of the most variable and complex conditions in medicine. Any number of different microbes could trigger it, each with its own specific PAMPs and pathogenic mechanisms. It could strike people of all ages, was influenced by vastly different host factors, and manifested as a chaotic array of signs and symptoms that varied from one patient to another.

This came as no surprise to some researchers. According to sepsis expert Dr. David Gilbert, during the 1970s and 1980s, many infectious disease experts conducted pathogen-specific research on sepsis.

Gilbert explains, "There were a lot of papers on meningococcemia, a lot of papers on endotoxemia. They didn't say 'sepsis.' It was more specific to the stimulus of the microorganism, whatever the microorganism du jour was for that particular investigator."

And while gram-negative endotoxic shock had its signature sepsis pattern, other infectious syndromes, such as meningococcal shock, had different expressions of sepsis.

Gilbert goes on, "The real experts say we should be saying 'bacteremic shock,' 'fungemic shock,' [or] 'endotoxic shock,' or '[cytokine] shock' if it's a virus."[42]

The host response could also manifest in different ways in different individuals, leading to hyperinflammation, immunosuppression, or some mixture of both states. We now know sepsis results when a severe infection triggers our body's defense system to behave erratically. Researchers have now dissected this response into its parts, finding layers of intricacy involving just about every system, with the complement system, cytokines, and the clotting cascade playing a central role. In fact, studies in mice have shown that over *one hundred* inflammatory mediators and metabolites are released during endotoxemia alone.[43] Similar studies of humans have shown that a low-dose injection of endotoxin alters the expression of 3,714 unique genes in circulating white blood cells![*][44] Combining this knowledge with all the possible kinds of patients, their inherent host factors, and all the different types of infections they could have, one can appreciate the diversity of "sepsis" that could be out there. Experts now believe that dozens, perhaps even hundreds, of varieties or phenotypes of sepsis exist. While they think it's possible to group some of these phenotypes into related clusters, it seems no two sepsis patients are truly alike.[45][†]

This prompts the question: if there are so many different sepsis patients out there, how can we be sure that they will respond similarly to a new drug? The short answer is that they probably *won't*. This brings us back to the central sticking point with patient selection. Like cancer, sepsis is what researchers call a heterogeneous disorder, meaning that a group of sepsis patients encompasses a wide array of different sepsis subtypes, each with its unique footprint. As

---

[*] In a 2014 opinion piece referencing the body's immune response mechanisms during sepsis, Marshall wrote, "It is improbable that modulating the activity of any one of these will have more than a modest effect on the clinical course of the illness." Another crucial factor is the kinetics or speed of the cytokine response, which occurs within minutes to hours. Once it happens, according to Gilbert, "the horse is out of the barn," thus further reinforcing the concept of treating sepsis early, before it gets out of hand.

[†] The most current terminology distinguishes sepsis *subphenotypes* as subgroups of patients who share clinical or biological features without necessarily sharing a common underlying pathophysiology, whereas sepsis *endotypes* refer to subgroups that do share a specific pathophysiologic mechanism.

a result, different patients will probably not respond the same way to some new and advanced sepsis therapy.

For instance, a clinical trial examining a new experimental therapy involving one hundred sepsis patients might produce a negative result, suggesting to researchers that the treatment didn't work. But because those one hundred sepsis patients might have represented twenty-five different subtypes of the syndrome, maybe the treatment only worked for a few of the subtypes while harming a few others.*[46] So, the *average* result misled researchers into thinking that the treatment had shown no overall benefit.[47]

This is exactly what some researchers started to see when they performed subgroup analysis, a method that reexamines the original pool of patients, focusing on subsets of patients within the group—for example, men older than sixty-five. When investigators reviewed the data, they found that some of these failed experimental treatments might have benefitted subgroups of patients with specific host factors or, in some cases, those with more severe illness. As it turns out, several secondary analyses have now shown that cytokine inhibitors can indeed benefit certain subgroups of sepsis patients.[48]

A significant net effect of this analysis of sepsis clinical trials was that it broadened awareness of the potential blind spots inherent to these studies. However, its *main* effect was to identify a critical flaw in how sepsis patients were being defined in the first place.

For the bulk of modern history, sepsis meant one thing to most doctors: bloodstream infection, usually with gram-negative bacteria and often involving shock. But that definition was missing a large swath of sepsis patients on the one hand, while on the other hand, it was vastly oversimplifying the definition and severity of sepsis for the patients it *was* counting. Moreover, because there weren't any standards or criteria for defining sepsis or its severity, it was difficult to apply the data from these trials to everyday patients. As different trials often used dissimilar definitions of sepsis, it was also hard to compare results from one trial to another, creating an apples-to-oranges comparison problem.

While the endotoxic shock model for sepsis was an inimitable catalyst in

---

* In a 2008 clinical trial called CORTICUS, which tested the efficacy of a corticosteroid called hydrocortisone in sepsis patients, investigators found higher rates of *secondary* infections and *new* sepsis episodes in patients in the steroid-treatment group. They suggested that this could have explained the lack of improvement seen with steroid therapy, as some of the patients may have actually fared worse with the steroids, nullifying any potential benefit in other patients.

expanding our comprehension of the disease, it also limited our understanding of its full scope. What about pneumonia, skin infections, and other pathogens, like viruses and fungi? These were left mainly as footnotes in the major review papers and textbooks. They were recorded as infrequent causes of sepsis, as the overwhelming case study was still considered gram-negative endotoxemia.[49]

Meanwhile, patients *known* to have sepsis were perishing in hospitals across the world as deaths from the syndrome continued to climb.* According to the US CDC, the number of patients suffering from sepsis in the United States had increased by almost two-and-a-half-fold between 1979 and 1987, with the most significant increase seen in patients sixty-five and older. Sepsis had also become the thirteenth leading cause of death in the US, with associated healthcare costs approaching ten billion dollars annually.[50]

US hospitals, particularly those in Western and Northeastern states, also experienced a surge in sepsis cases and deaths in males aged fifteen to forty-four years. Although mysterious at the time, it was later attributed to the rise in HIV infections beginning in the early 1980s. As doctors lacked effective antiretroviral therapy at the start of the HIV epidemic, many of those patients developed acquired immunodeficiency syndrome (AIDS), which was associated with a high risk of secondary infections and sepsis related to immune system compromise.[51]

Additionally, dangerous drug-resistant pathogens were becoming regular fixtures in hospitals in the US and worldwide. By the late 1980s, there were an estimated one *million* hospital-acquired infections involving antibiotic-resistant bacteria each year in the US alone. It was becoming all too common for doctors to see sepsis from resistant superbugs like MRSA, vancomycin-resistant *Enterococcus* (VRE), and extended-spectrum beta-lactamase-producing *Enterobacteriaceae* (ESBL). Data showed that between 1986 and 1992, the rate of MRSA strains increased from 8 to 40 percent in large teaching hospitals, while it slowly climbed to 20 percent in smaller community hospitals.[52] Meanwhile, rates of VRE strains in US intensive care units increased twentyfold during that period. This trend would continue for decades, with a public health report published in 2007 estimating that from 1997 to 2006, the number of patients hospitalized with antimicrobial-resistant microbes increased by over three and half times.[53]

---

* Surveillance bias may have also been a factor. This occurs when increased detection results from more aggressive screening rather than an actual rise in the incidence of a disease.

Community pathogens were no different. By 1985, tuberculosis cases were on the rise again in the US, with outbreaks of multi-drug-resistant strains reported in thirty-five states.[54] As for *S. pneumoniae*, by the late 1980s, penicillin resistant strains were increasingly reported, and by the early 1990s, some were even beginning to show resistance to newer cephalosporin antibiotics.[*][55]

There was also something ominous about the sepsis case counts in the 1980s. By then, gram-negative bacteremia had become the most well-understood model for sepsis. The terms "sepsis," "septic shock," "septicemia," and "bacteremia" had blended into an amalgam of four interchangeable diagnoses. To many, the broader term, "sepsis," was still synonymous with blood poisoning or the presence of bacteria or bacterial toxins in the blood. This meant that many doctors weren't even considering sepsis unless there was clear evidence of bacteremia or shock.[56] Many patients likely died during those years from sepsis due to other infectious causes without any record of ever having it.

In other cases, even if sepsis was identified as the cause of death, the death certification process would obfuscate this fact. When certifying a death, physicians and medical examiners are required to conform to a rigorous format in which they report a chain of events leading from a specific underlying disease or injury, like appendicitis, to the immediate cause of death, like septic shock. Meanwhile, historical public death records might only capture the *underlying* cause of death. So, even if a patient with appendicitis died of overwhelming septic shock, a retrospective review of the data might only identify appendicitis as the cause.[†][57]

However, the one place where the US data *were* clear was the overall trend in infectious disease mortality. By 1980, the historic eight-decade-long decrease in infection death rates had not only leveled off—the rates were *increasing* for the first time since the beginning of the century.[58] With each passing year, more people were dying from infections—and not just due to the AIDS epidemic. Infection-related deaths were rising among all adults, particularly those aged

---

[*] Today, more than two in five *S. pneumoniae* infections involve strains resistant to at least one antibiotic.

[†] Studies also show that physicians often receive little to no training on how to complete a death certificate. One survey of New York City medical residents showed that only 40 percent obtained formal training in death certification. One could imagine how, when placed against a frontline physician's time constraints, this could easily result in significant errors and omissions in death records. In fact, studies comparing autopsy records to death summaries have shown significant discrepancies between the cause of death in 12 to 29 percent of cases.

sixty-five and older. And sepsis likely had a hand in most of these deaths.

———

On November 1, 1982, a research group working out of Rush-Presbyterian-St. Luke's Medical Center in Chicago, Illinois, launched a sepsis clinical trial involving nearly four hundred patients across nineteen US medical centers. The trial's objective was to settle what had become a seesawing debate over whether corticosteroids could prevent shock and/or death in sepsis patients.[59]

From the outset, the trial had a robust design and adhered to rigorous scientific methodology. The lead investigator, Dr. Roger Bone, was an extraordinary researcher who had emerged as one of the most prominent sepsis experts in the world. He had also become a regular fixture on television, hosting Lifetime Medical Television's *Internal Medicine Update* and using his platform to spotlight sepsis—becoming one of the first physicians to speak publicly about the syndrome on the national stage.[60]

Before the 1980s, investigators relied on the gestalt of frontline clinicians to identify sepsis patients for experimental trials. However, waiting for a physician to *see* sepsis in the contemporary sense—by observing shock, bacteremia, or an otherwise "toxic" appearance in the patient—could take many hours or, in some cases, days.[61]

Such vagaries weren't acceptable to Bone.[62] Having grown weary of the older way of looking at sepsis, he had set his sights on a more objective and systematic sepsis definition—one that reflected the latest science of the inflammatory response rather than relying solely on bacteremia or shock as its defining characteristics.

This idea finally came to fruition in 1980, not within the prestigious halls of the academe, but in a Las Vegas hotel room, where Bone and colleagues spent an entire day spitballing a diagnostic framework to help them quickly identify sepsis patients.[63] They called it the "sepsis syndrome," and it required *some* clinical evidence of infection combined with signs of a system-wide inflammatory response: fever (or hypothermia), tachycardia, and an elevated respiratory rate.[*64]

---

*   This part of the story has become a source of consternation for some researchers, who remain incredulous that the entire sepsis framework was based on a freeform idea session in Vegas, which, in the words of one expert, "was completely unencumbered by data."

Bone and colleagues also noted that prior animal studies showed steroids to be particularly beneficial when administered before or immediately after the onset of septic shock. Either way, treatment success was *time*-dependent, with preventive and early treatments producing the best results.[65]

The study randomized patients to treatment with a corticosteroid called methylprednisolone at the first sign of shock, or even when shock appeared imminent. To accomplish this, they broadened the inclusion criteria to include evidence of organ dysfunction, such as altered mental status or impaired kidney function, without necessarily requiring low blood pressure.

This is an important point. Let's say we had enrolled Rosaria in Bone's study. According to the protocol, our team would have started aggressively treating her infection at the *first* sign that her body was exhibiting a harmful response during our initial visit with her in the emergency room. We wouldn't have waited until later in the afternoon when she'd developed septic shock.

The trial centered on rapidly identifying patients who met early sepsis criteria and treating them within two hours. The control group received the standard of care for sepsis at the time: antibiotics, intravenous fluids, and vasopressor medications for low blood pressure. The treatment group received intravenous methylprednisolone in addition to standard therapy.

The results after three years were disappointing: there was no difference between the two groups. Methylprednisolone didn't decrease the chance of developing shock or reduce the risk of death compared to standard therapy, whether it was given before the appearance of septic shock or shortly afterward. In fact, if anything, the steroid appeared to *increase* the risk of death in the treatment group.[66] Some in the clinical research community would conclude this was a *negative* clinical trial.

However, careful analysis of the results led to some important insights, some of which Bone and his colleagues summarized in a now iconic 1987 paper published in *The New England Journal of Medicine*. For one, the overall death rate in both groups, *including* the control group, was much lower than what doctors were typically seeing in hospitals at the time. While the average death rate for sepsis patients around the nation was 40 to 50 percent, in Bone's study, it was closer to 30 percent.[67] Bone felt that the most important reason for this improved mortality was "early identification and aggressive treatment" of patients enrolled in the study.[68] In his view, investigators achieved better results in both groups by capturing patients as soon as possible and treating them quickly and deliberately.[69]

The results also challenged conventional wisdom regarding sepsis patients at the time. Contrary to commonly held beliefs, bacteremia was present in only about half of the sepsis patients in the study. Furthermore, only two-thirds of these bacteremic patients had gram-negative bacteria in their blood.*[70] Thus, sepsis could no longer be exclusively associated with bloodborne infections, as it could clearly be seen in a wide array of infections.

Data also showed that certain factors could *predict* sepsis. For example, one marker of kidney organ dysfunction—the blood creatinine level—was strongly linked to an increased risk of developing septic shock and death.† So, there were now measurable blood biomarkers that could herald the onset of septic shock before it was too late.‡[71]

Bone concluded that by objectively identifying sepsis patients early and then rapidly treating them with antibiotics and supportive care, doctors could significantly reduce their death rates. Others could now employ this strategy to recognize the sepsis syndrome *before* patients developed shock. Moreover, data showed that the sepsis doctors were seeing in hospitals entailed far more than just gram-negative bacteremia. It accompanied a wide array of infections. Finally, patient characteristics and detectable blood markers could predict how sick a sepsis patient *might* get. Armed with these insights, Bone and colleagues began reimagining their approach to the syndrome.

Looking back, some experts believe that Bone's conclusions were overzealous and that any number of factors may have contributed to the improved mortality outcomes in both groups. It was probably a stretch to attribute the results solely to early treatment. For example, Bone may have selected patients who were less likely to die than average sepsis patients being seen in US hospitals at the time. Also, by the 1980s, supportive care for sepsis had improved considerably, particularly in large academic centers.[72] It's now well known that clinical trial patients have lower sepsis mortality than those in the community, reflecting

---

*   The inverse is also true. Not all patients with bloodstream bacteria end up with sepsis. Studies have shown that even the simple act of toothbrushing can lead to transient episodes of bacteremia.

†   Recall that Rosaria from chapter one had an abnormal blood creatinine level on arrival at the emergency room.

‡   Additionally, shock wasn't just an early development in many patients. It could still develop up to seventy-two hours *after* patients had been enrolled in the study. This effectively widened the period during which doctors needed to remain vigilant while caring for these patients.

differences in their baseline characteristics, the location in which they receive care, and a lack of exclusionary comorbidities. An academic purist would say that this study demonstrated only one thing: steroids were not effective at reducing the risk of shock and/or death in a diverse group of sepsis patients.[73]

Moreover, the results revealed another important clue: the mortality rate in the treatment group was actually *higher*. As Marshall explains, "This trial showed very nicely that high-dose methylprednisolone given to a heterogeneous population characterized by the sepsis syndrome was more likely to result in harm."[74] Thus, while steroids may have helped *some* sepsis patients, they clearly harmed others. We can now speculate that within the *average* results of numerous steroid trials lay a complex mix of patients with widely varying responses to the particular therapy. This concept, known now as the heterogeneity of treatment effect, would continue to impact sepsis clinical trials and treatment recommendations for decades.*

By the 1990s, sepsis had emerged as a bewilderingly heterogeneous disorder. Like the mythical Hydra, it had multiple heads—each one monstrously deadly. At the same time, it seemed impervious to cutting-edge therapy or examination by clinical trial.

Sepsis defied the average physician's intuition, contradicting common wisdom at every turn. Meanwhile, it hijacked multiple systems, spinning them into a self-destructive cascade, growing stronger with each passing hour. By the time it revealed itself, it was often too powerful to stop, the patient too far gone to be saved.

Yet, amid the uncertainty, something new was beginning to emerge—a system with the power to spot danger early and offer doctors a chance to change the course of illness.

As we would come to learn, it was a concept marbled with both merit and misunderstanding. We had entered the battle, but the shape of the enemy was only just coming into view.

---

* As of today, expert guidelines still recommend steroids in certain sepsis patients, including those with shock, ARDS, and severe bacterial pneumonia.

CHAPTER EIGHT

SIRS

Early recognition of impending circulatory compromise in patients with sepsis may improve survival through rapid and aggressive therapeutic intervention . . . in the future, we will be able to begin therapy at an early stage in the disease process, before the onset of shock and multiorgan failure.

—ROGER BONE, February 15, 1991[1]

IN THE SUMMER OF 2006, a nineteen-year-old man named Miguel lost control of his motorcycle, skidded across the asphalt, and slammed into a highway barrier. The impact launched him forty feet through the air before he crashed onto the road.

Paramedics responded quickly, rushing him to the emergency department. There, he was found to have a traumatic brain hemorrhage, a large open fracture in his right leg, and extensive road rash over his body.

The trauma team worked quickly and intently. After stabilizing his vital signs, they whisked him to the operating room, where neurosurgeons evacuated blood from his brain, leaving a surgical drain in his skull. Meanwhile, orthopedic surgeons reduced (realigned) his broken leg, cleaned the wound around his fracture, and placed his leg in an external fixator. He was then admitted to the trauma-surgical intensive care unit for close monitoring.

Three days later, I was covering the hospital's internal medicine service when I received a consultation request from one of the trauma surgery residents. That morning, Miguel's heart had begun racing at 140 beats per minute. His

EKG showed sinus tachycardia, a relatively nonspecific heart rhythm. Aside from an elevation in his blood creatinine level (a marker of kidney dysfunction), the rest of his workup was unremarkable. This left the surgeons baffled, and they hoped I could solve the case.

As I approached the trauma-surgical intensive care unit, Miguel was lying calmly in room 2, still on a ventilator. Aside from his abnormal creatinine level, there were no other obvious findings. His respiratory parameters also appeared stable. His heart rate, however, was alarmingly high.

I knew that persistent tachycardia in this situation indicated something serious, but it wasn't clear what it was.

————

Revelations from his historic 1987 steroid trial left Roger Bone determined to clarify what had been decades, if not centuries, of ambiguity surrounding sepsis. Over the next several years, he wrote numerous papers and letters to prestigious medical journals, challenging doctors to reimagine its definition.[2]

In August 1991, Bone led representatives from two major medical societies—the American College of Chest Physicians and the Society of Critical Care Medicine—as they convened in Northbrook, a quiet suburb outside Chicago, Illinois, for a historic sepsis conference. There, he teamed up with other prominent experts, like Canadian William J. Sibbald and American–Israeli Charles L. Sprung, to help refashion the sepsis definition into one that could help frontline doctors and clinical researchers more rapidly identify and treat patients.[*][3]

By the 1990s, experts understood sepsis as the body's severe response to infection—a frenzy of cytokines flooding the body, resulting in organ injury. It was one that could be triggered by a wide variety of infectious pathogens.

During this time, there were many discussions among experts centered around cause and effect. For instance, they knew that a microbial invasion could cause sepsis, but it could just as easily cause mild symptoms, or no symptoms at all. On the other hand, the body's observed inflammatory response could also be triggered by noninfectious insults, such as severe burns, trauma, and even pancreatitis.

---

[*]   The conference resulted in a landmark paper published in 1992 titled "Definitions for Sepsis and Organ Failure and Guidelines for the Use of Innovative Therapies in Sepsis."

Thus, the critical insight was to see the infection and the body's response as two separate but intertwined components.[4]

And as the body's response was clearly something in and of itself, it needed its own name and a set of defining characteristics—one that captured its essence as a distinct process, tied to the injury or infection that triggered it.

It was here, in a heated brainstorming session during a conference committee meeting, that Sibbald's protégé, a young Canadian researcher named John Marshall, blurted out, "What about systemic inflammatory response syndrome, or SIRS?"[5]

The idea quickly caught on with another committee member, who immediately sketched the Venn diagram depicted in Figure 8.1.

Some, including Bone, believed that physicians and investigators could use objective criteria to identify the body's response to infection (and other insults). In theory, it could be detected before patients developed shock, enabling doctors to start treatment sooner, which could, in turn, improve survival rates. This idea resonated with many experts, researchers, and, in particular, representatives from the pharmaceutical industry, who were clamoring for more explicit standards to aid them in designing clinical trials for sepsis drugs. And while those in the definitions committee knew there was limited data supporting any such framework, they nevertheless proposed a set of standardized criteria to define SIRS, with the hope that they could refine it as our understanding of the response evolved.[6]

What they came up with continues to be the standard by which we define SIRS today, as the confluence of the body's severe response to infection and injury. Its criteria include four components, each with thresholds: a body temperature either greater than 100.4°F (representing fever) or less than 96.8°F (signifying hypothermia); a heart rate greater than 90 beats per minute; a respiratory rate greater than 20 breaths per minute; and a white blood cell count either greater than 12,000 or less than 4,000.*† In addition, the white blood cell count is considered abnormal if the percentage of immature white blood cells, called bands, is above 10 percent. (We'll discuss bands in more detail shortly.[7]) If two or more of the four SIRS components are abnormal, the patient is considered to have "positive SIRS criteria" or to be "SIRS positive."

---

*   Recall from chapter six that a *low* white blood cell count can be a sign of sepsis as well.

†   Ninety beats per minute is a level shy of the official threshold for tachycardia (100), to make it a more sensitive indicator of a hyperactivated state.

This new definition of sepsis—"Sepsis 1"—became infection *plus* SIRS.[8] For example, if a pneumonia patient had a fever and an elevated heart rate—two of four SIRS criteria—we would say they were "SIRS positive." Hence, they would have pneumonia *plus* SIRS, translating further to "pneumonia *with* sepsis."

According to Sepsis 1, doctors treating any infected patient or researchers studying a group of infected patients could now quickly and objectively identify those who had sepsis. Instead of waiting for shock, a positive blood culture, or some vaguely defined concurrence of findings, they could look for SIRS criteria. It was a massive overhaul of a centuries-old concept: an objective system designed to spot sepsis, no longer leaving it solely to clinical experience or gestalt. (See Figure 8.1.)

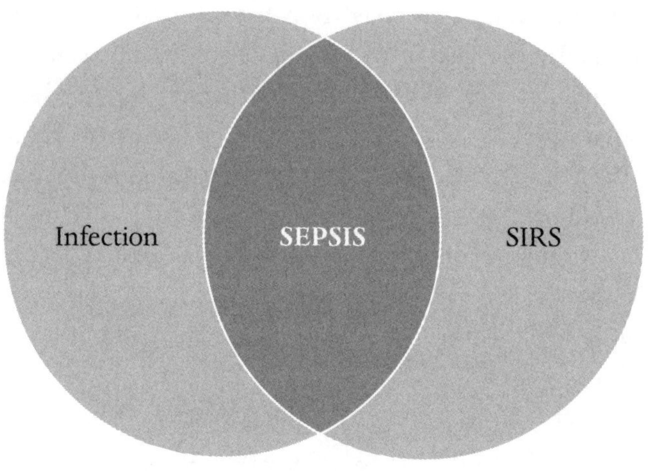

Figure 8.1: The 1992 definition of sepsis.[9]

Committee members also agreed that septicemia, or "blood poisoning," was an antiquated concept. The body's *response* to infection caused sepsis, not the microbes or their toxins seething throughout the blood. In fact, studies showed that sepsis didn't require a bloodstream infection at all.*[10]

Despite its apparent elegance, in the eyes of its critics, SIRS was fundamentally broad and nonspecific: its criteria, like fever and elevated heart rate, were generic and often *expected* physiologic responses to infection. For example, a

---

* "Septicemia" was not officially retired from the medical coding language until 2013, over twenty years later!

child with the flu might have a fever and an elevated heart rate, yet in no way have sepsis. Considering the SIRS framework, how would a physician then be able to distinguish between a normal and an abnormal response? A sick and a not-sick patient? As one might expect, the medical community didn't universally embrace the concept.*[11]

Members of the nation's premier society of infection doctors, the Infectious Diseases Society of America (IDSA), were nervous about the SIRS concept because they felt it could lead to sepsis overdiagnosis. While there was no doubt that SIRS criteria could indicate infection, they weren't convinced that SIRS was capturing the incipient stages of sepsis itself. They worried that relying on the SIRS framework could result in a rush to judgment and overprescription of antibiotics.[12]

Such concerns would begin a decades-long debate over the difference between sepsis and so-called uncomplicated infection.

What's more, many infectious disease researchers had studied the unique syndromes associated with different infections for decades and understood sepsis to be a vastly heterogeneous disorder. Like cancer, it was made up of a virtual library of syndromes depending on the causative pathogens. They worried that using the term "sepsis" too broadly ran the risk of creating a "mishmash."[13] After all, there were dozens of distinct pathogenic diseases causing sepsis-like syndromes. Weren't we losing something by lumping them together?

That said, many sepsis experts believed the status quo at the time—waiting for obvious signs of shock or a toxic-appearing patient—was unacceptable. A system was needed to identify the syndrome much earlier.

Looking back at Rosaria's story from chapter one, while she didn't initially *look* "septic" to me, she had three out of four SIRS criteria: fever, elevated heart rate, and a high white blood cell count. Based on the Sepsis 1 definition, we could have diagnosed her with sepsis right then and there. As for Janet in chapter three, it's the same thing; Tom from chapter four? You guessed it. They all had early evidence of SIRS, which could have prompted more attention and aggressive treatment. Could SIRS have altered their courses or saved Tom's life? Intuitively, one would say yes, and some preliminary data suggested as much.

---

*   According to John Marshall, task force members felt uneasy about the SIRS concept given that SIRS by itself did not adequately differentiate between an uncomplicated infection and sepsis, while the SIRS criteria themselves were somewhat arbitrary and not data-driven.

———

I sifted through Miguel's chart until I spotted something his surgeons had over-looked. While his white blood cell count appeared normal, the surgical team hadn't ordered a differential—a breakdown of the numbers and percentages of each white blood cell type in the blood.

The most abundant white blood cells in the body are neutrophils. Named for their affinity for neutral-charged dyes during microscopic staining, they are engineered for one purpose: to seek and destroy pathogens.

Each neutrophil carries a potent arsenal of weapons. During an infection, they unleash a barrage of chemical attacks, including granules—little bomb-like packets filled with enzymes capable of destroying microbial cells. They also deploy neutrophil extracellular traps (NETs), web-like DNA fibers that capture and kill large bacteria.[14] In a grislier example, they engulf germs through phagocytosis and then liquify them inside vesicles called phagolysosomes. But as effective as they are at containing and destroying microbes, these attack mechanisms can also inflict unintended collateral damage on surrounding cells and tissue.[15]

Neutrophils are continuously manufactured in the bone marrow—about one hundred billion per day. Afterward, they are slowly released into the blood circulation, where they live a remarkably short existence of only about a day or two.[16] Normally, only 1 to 2 percent of neutrophils in the body circulate in the bloodstream at any given time. The rest of them remain in the bone marrow as reserves or hang like bats from the inner lining of the blood vessels using specialized sticky protein anchors called selectins. The body tightly controls neutrophil circulation through a complex interplay of selectins, hormones, and cytokines.[17]

During a fight-or-flight response, stress hormones like adrenaline quickly unglue neutrophils from blood vessel walls by downregulating selectins. This releases white blood cells into the bloodstream via stress demargination. We see this all the time in patients suffering from non-infection-related conditions such as trauma, heart attacks, and strokes, and even after routine surgeries. The response is so powerful that it can double the number of circulating neutrophils within minutes.[18]

During infection, pro-inflammatory cytokines trigger neutrophils to demarginate, detaching from the vessel lining into the bloodstream.* Once released, they race through the circulatory system like bloodhounds tracking a scent, chasing chemical signals that guide them toward the infection. Upon arrival, they grasp, cartwheel, and squeeze their way through leaky blood vessel walls, infiltrating the tissue space to launch their counteroffensive.[19]†

Meanwhile, cytokines also stimulate the bone marrow to accelerate neutrophil production, flooding the circulatory system with reinforcements. In severe infections, such as bacteremia, the bone marrow can unleash a massive wave of these immune soldiers—along with immature neutrophils called bands.

Named for their underdeveloped band-like nucleus structure, bands are the junior cadets of the immune system, conscripted for the battle of their lifetime. A surge in circulating bands is often a sign of a severe bacterial infection—an all-hands-on-deck moment signaling that inflammatory cytokines are pushing the bone marrow to release everything available.

Neutrophils are the most abundant white blood cells, so when their numbers rise, the *total* white blood cell count (WBC) increases too. This phenomenon, leukocytosis, is often the first clue that neutrophils are elevated. This is one of the first things clinicians notice when reviewing a patient's lab results, as most electronic medical record (EMR) systems automatically flag it as abnormal.

However, a normal total WBC count is not always reassuring. Hidden within a "normal" total count may be a high percentage of neutrophils or even bands, making it essential to check the differential rather than relying on the total WBC alone.

Furthermore, while an elevated neutrophil count isn't by itself highly specific for infection, an increased *band* count can be. Studies consistently show that an elevated band count significantly raises the likelihood of a bacterial infection. In one study, for example, a bacterial infection was five and a half times more likely when the proportion of bands exceeded 10 percent.[20] Simply incorporating this detail into clinical assessment can substantially improve a doctor's ability to identify sepsis patients earlier.

---

*   This is simplified; see the first footnote in chapter six. Immediately after bacterial intrusion into the bloodstream, the circulating neutrophils may decrease sharply due to margination. Afterward, the neutrophil count increases again. Additionally, in severe cases of sepsis, the neutrophil count may decrease later due to the suppression of bone marrow production.

†   During sepsis, neutrophils have also been observed to be hypofunctional.

———

I immediately called the lab and requested a differential on Miguel's blood count from that morning. An hour later, the results came back: his band percentage had skyrocketed to 30 percent, *three times* the normal limit. This made a severe infection much more likely. More critically, Miguel's elevated band percentage and rapid heart rate now met two of the four SIRS criteria, suggesting he could be showing early signs of sepsis.

It was all making sense. As a trauma patient, Miguel was susceptible to any number of hospital-acquired infections. His system was vulnerable; his road rash had severely compromised his skin barrier, and he had undergone multiple surgeries. Beyond that, he had an external ventricular drain in his skull, hardware drilled into his bones, and various tubes and lines invading his body—each one a potential gateway for infection.

"You'll know it when you see it," they said.

In medical school, we were taught the classic textbook features of sepsis— many of which were based on studies from around the 1950s and inherited from centuries of medical understanding. It was ingrained in many of us that "sepsis" required an obvious presentation. Miguel was critically ill, yet at first glance, neither the surgeons nor I recognized it as sepsis. It's hard to say how much longer his diagnosis might have been delayed without a tool like SIRS to guide me.

In the end, sepsis was the most likely explanation for Miguel's unusual presentation. I now had to convince the trauma team, help them find the source of infection, and ensure treatment started before it was too late—so I rushed to the surgical intensive care unit.

———

One of the earliest concepts of intensive care medicine was born in 1854, during the Crimean War, when English nursing pioneer Florence Nightingale thought to organize injured soldiers by illness severity.[21] This provided them the additional attention they needed, dramatically reducing their mortality.[22]

A hundred years later, the first intensive care unit (ICU) was formed in the Blegdams Hospital in Copenhagen to provide ventilatory life support to victims of the 1952 polio epidemic.[23] By 1958, the Czech–Austrian anesthesiologist

Peter Safar opened the first physician-run, multidisciplinary American ICU in Baltimore City Hospital.[24] Safar, also a pioneer in cardiopulmonary resuscitation (CPR), developed the world's first intensive care medicine training program and established the first prehospital emergency medicine ambulance service in the US.[25]

In just a few decades, demand for intensive care treatment in hospitals surged, and by the 1980s, ICU care accounted for nearly 2 percent of the US gross domestic product.[26] As a result, hospital resources became increasingly constrained, with sicker patients and complex medical cases crowding ICUs in the US and around the world. At the same time, hospitals were admitting and housing patients whose conditions could deteriorate rapidly—sometimes unexpectedly—leading to death.

This meant that physicians needed the ability to predict which patients were at risk of deteriorating or dying while also determining who required high-level ICU care. Beyond that, they were often expected to decide whether a particular medical treatment was indicated, contraindicated, or, in some cases, futile.[27] At times, placing this immense burden on individual clinical judgment felt precarious, especially when it came to end-of-life prognostication. To put it plainly, how could one doctor be certain of a patient's true odds of survival?

At the same time, doctors were learning to use objective vital signs and laboratory measurements to accurately track the progression of severely ill hospital patients. They also began to integrate this data into complex mathematical models designed to predict outcomes.[28] Experts later refined these models into advanced clinical tools that could enable physicians to assess illness severity and estimate a patient's risk of death more accurately. In theory, such tools could help anticipate and prevent deterioration while helping physicians and hospital administrators allocate what had become a precious resource: ICU beds. These models also showed promise in assisting physicians in end-of-life care discussions, offering objective insights to support prognosis and decision-making.

Meanwhile, the existing classification systems for medical diagnoses weren't reliable predictors of patient outcomes—they were primarily oriented toward utilization and billing.[29] Sizeable healthcare administrators, like the Centers for Medicare and Medicaid Services (CMS), had evolved to use large documentation schemes like the Diagnosis Related Group (DRG) system, which clustered patients with similar patterns of diagnoses to manage cost more efficiently.

For example, instead of submitting a line-item bill for the hundreds of events, procedures, and physician assessments that encompassed a single hospital stay for "septicemia," its DRG represented a single bundled average cost figure for a typical septicemia admission, regardless of the variation between encounters.* As a result, healthcare payers could expect to pay a similar amount for the septicemia DRG, reducing the individual variation between hospitals.[30]

When it came to assessing outcomes such as mortality, relying solely on individual diagnoses and DRGs was problematic. These classifications didn't provide enough detail to accurately assess a patient's risk of dying. For example, most doctors could ascertain that a sepsis patient like Miguel was "sick," but *how* sick? Remembering that no two sepsis patients are alike, simply having a sepsis diagnosis didn't necessarily reveal their actual risk of dying. Determining severity and whether a patient required ICU admission often fell to individual clinical judgment or gestalt. Moreover, researchers faced similar challenges when conducting clinical trials. Grouping patients by DRGs made it difficult to differentiate apples from oranges—a DRG like "septicemia" often produced a heterogeneous group of sepsis patients with widely varying mortality.

By the 1970s, this had sparked an interest in so-called severity of illness scoring systems, mathematical formulas or algorithms that used biometric data to calculate a patient's mortality. Such systems could provide doctors with predictive information when caring for critically ill patients at the bedside while allowing researchers to classify disease severity more objectively in clinical trial patients. In 1978, a group from George Washington University led by William Knaus secured funding from the US National Center for Health Services Research (now known as the Agency for Health Care Research and Quality, or AHRQ) to develop one of the first comprehensive severity of illness scoring systems: the Acute Physiology and Chronic Health Evaluation Score (APACHE), followed shortly by the more user-friendly and refined APACHE II.[31]

The APACHE II was a high-tech concept for its time—one could even call it an early attempt at an artificial intelligence (AI) system for doctors. By inputting a handful of patient data points into a simple algorithm, one could quickly generate a score linked to a mortality prediction. For example, a patient with appendicitis and an APACHE II score of 20 would have an estimated mortality risk of 30 percent after surgery. In comparison, the same

---

* This is simplified. The DRG system is quite complex with grouper logic, DRG modifiers for specific diagnoses, etc.

patient with a score of 35 would have a mortality risk of 88 percent.[32] It was also remarkably accurate, with studies showing that it could correctly predict mortality rates up to 86 percent of the time.[33]

Severity-of-illness scoring systems proved especially useful when looking at groups of patients. In the 1980s, researchers like Knaus began using them to assess the quality of care across multiple hospitals.[34] By comparing a hospital's actual and predicted mortality rates, an investigator could determine how the facility was performing relative to expectations.

The statistic that comes out of this comparison is called the mortality ratio, calculated by dividing actual mortality by predicted mortality. For example, if the APACHE II predicted twenty-one deaths for one hospital, and twenty-one patients *died*, then the mortality ratio would be 1.0. A mortality ratio below 1.0 would suggest the hospital outperformed expectations, while a ratio above 1.0 would indicate worse-than-expected outcomes.

Researchers could also calculate an overall average or standard mortality ratio across hospitals to use as a benchmark for comparison. When Knaus's team applied this method to thirteen centers, they found that most hospitals had mortality ratios close to 1.0. However, two outliers—ranked #1 and #13—deviated significantly, with mortality ratios of 0.59 and 1.58, respectively.[35]

In the research world, outliers can sometimes hint at an underlying phenomenon worth exploring. Most of the thirteen hospitals performed similarly, yet two stood out. Additionally, when researchers compared patient diagnoses and average APACHE scores, both hospitals appeared to be treating a similar mix of patients with comparable disease severity.[36]

To determine what was different about these outlier hospitals, you had to look at how they ran their ICUs. While most ICUs had full-time physician directors, top-performing hospitals, like Hospital #1, gave the directors more autonomy over admission, discharge, and treatment decisions while also providing dedicated, 24-7 coverage. Higher-performing hospitals were also more likely to utilize standardized treatment protocols and invest in comprehensive nursing education led by clinical nursing specialists. Moreover, top centers fostered regular communication between nurses and physicians regarding patient care and administrative issues. Finally, high-performers carefully guarded nursing staffing. For example, Hospital #1 empowered charge nurses to cancel elective surgeries whenever nursing staffing levels were insufficient, ensuring that patient safety remained a top priority.[37]

Knaus's study, and others like it, suggested that variations in hospital mortality could be attributed to how each center was structured and administered. This meant hospitals could improve patient outcomes by improving their internal systems and processes. Moreover, the research revealed that the best-performing hospitals were ones that used clinician-designed treatment protocols and had institutional cultures that prioritized adequate physician and nursing staffing, promoted autonomy, and fostered communication and teamwork.

Like any system, the APACHE II had its limitations and criticisms. Aside from its computational accuracy, it had significant blind spots. For instance, it could overestimate mortality risk, predicting that a patient undergoing routine heart bypass surgery had a risk five times higher than reality.[38] Similarly, it could equate the risk of death of a young, otherwise healthy asthma patient to that of a medically complex patient dying from septic shock. This highlighted a fundamental limitation of computational predictive tools: they could analyze data but lacked real-time clinical awareness. Another concern was that the original patients calibrating the score might not have been relatable or "generalizable" to patients in different hospitals worldwide.[39] There was also a major technical hurdle: the APACHE system faced interoperability issues with existing electronic health record systems, making it difficult for many hospitals to integrate the tool into their existing EMR infrastructure.[40]

There was also a backlash from clinicians, who felt these tools infringed on physician autonomy. Some even felt that adding negative prognostic information too early in a patient's course could influence providers into believing that no intervention could reverse their outcome—a form of self-fulfilling prophecy known as confirmation bias.[41] This was particularly relevant when ICU physicians provided prognoses to patients and families, where a dire APACHE II forecast could bias a physician into recommending a less aggressive medical course.

Perhaps the most significant barrier to adopting these early risk tools was the widespread belief that computers and algorithms could never replace an experienced physician's gestalt.

As my mentor, Dr. David Schmidt, explains, "The brain of an experienced human doctor can integrate and assign weight to more data points than the APACHE."[42]

In other words, no physician can rely solely on an APACHE score—or any algorithm, for that matter—to make clinical decisions. Doctors consider far more variables, assessing each patient as a whole, not just a collection of data points.[43]

The academic medical community also examined this question scientifically. In the late 1980s, studies comparing physician clinical judgment to risk tools consistently showed that physician judgment was equal to or better than algorithmic risk tools. One group led by Dr. Mary Charlson out of Cornell University found that, out of all the potential factors leading to an admission decision, a physician's assessment of a patient's illness severity was the most predictive of in-hospital death. Interestingly, the relationship between physician assessment and mortality wasn't linear, suggesting there was something decidedly *non*-computational going on in physicians' minds when making these decisions.[44] When another group out of Wayne State University in Detroit compared physicians and nurse assessments to the APACHE II, they found no significant differences in accuracy in predicting mortality.[45]

Before 1991, for most mainstream doctors, there were usually only two settings for sepsis severity: not sepsis and *oh, crap*.*[46] While many sepsis experts and researchers were beginning to understand that sepsis had levels of severity, it would take much effort and many decades for this insight to make it to medicine's front lines. In addition, although there was some delineation among "sepsis," "septicemia," and "septic shock" in the literature, these terms were used so interchangeably throughout most of the twentieth century that it was difficult to assign any validity to the distinction before 1991.[47]

Until the Sepsis 1 conference, there had been no clear framework for correlating the definition of sepsis with illness severity. While sepsis patients were more likely to die, just *how* likely was a different matter. Before the 1990s, mortality rates for patients diagnosed with "sepsis" or "septicemia" were all over the map. Reviews on the subject cited wildly varying mortality figures, ranging from 20 to 50 percent for sepsis and 40 to 90 percent for septic shock.[48]

This made it difficult for frontline doctors to tailor their treatment to each patient. At the same time, they were often caught off guard when sepsis patients deteriorated rapidly and unexpectedly. Meanwhile, clinical investigators struggled to identify which patients were sick enough to be included in advanced sepsis therapy trials.[49] With no reliable means of estimating mortality risk,

---

*   In one of the earlier steroid sepsis trials in 1976, researchers identified three different levels of septic shock severity: mild, moderate, and severe, based on the duration of hypotension and the levels of certain biomarkers measured in the blood. However, this method wasn't widely practiced or taught.

they were often forced to treat all patients the same—a limitation that could impact trial results, averaging outcomes to show no benefit.

Shortly after the Norfolk meeting, Knaus assembled a team out of George Washington University to apply the SIRS definition to sepsis patients being treated in hospitals. They mined an extensive patient database, pulling 519 charts with a physician's diagnosis of "sepsis" upon admission and determining how many met SIRS criteria. Their results showed that SIRS identified an impressive *97 percent* of sepsis patients on day one.[*][50]

When they applied the APACHE risk tool to the 519 sepsis patients, they generated a graphic similar to Figure 8.2 that showed an almost even distribution in predicted day-one mortality risk, from less than 10 percent to 90 percent.

While the SIRS framework was excellent at identifying sepsis patients, it couldn't predict which ones were more likely to die. The only thing you could say, looking at the numbers, is that if a patient *didn't* have SIRS, they were probably okay.

Day One ICU Mortality Estimate

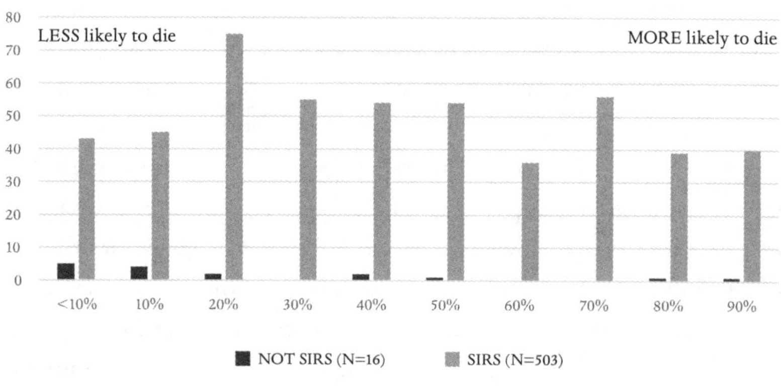

Figure 8.2: Distribution of APACHE-predicted mortality for sepsis patients meeting SIRS criteria. The horizontal axis represents predicted mortality, and the vertical axis defines the number of patients.[51]

But when we look at Figure 8.3, which plots day-one APACHE-predicted mortality against *actual* mortality at discharge, we see a linear relationship.

---

[*] When Knaus's group applied the sepsis criteria Bone used for his 1987 steroid trial, they found that Bone's criteria only identified 308, or 59 percent, of the patients on day one.

When the risk score predicted high mortality, patients died; when it predicted low mortality, patients survived. By simply adding the second step—assessing the severity of illness in SIRS-identified patients—investigators could reliably predict which sepsis patients were most likely to die.

Actual Hospital Mortality vs. Day One ICU Mortality Estimate

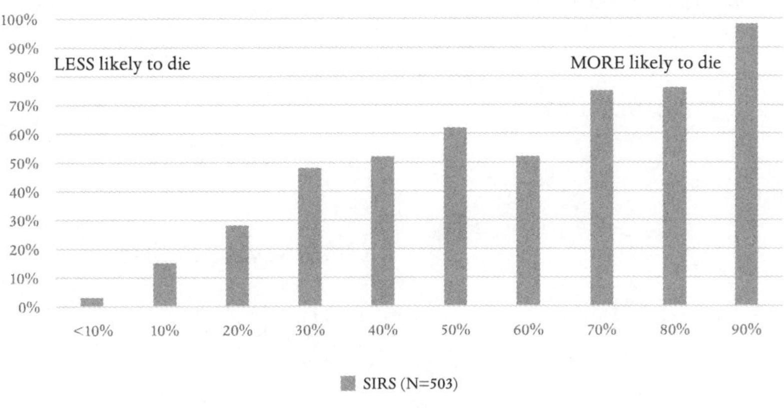

Figure 8.3: Predicted mortality (horizontal axis) vs. actual mortality (vertical axis) for sepsis patients with SIRS.[52]

Not surprisingly, this resonated with Bone and his colleagues. This is especially true as they faced a real challenge with SIRS and its inability to identify truly "sick" patients. They concluded that diagnosing sepsis should follow a two-step approach: first, identify the inflammatory SIRS response, *then* assess the severity. To simplify this framework, they created three levels of severity: sepsis, severe sepsis, and septic shock. *Sepsis* represented the primary cytokine-driven inflammatory response, the earliest sign that it was taking hold of the body. *Severe* sepsis included the same inflammatory response but with evidence of inadequate blood perfusion, organ injury, or dangerously low blood pressure—signaling that the response was spiraling out of control, disrupting circulation, and impairing organ perfusion and function. Septic *shock* marked the final stage, when the cardiovascular system was collapsing, requiring vasopressor life support to maintain blood pressure.*[53]

---

* According to Marshall, while elegant, this interpretation may be too generous. In reality, the sepsis severity schema was an awkward concept attempting to reconcile the fact that

The group recommended moving away from dualistic language and instead viewing sepsis as a continuum, with SIRS as the entry point and death as its end. (See Figure 8.4.) To emphasize the progressive nature of sepsis-related organ injury, they introduced the term "multiple organ dysfunction syndrome" (MODS). This concept highlighted the progressive injury inflicted by sepsis on interdependent organ systems, such as the brain, kidneys, and cardiovascular system.

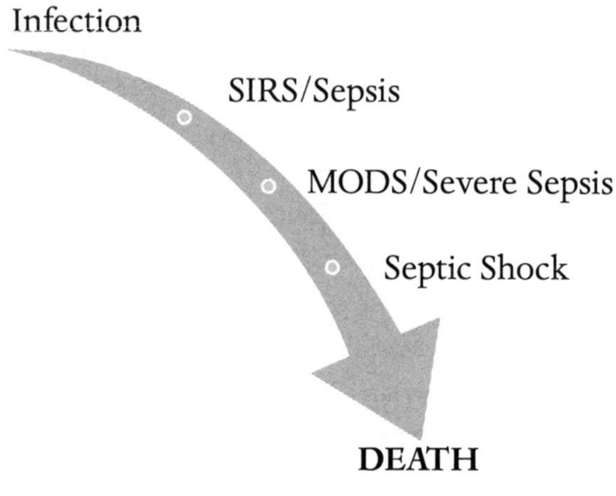

Figure 8.4: The 1992 concept of the sepsis spectrum, from infection to death.[54]

To my chagrin, when I arrived at the ICU, the trauma team was in the middle of afternoon rounds—meaning I'd have to face Dr. Emory, the trauma attending, in front of the entire team.

Dr. Emory was a seasoned, no-nonsense trauma surgeon and a retired Army colonel. On call, he often wore a "U.S. Army"-emblazoned baseball cap, and to be honest, he intimidated the hell out of me. Yet beneath his tough exterior, he had a heart of gold and was one of the best surgeons I had ever known.

"So, you think this is septicemia?" Dr. Emory said with a half-grin.

"That's . . .Yes, that's what we're thinking," I replied, mustering as much

SIRS was considered by many to be a physiologically inaccurate depiction of sepsis.

confidence as I could.

"And you've staffed this with your attending?"

"Yes, sir," I replied.

"I think you're probably right. Thanks for the input."

He turned to one of the surgery interns and said, "Let's get a urinalysis and urine, blood, and drain fluid cultures."

I had expected more resistance, but in all his years of experience, Dr. Emory had no doubt seen stranger things. As a military trauma surgeon, he may have understood sepsis better than the rest of us. After a quiet sigh of relief, I left the surgery team and returned to the medical ICU to continue following Miguel's case alongside the surgeons.

Overnight, preliminary blood culture results came back positive for bacteria. The on-call surgery resident immediately started Miguel on broad-spectrum antibiotics. By the next morning, his heart rate had improved. Later that day, the lab confirmed the presence of MRSA. After further investigating, the surgeons determined that one of the metal half-pins on Miguel's external fixator had become contaminated with the microbe—likely during or after his initial surgery.

The next step was source control: surgically removing the source of infection. The orthopedic team took him back to the operating room to extract the infected pin. Following the procedure, his condition steadily improved. When I checked on him a few days later in the surgical ward, he was doing well. The orthopedic surgeons planned to take him back to surgery in a couple weeks to remove the fixator and repair his fracture. In the end, Miguel made a full recovery.

———

The Sepsis 1 framework marked a radical departure from tradition. It contested the long-held practice of relying on clinical gestalt or waiting for the obvious demise of a patient in shock before diagnosing sepsis. With SIRS, we now had a system that could enhance our ability to identify sepsis patients *before* they deteriorated, potentially giving doctors a crucial advantage.

SIRS was objective and methodical; unsurprisingly, it captured the attention of many experts at the time. Some now associate that era with a certain euphoria, as doctors finally felt empowered to apprehend a historically enigmatic foe.[55]

However, while it could help identify sepsis patients earlier and draw greater attention to the syndrome, SIRS was not physiologically accurate, nor did it resolve the heterogeneity problem. Some would even argue that it exacerbated the issue by further generalizing sepsis diagnoses under one broad umbrella. This would set the stage for a decades-long debate focused on the criteria—something that would prove to be a major setback for sepsis research and quality improvement work.[56]

Beyond that, mobilizing the medical community to rapidly and *reliably* identify and treat sepsis patients would require more than just a new way of thinking about the syndrome—it would demand a fundamental transformation of our healthcare system.

CHAPTER NINE

The Golden Hour

*The first hour after injury will largely determine a
critically injured person's chances for survival.*

—R. ADAMS COWLEY, 1975[1]

ON JANUARY 4, 2007, EDUARDO, a fifty-six-year-old father of seven,
scraped his leg on a piece of metal in the garage. The next day, he awoke to
a leg that was swollen, red, and throbbing in pain.

Eduardo was stoic—a man who accepted his fate without grievance. As
his family's primary breadwinner, he worked tirelessly, often at the expense
of his own health.

Convinced the leg would heal on its own, he brushed off the pain, got
dressed, and headed straight to work.

The following morning, his wife, Anita, sensed that something was wrong.
She went to check on Eduardo and found him in bed, shaking with rigors and
too weak to move. She called for help. Their son, Jaime, came right away, and
they took Eduardo to the hospital.

When they arrived at the emergency room, they were met with chaos—a
waiting room full of patients and a registration line out the door. Even after
they'd checked Eduardo in, it took hours for the triage nurses to see him. By
then, he had developed a fever and become lethargic and confused.

His nurse notified the charge nurse, Jason, who placed him on a hallway
stretcher by the central nurses' station. Jason also flagged down one of the
ER physicians, Dr. Thomas, who diagnosed Eduardo with cellulitis—a skin

infection of the leg.* Dr. Thomas ordered an antibiotic and contacted internal medicine for further evaluation. Moments later, a high-priority trauma call came in over the dispatch radio, diverting Dr. Thomas, Jason, and several other staff members to the trauma bay.

An internal medicine resident arrived two hours later and noticed that Eduardo's antibiotics had yet to be administered. He alerted a nearby nurse, who administered the antibiotic and repeated his vital signs. Eduardo's blood pressure had dropped to 80/40. His bloodwork revealed a high white blood cell count of 20,000 and an elevated creatinine level, indicating kidney dysfunction. Concerned, the resident ordered a one-liter bolus of intravenous fluid, which helped raise Eduardo's blood pressure. Satisfied with the initial response, he noted "condition stable" in the chart and admitted Eduardo to the step-down unit.

Later that evening, Eduardo's condition worsened—his fever spiked, his blood pressure dropped again, and he became increasingly lethargic. Worried, his nurse, Maria, paged the on-call general medicine intern, who gave her a verbal order for a fluid bolus and said he would be up to evaluate Eduardo shortly. Ten minutes later, Maria was urgently called next door to help a colleague get another patient back into bed. When she returned to Eduardo's room, he was no longer responsive.

———

In 1819, French physician René Laënnec, best known for inventing the stethoscope, described sudden circulatory collapse and death in patients with *péripneumonie*—the extension of pneumonia into the pleural space surrounding the lung, a condition we now recognize as an *empyema*.[2] Just over half a century later, in the throes of the Spanish–American War, "septic shock" had become widely used to describe the disastrous complication of infected wounds and gangrene suffered by soldiers on the battlefield.[3] It was known to cause ruinously low blood pressure, disorder of the body's vital systems, and, in many cases, death. Yet its underlying mechanism remained a mystery.

Meanwhile, for nearly a century, another syndrome was vexing field surgeons, claiming the lives of countless soldiers on the battlefield. Many died without any signs of infection or bleeding—often following a slow and steady decline

---

*   Cellulitis is often caused by *Streptococcus* or *Staphylococcus*.

in blood pressure. Experts named this perplexing syndrome "traumatic" shock, while some referred to it as "secondary" shock owing to its delayed onset. The condition drew significant attention as it rose to one of the leading causes of death among soldiers during World War I.[4]

Like septic shock, traumatic shock was a profoundly cryptic process. At first, it revealed no obvious mechanism. This led Dr. Alfred Blalock, a pioneer in shock physiology, to describe it as a "deep mischief lurking in the system."[5]

It wasn't until the 1930s that Blalock, working closely with his laboratory assistant, Vivien Thomas, demonstrated that traumatic shock resulted primarily from massive losses of blood and fluid, most of it leaking into injured tissues. Through a series of meticulously designed experiments, Blalock, guided by the crucial, often uncredited, experimental ingenuity of Thomas, connected *all* the shock syndromes—including septic shock—to one common thread: the flow and pressure of circulating blood volume.[6]

———

To understand how blood volume impacts sepsis patients and the mechanisms behind their treatment, we need to take a brief tour of cardiovascular physiology. If you prefer to skip a scientific deep dive, feel free to gloss over this section.

The cardiovascular system consists of the heart and blood vessels. Its primary function is to deliver oxygenated, nutrient-rich blood to vital organs while returning deoxygenated blood to the lungs for replenishment.[7]

To achieve this, the heart rhythmically fills and contracts, propelling blood through a sequence of large muscular arteries, medium to small arterioles, and ultimately through a microscopic network of thin-walled capillaries, where organs extract oxygen and nutrients. The heart has two phases. During "diastole," it is relaxed and its chambers fill with blood, while in "systole" it contracts, ejecting blood into the circulatory system. Deoxygenated blood returns to the heart through the venous system, a series of less-muscular blood vessels, after which the heart pumps the blood back to the lungs.

The venous system also serves as a reservoir, holding most of the blood volume.

The heart functions as a dynamic pump, adjusting its force of contraction based on the amount of blood volume filling its chambers at the end of each cardiac cycle, which is also known as the "venous return."* Generally, a greater blood volume returning to the heart leads to a stronger contraction. This principle, known as the Frank-Starling Law, was first described by physiologists Otto Frank and Ernest Starling.

A helpful analogy is to think of the heart muscle as an elastic band. Up to a point, the more it's stretched or "loaded," the more forcefully it recoils or pumps. The blood returning from the venous system stretches cardiac muscle fibers as it fills the heart, much like pulling on a slingshot. We refer to this effect as "preload." If the heart has more preload, its force of contraction becomes more vigorous, but only to a point; once its muscle fibers are overstretched, it can no longer contract effectively.

Doctors can raise the preload by increasing the blood volume through blood transfusions or intravenous fluid administration. Some people use the analogy of "filling the tank" when describing this effect.

The relationship between preload and force of contraction also depends on the heart's intrinsic condition. In a failing heart, such as one in cardiogenic shock, an increase in preload fails to generate a strong contraction. In contrast, a stimulated heart—for example, one exposed to hormones like adrenaline or drugs called inotropes—experiences enhanced contractility, improving its response to preload. (See Figure 9.1, which shows three different Frank-Starling "curves.")†

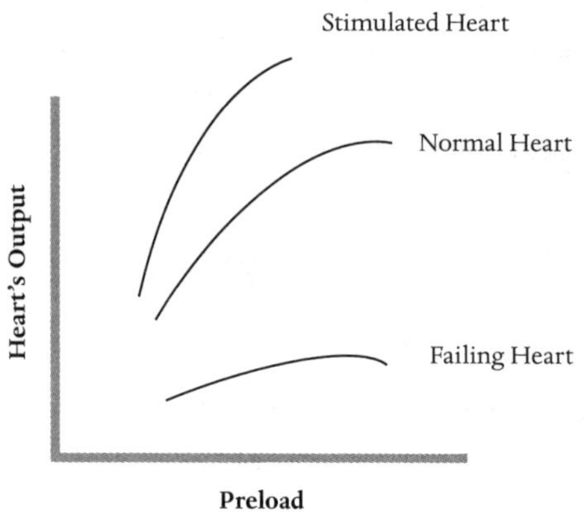

Figure 9.1: The Frank-Starling Law. The more the heart fills with returning venous blood (also known as preload), the stronger the contraction force until the heart muscle becomes overstretched. Figure 9.1 illustrates a normal heart in comparison to a failing heart and a stimulated heart (inotrope).

---

* This is simplified, as venous return refers specifically to the volume of blood returning to the heart's right atrium per unit time—not the end-diastolic volume itself. However, the venous return largely determines the end-diastolic volume by influencing how much blood fills the ventricles during diastole.

† The relationship between preload and cardiac output also depends on the "afterload," which is the pressure the heart must overcome to eject blood into the aorta and pulmonary artery during contraction.

The term "cardiac output" represents the heart's overall performance—the volume of blood (in liters) pumped per minute. It's calculated by multiplying stroke volume (the volume of blood ejected per heartbeat) by the heart rate (in beats per minute). Under normal conditions, cardiac output averages around five liters per minute.*[8]

The equation *mean arterial pressure equals cardiac output multiplied by systemic vascular resistance*, or *MAP = CO x SVR*, represents how doctors understand the relationship between the heart, blood vessel resistance, and the average blood pressure.† Simply put, blood pressure rises when the heart pumps more forcefully or when the resistance to blood flow increases, and vice versa.

Blood flow resistance is primarily determined by the diameter of blood vessels—the narrower the vessel, the greater the resistance. The total resistance within the circulatory system is referred to as the systemic vascular resistance (SVR). When blood vessels constrict, SVR increases, leading to a rise in mean arterial blood pressure (MAP). The opposite happens as they dilate.

Individual organs, like the brain and kidneys, regulate their own blood flow by dilating or constricting the blood vessels that supply them. Under normal conditions, this autoregulation ensures a steady blood supply to these vital organs, regardless of the MAP. However, this system breaks down once the MAP drops below 60 to 65 mmHg. In older adults with hardened arteries or those with hypertension, this threshold may be even higher, making them even more vulnerable to lower blood pressures since their bodies are accustomed to operating at higher pressures. All in all, this makes it crucial to maintain arterial blood pressure above a certain level, which can vary from individual to individual.

In septic shock, a flood of cytokines and other chemical mediators triggers widespread blood vessel dysfunction, causing the vessels to lose their muscle tone and become porous and leaky. This can lead to a severe drop in vascular resistance, leaving vessels limp and unable to conduct blood flow effectively. As vascular resistance drops, so can arterial blood pressure, potentially reducing blood flow to vital organs. At the same time, venous pressure decreases, leading to reduced venous return, aka preload, to the heart. With less blood returning to the heart, preload decreases and cardiac output declines, causing

---

*   Athletes can raise their cardiac output to almost forty liters per minute during exercise.

†   MAP = diastolic blood pressure + 1/3 (systolic blood pressure – diastolic blood pressure). Recall from chapter one that normal MAP is 65 mmHg or higher.

a further drop in arterial pressure.

Additionally, fluid leakage from capillaries creates a low-volume state, similar to the traumatic shock seen in wounded soldiers throughout the nineteenth and twentieth centuries. This further reduces preload, exacerbating the situation.*

Complicating matters, many sepsis patients are too ill to drink fluids while fever and perspiration increase fluid loss. As a result, blood volume decreases even further from dehydration.

And if that weren't enough, sepsis can *directly* impair heart function, adding a third component known as sepsis-induced myocardial dysfunction (SIMD). This is compounded by the fact that sepsis can also injure the brain, kidneys, and adrenal glands, disrupting their ability to coordinate an adequate stress response and maintain homeostasis.†

———

I was the hospital's senior ICU resident on call the night Eduardo was admitted. My intern, Alex, and I were in the emergency room, finishing another admission, when the hospital intercom system blared:

"CODE BLUE, SDU, ROOM 16 – CODE BLUE, SDU, ROOM 16 – CODE BLUE, SDU, ROOM 16."

Alex and I looked at each other, grabbed our papers, stuffed them in our coat pockets, and raced to the main hospital's step-down unit, where we joined the rest of the ICU code team.

A "code blue," or "code," is the five-alarm fire of the hospital—a call for immediate action when a patient suffers a severe catastrophic event such as a cardiopulmonary arrest, when the heart and lungs suddenly stop functioning. What follows is a race against time to revive the patient before irreversible brain damage occurs from lack of blood flow. Every second counts, and when a code blue is called, people come running. Most hospitals have dedicated code teams staffed by personnel trained to respond to urgent hospital conditions. These teams are typically led by the senior ICU resident on call—in

---

*   The leakage described here involves escape of blood plasma, which doesn't contain red blood cells, through tiny spaces between the cells lining the blood vessel wall. It is not the same as bleeding, which involves leakage of the entire blood volume, including red blood cells, through larger tears or holes in the blood vessel.

†   Sepsis-induced myocardial dysfunction (SIMD) is partially related to the effects of inflammatory cytokines, but as we'll see shortly, there are other mechanisms involved.

this case, me.

When we arrived, as was usually the case with codes, there was a large gathering of first responders and spectators around room 16. Alex, the ICU team, and I pushed through the crowd to the bedside and asked Eduardo's nurse, Maria, for a synopsis.

"Fifty-six-year-old diabetic man with cellulitis, now unresponsive. We just started a round of compressions. Respiratory's got the airway," Maria responded nervously.

I took the lead, running through the advanced cardiovascular life support (ACLS) algorithm—the American Heart Association's step-by-step, evidence-based approach to managing cardiopulmonary arrest. Eduardo's heart monitor showed sinus tachycardia—an organized rhythm—but he had no blood pressure or palpable pulse. Given the history, I was worried about septic shock, but we also needed to rule out other potential causes. Most urgently, we had to get his circulation back—fast.

Shortly after, Raj, an anesthesia resident, arrived and inserted a plastic endotracheal tube down Eduardo's throat, securing his airway before connecting him to a bag valve mask ventilator.* Meanwhile, Bill, a burly ICU nurse, delivered forceful chest compressions.

"What's the time?" I asked.

"Two minutes. We're ready for a rhythm check," Alex responded.

"Okay. It still looks like sinus tach. Do we have a pulse?"

"Still no pulse!" Bill yelled after palpating Eduardo's carotid artery.

"Let's give one milligram of epinephrine and resume compressions," I said.

———

Shock was uniformly fatal throughout most of history. Homer noted that, during the Trojan War, only one in four wounded soldiers survived their injuries.†[9] Such tragic outcomes continued to pile up until the twentieth century. It wasn't until doctors understood the intricate relationship between shock and blood volume that they could begin to use rational methods, such as blood and fluid replacement, to treat wounded soldiers on the battlefield

---

*   A bag valve mask is a handheld device used to ventilate the lungs during CPR.

†   This is an extrapolation based on an analysis of battles described in the *Iliad*.

and critically ill patients in civilian hospitals.

In 1665, English physician Richard Lower at Oxford performed the first recorded blood transfusion between two dogs—an experiment that successfully revived canines suffering from shock and established the principle of intravenous blood replacement. Two years later, French physician Jean-Baptiste Denis in Paris attempted the first animal-to-human transfusion, using lamb's blood, an effort that ended in disaster and led to official bans across Europe by 1669. The practice would remain dormant until 1818, when British obstetrician James Blundell reported the first human-to-human transfusion while treating postpartum hemorrhage.[*][10]

The first clinical use of intravenous *fluids* dates back to 1832, when Scottish physician Thomas Latta used such therapy while treating severely dehydrated patients during the second cholera pandemic.[†][11] Despite its success, the method was not initially embraced by the wider medical community. Many physicians were skeptical about the concept, and the lack of infrastructure and technology made widespread intravenous fluid administration impractical.[12] It would thus take many decades before intravenous fluid therapy became the standard of care for shock and other critical conditions.

During World War I, field surgeons recognized that delays in fluid administration and the resulting dangerously low blood pressure were associated with markedly higher rates of death. French surgeon Paul Santy noted, for instance, that the mortality rate of shock victims increased substantially as treatment was delayed beyond the first hour, to as high as 75 percent by the eighth hour.[13]

By the Second World War, there was greater attention to fluid replacement and blood pressure management in shock, and this practice reached the corridors of civilian hospitals in the 1940s.[14] The combination of better blood transfusion techniques and commercially available intravenous fluid solutions meant that doctors also had more options.[15] Interestingly, despite the central role of hypotension in septic shock, fluid and blood therapies were considered supportive, not primary treatment. One consequence of this was significant

---

[*]   Blundell was ignorant of blood types and aseptic technique. It wasn't until 1901 that Austrian-American Karl Landsteiner modernized the practice by discovering the ABO blood antigen system, which also earned him the Nobel Prize for Medicine and Physiology.

[†]   His method was based on a theory proposed by an Irish physician, William Brooke O'Shaughnessy, who thought of replacing the electrolyte-containing fluids lost during severe diarrhea suffered by patients during their illness.

variation in the use of these therapies from one physician to another.[16]

With the advent of vasopressor drugs in 1900 with epinephrine, a synthetic form of the hormone adrenaline, doctors could effectively raise the resistance in the circulatory system by causing the blood vessel walls to contract and tighten, helping them quickly raise blood pressure in shock.

However, vasopressors presented certain challenges. During World War I, their use on patients with hemorrhagic shock often resulted in devastating complications. As these patients often had insufficient overall blood volume due to external or internal losses, tightening their medium to large blood vessels with drugs like epinephrine effectively cut off the remaining blood flow in arterioles and capillaries, leading to organ damage, limb necrosis, and sometimes even death. Such adverse reactions created a lasting memory in medical culture, associating vasopressors with limb loss and other tragic outcomes.[*][17]

It eventually became common wisdom to administer intravenous fluids, increase the preload, and "fill the tank" before starting vasopressor therapy to reduce the risk of such complications. By the time I was in residency, we used sophisticated pressure-measuring catheters in the large central veins to measure the central venous pressure (CVP), which we thought was a good indicator of the preload. In fact, by the early 2000s, it was considered standard of care to target a CVP of 8 to 12 mmHg. (Evidence would later show that CVP is an unreliable measure of the body's fluid volume status.)

By the mid-twentieth century, vasopressors had become a regular component of septic shock treatment, though their use varied from physician to physician.[†] Clinical studies during this time also showed that, in many cases, by the time a patient needed vasopressors, they were of little benefit in improving their chances of survival.[18]

Conspicuously absent from this early septic shock history is any mention of systems, protocols, or guidelines to expedite treatment or any attempt to provide a general approach to therapy. Although different treatments were reported during the first half of the twentieth century, there is little evidence of a synthesis of these methods into a consistent standard of practice.[19]

Equally evident during this time were horrendous patient outcomes, with

---

[*] Even as recently as the Vietnam War, some field surgeons gave the modern vasopressor Levophed the nickname *"Lethophed."*

[†] By then, additional vasopressors had entered the field, such as ephedrine in 1920, phenylephrine in 1927, and norepinephrine (Levophed) by 1953.

mortality rates for diseases such as *Staphylococcus* sepsis no better than 50 percent in the best of cases and exceeding 80 percent at worst. Reports from the 1941 *Archives of Internal Medicine* paint a chilling picture of patients quickly overcome with bacterial shock and doctors virtually powerless to stop its relentless assault: a boy, age eight, perfectly healthy six days prior, with the sudden onset of groin pain, fevers, and shock, dying within two days of being hospitalized, with the only sign of infection blood cultures positive for *S. aureus*; a forty-six-year-old healthy man with an infected carbuncle of the neck who developed sudden chills, shock, and multiple bacterial abscesses all over the body, ultimately dying six days later; a seventeen-year-old girl with an infection of her right tibia, bacteremia, and shock, dying after a heartbreaking monthlong battle involving multiple rounds of antibiotics, antitoxin therapy, and blood transfusions.[20]

Anyone who has worked in an ICU will tell you there is nothing more demoralizing than trying to save a septic shock patient once their system is barreling toward shutdown. The convergence of so many insults to the body, particularly the cardiovascular system, makes sepsis daunting to treat, particularly when it's been running amok for hours or days. A process that mercilessly attacks the body's core infrastructure creates a chain reaction that can rapidly cycle out of control. This damage can injure the organs, leaving them dysfunctional and incapable of maintaining homeostasis, compromising the system further and making it harder to reverse.

Sepsis begins with a dysregulated host response to infection and, all too often, ends in death.

———

After two more cycles of chest compressions, Eduardo showed no signs of life. Panic set in as my stomach twisted in knots. I tried to keep my composure as I requested another dose of epinephrine and instructed the team to continue CPR. I hoped that we could generate enough pressure to jump-start his system by tightening his arteries with the vasopressor.

Less than a minute later, midway through the next round of compressions, Eduardo suddenly moved toward Bill as if trying to fight him off.

Bill jumped back, yelling, "He's awake!"

A rush of gratitude and exhilaration hit me as a smile spread across my face.

Meanwhile, Eduardo's eyes were now wide open. He looked terrified as he struggled to get out of bed, trying to pull at his endotracheal tube. The respiratory therapist, Sandra, attempted to calm him down as I moved to the head of the bed, held his hand, and rubbed his shoulder. After explaining what had happened to him, I ran through a basic neurological assessment. His brain appeared intact, and he was able to follow directions. I explained what would happen next and that we would take good care of him. He seemed to relax a bit after that.

Lab data trickled into the computer as the code team prepared to move Eduardo to the ICU. His white blood cell count was now almost 30,000, indicating an intensifying response to his infection. His blood acid level had also severely increased—something called lactic acidosis—a strong marker of illness severity. Meanwhile, his blood platelets had plummeted, suggesting that his blood clotting system was malfunctioning.

This was clearly septic shock from his leg infection, and his system was now tumbling into disarray. We immediately broadened his antibiotic regimen to cover a wide array of bacteria, including MRSA. We also consulted the general surgery team on call, and after a thorough examination, including a bedside ultrasound, the surgeons concluded that there was no abscess or necrotic tissue infection requiring surgical debridement.

As we reviewed Eduardo's admission paperwork, it became clear that his initial blood pressure in the emergency room had been dangerously low. In sepsis, even transient hypotension can be a harbinger of catastrophe. A 2009 study found that just the presence of low blood pressure upon arrival in the emergency department tripled a sepsis patient's risk of death.[21] Yet many of us had been conditioned to focus only on persistent or obvious warning signs—*sustained* hypotension, shock, or cardiac arrest—while fleeting clues often went unnoticed. And while we fixated on obvious vital signs, beneath the surface, a patient's bloodstream was already seething with invisible biomarkers, foreshadowing calamity.

———

In 1780, Swedish chemist Karl Wilhelm Scheele isolated an organic acid in sour milk, which he called lactic acid.[22] Almost three decades later, another Swede named Jacob Berzelius discovered the consistent buildup of lactic acid in muscles during exercise. Over time, investigators observed that lactic acid built up as exercised muscles used up their oxygen supply, and when they were exposed to oxygen again, it disappeared.[23]

Shortly after Berzelius's discovery, a physician named Johann Joseph Scherer discovered high levels of lactic acid while analyzing the blood of seven young women who had died during an epidemic of puerperal sepsis in Würzburg, Germany. One of the women, twenty-three-year-old Eva Rumpel, had just given birth to her first child on January 9, 1843, when she suddenly developed severe abdominal pain, fevers, and delirium. She deteriorated rapidly and died only thirty-six hours after the onset of her fever. Scherer concluded that high blood lactic acid levels resulted from bodily deterioration during severe illnesses.[24]

By the 1920s, two groups led by British physiologist Archibald V. Hill in London and German–American biochemist Otto Meyerhof in Berlin integrated decades of science into a unifying theory of energy metabolism, which stated that in the absence of oxygen, muscles and other tissues shifted to an anaerobic metabolic pathway—the lactic-acid cycle—which produced lactic acid as its byproduct.

By the second half of the twentieth century, biochemists had also realized that, at the body's normal pH, lactic acid exists almost entirely in its dissociated form—one positively charged hydrogen ion (H+) and one lactate anion; thus, from here on, we will refer to it simply as "lactate."

We now know that, during metabolism, skeletal muscle and other tissues convert glucose—the body's primary fuel— into an intermediate molecule called pyruvate. During aerobic metabolism, which occurs in the presence of oxygen, pyruvate enters the mitochondria—the cell's energy factories—and is converted to a substance called acetyl-CoA. Acetyl-CoA is then run through a complicated chemical pathway called the citric acid cycle, which generates large amounts of a usable energy molecule called ATP that powers most cellular functions. Aerobic metabolism is impressively efficient, capturing up to 40 to 45 percent of the usable energy stored in glucose, comparable to a high-performance automobile engine.[25]

Under certain conditions, the aerobic metabolic pathway slows or shuts down and the anaerobic energy pathway kicks in. This alternate pathway generates a much smaller energy cache while converting pyruvate directly into lactate. Anything that interferes with the normal aerobic metabolic pathway or compromises cellular oxygen supply can shift metabolism toward lactate production. For example, when you exercise past your anaerobic threshold, oxygen delivery to the organs through blood flow can't match demand, and your muscles begin generating lactate. In fact, it is the hydrogen ions generated from this reaction that create the burning sensation in your muscles during strenuous exercise. During shock, lack of oxygenated blood to vital organs, such as the liver and kidneys, also results in increased lactate production.*

Lactate elevation in sepsis is complex and relates to impaired blood and oxygen perfusion to organs, as well as the shifting of energy metabolism toward the anaerobic pathway through both adaptive and maladaptive influences on the metabolic enzymes themselves.

As you can imagine, lactate is not specific to sepsis either. There's an extensive list of causes of lactate elevation, including any cause of shock, heart failure, alcohol poisoning, certain diabetic medications, seizures, excessive work of breathing, liver failure, cancer, and deficiency of a B vitamin called thiamine, to name a few.

In 1964, Swiss–American physician Max Henry Weil published a study showing that as blood lactate levels increased during shock, patients were more likely to die.[26] Weil, often credited as the "father of critical care medicine," opened one of the earliest ICU prototypes—a four-bed "shock ward" at Los Angeles County/University of Southern California Medical Center in the early 1960s.[27] He concluded that lactate was a severity of illness measure, with a level greater than 4 mmol/Liter representing a critical threshold, after which the risk of death increased sharply.† This provided an objective blood measurement that doctors could use to supplement their gestalt on how sick a patient was when suffering from shock. In addition, as experts gained greater insight into the underlying sepsis inflammatory response, they connected it to the precise metabolic derangements that could lead to elevated lactate. Lack of oxygen delivery wasn't a prerequisite for lactate production. The dysregulated sepsis response was enough to shift the body into anaerobic metabolism by both interfering with metabolic enzymes in the mitochondria and ramping

---

* Lactate is a complex molecule and is not inherently toxic. It serves as an energy source and may be adaptive. However, concerning infection and sepsis, lactate is a *marker* of how sick a patient is.

† Mmol/Liter represents a concentration or amount of a substance per unit volume of blood.

up the anaerobic pathway through direct stimulation by stress hormones.*[28] Moreover, though an *early* sepsis response might be too subtle for a doctor to pick up just by looking at a patient's vital signs or usual laboratory values, a measurably high lactate level, on the other hand, could reveal a looming catastrophe within the body.

At the same time, another chemical pathway slowly came into view as a crucial player in the body's septic response. As early as the 1970s, experts knew that sepsis caused widespread dilation of the blood vessels, but it was unclear how this happened. The mystery was solved a decade later when American biochemist Robert Furchgott showed that the inner lining of the blood vessels, called the endothelium, released a muscle-relaxing chemical in response to certain stimuli. He named this intermediary substance endothelial-derived relaxation factor (EDRF). Meanwhile, other researchers studying the effects of the powerful vasodilating medication nitroglycerin had realized that instead of working directly on the blood vessel's smooth muscle, it generated an intermediary chemical messenger, which they named nitric oxide. Follow-up experiments showed that EDRF and nitric oxide were one and the same.[29]

We now know that nitric oxide is a significant player in the pathophysiology of sepsis. Under normal conditions, it's an essential signaling molecule that helps regulate endothelial function, blood clotting, and immune system activity.[30] During sepsis, this system gets dysregulated, resulting in excess nitric oxide production, which can wreak havoc on the cardiovascular system by excessively dilating blood vessels and decreasing vascular resistance while also inhibiting platelet aggregation and disrupting white blood cell function.[31] In addition, nitric oxide directly depresses heart muscle function, further impairing cardiac output, resulting in a drop in blood pressure and reduced organ perfusion. Furthermore, it can severely disrupt mitochondrial activity, resulting in widespread cellular metabolic dysfunction and—you guessed it—elevated lactate.†

---

* In sepsis, the body's fight-or-flight response also releases epinephrine, which stimulates the breakdown of glycogen into pyruvate, which is then converted to lactate, thus increasing lactate levels further. This is considered an adaptive response.

† Many experts now believe that sepsis is predominantly a disorder of microvascular and cellular dysfunction.

———

Back in the ICU, Alex and I hovered nervously around Eduardo's room, waiting for the nursing team to get him settled in. Sandra had just performed a rapid point-of-care lactate test at the bedside, which showed a blood lactate of ten mmol/Liter—*five* times the normal level—indicating that Eduardo's body was experiencing a massive sepsis response.

Just then, Deb, the charge nurse, turned to me and said, "The MAP's dropped to 50. Do you want to give more fluid? We're going to need a central line, you know."

"What do you want to do?" I asked Alex.

"I think we should give him an IV fluid challenge now and get set up for central line so we can start vasopressors and monitor his CVP," he responded.

"That sounds like a good plan. What would be your initial target for his MAP and CVP?"

"Sixty-five for the MAP and 8 to 12 for the CVP," Alex replied.

"Sounds good."

———

The expression "critical care happens at the bedside" is one of the oldest ICU proverbs. It refers to the notion that intensive medical care, like that seen with a septic shock patient like Eduardo, is unpredictable and subject to moment-to-moment fluctuations in an array of biological parameters. It requires a near-constant level of vigilance and intellectual agility. While one patient may need an intravenous fluid bolus, another patient might be on a different point on their Frank-Starling curve or even have a "flat" curve due to a failing heart; the situation could also change for the same patient, requiring a mid-treatment course correction. There's currently no way to replace a physician's ability to account for all these variables. At the bedside, medicine becomes both science *and* art.

Critical care has always been taught through mentorship and hands-on clinical experience. "See it, do it, teach it" is a mantra still echoing in the hallways of teaching hospitals today. There's something intangible about medical training that lives outside the textbooks, requiring thousands of hours of carefully mentored bedside experience.

However, behind every clinical intuition lies a framework rooted in decades of scientific discovery. In 1964, while studying disease models in the laboratory, vascular surgeon Edward Frank of Beth Israel Hospital in Boston contributed early insights into septic shock, emphasizing the importance of restoring blood volume, controlling infection, and stabilizing blood pressure. These principles—while expanded upon significantly in later decades—laid part of the groundwork for what would become modern septic shock management.[32]

Frank described sepsis as an unpredictable condition requiring a near-constant level of bedside attention, continuous monitoring of arterial and venous pressure, and regular blood tests that measured the body's consumption of oxygen and nutrients. He helped crystallize decades of past knowledge and experience into a structured approach to septic shock. While his methods have since been refined and expanded, the principles he emphasized remain central to critical care today—practices that have been passed down through generations of physicians, taught hands-on at the bedside, almost like tradition.

By the time I was in training, we understood the general goals of septic shock management: treat infection and restore blood perfusion to the organs. This generally meant a few significant objectives: administer antibiotics, improve blood pressure, restore aerobic metabolism, and see evidence of improved organ perfusion. Yet in practice, there was a lot of variation in how physicians accomplished this. Each clinical instructor interpreted the scientific landscape differently. When I was training, the seasoned residents and fellows even knew to adjust their treatments based on which attending was on duty.

But there was one constant when it came to sepsis patients: they were often so ill by the time they reached the ICU that many still died despite our best efforts.

By the 1960s, clinicians used sophisticated tests to measure and calculate variables, such as blood oxygen level and cardiac output, while caring for shock patients. Max Weil had effectively proven the link between higher lactate levels and death, so many doctors realized that the key to saving patients with shock was to quickly improve the delivery of oxygen and other nutrients to the vital organs before they were irreversibly damaged.

In a series of studies conducted between 1967 and 1973, a group led by American surgeon William Shoemaker out of Cook County Hospital in Chicago showed that the body's adaptive response to traumatic shock immediately increased cardiac output. Shoemaker theorized that this adaptation was not merely about restoring blood pressure, but about preserving oxygen delivery to vital organs—including the heart itself. His findings helped shift clinical thinking toward monitoring and optimizing oxygen delivery as a central goal in the management of critically ill patients.[33]

They also found that blood *volume* was critical in determining the heart's ability to increase its output.[34] Patients with ample blood volume, such as those rapidly resuscitated with blood and fluid infusions, were observed to more readily increase their cardiac output in response to shock and thus maintain organ perfusion. They were also far more likely to survive.[35] On the other hand, those with insufficient volume couldn't raise their cardiac output, causing inadequate blood flow to their organs, resulting in severe organ dysfunction, lactate elevation, and a rapid death spiral. In their final moments, many of these unfortunate patients experienced a collapse of their cardiac output and blood pressure as their hearts effectively gave out.[36]

Meanwhile, during the 1970s, American surgeon R. Adams Cowley, often called the "father of trauma medicine," introduced the world of trauma surgery to the concept of the "golden hour": the critical timeframe in which a trauma patient needs to be stabilized before their body becomes unsalvageable.

As Cowley explained in 1975, "There is a golden hour between life and death. If you are critically injured, you have less than sixty minutes to survive. You might not die right then; it may be three days or two weeks later—but something has happened in your body that is irreparable."*[37]

As early as 1973, Shoemaker and colleagues suggested that, once in the hospital, a rapid, goal-directed strategy could be beneficial in treating traumatic shock patients. This would involve a mixture of therapies and practices to intentionally raise and maintain the cardiac output to so-called supranormal levels—30 to 80 percent higher than a normal resting heart's output. Such therapies included blood and intravenous fluid infusions to increase the heart's preload and inotropic drugs to enhance its force of contraction. They also took regular blood measurements to ensure adequate oxygen delivery to the vital organs. Having carefully analyzed the parameters and outcomes of hundreds of traumatic shock patients, his group proposed the therapeutic ranges that would likely ensure adequate organ perfusion, allowing future doctors to

---

* Cowley founded one of the first trauma units in the United States at the University of Maryland Medical Center, which would later become the internationally renowned Shock Trauma Center.

calibrate their treatment to meet those targets. By the 1980s, they had used this technique to improve the surgical outcomes of trauma patients.[38]

Other groups scrambled to reproduce Shoemaker's results while applying his goal-directed strategy to a broader base of critically ill patients, including those suffering from septic shock. These follow-up studies would produce mixed results, foreshadowing a decades-long debate in the medical community about the efficacy of so-called protocolized shock treatment.[39] Like the sepsis immunotherapy trials, many of these studies faced the problem of heterogeneity, which averaged the overall effect across different patient subgroups, resulting in a negative study. Investigators also noted that it was much more difficult to consistently increase cardiac output in older, more chronically ill sepsis patients.[40]

———

Eduardo's blood pressure failed to respond to one fluid bolus, then another, and another. We instructed his nurse, Jenny, to start a vasopressor called dopamine while Alex and I prepared to place a central venous catheter in Eduardo's internal jugular vein.*

I steadied my nerves as I watched Alex carefully move through each step of the procedure with novice hands. After locating the jugular vein with an ultrasound probe, he advanced the needle and drew a flash of dark, deoxygenated venous blood. He then threaded the guidewire, dilated the tract, and slid the catheter in place.

"Looks good," I said, letting out a sigh of relief.

I exchanged a thumbs-up with Jenny as we finished. Deb popped her head into the room, informing us that Eduardo's family had arrived.

Eduardo's family filled the waiting room—his wife, Anita, their children, and several of his siblings, all anxiously awaiting my update. After introducing myself, I pulled Anita aside to explain what had happened. There was no way to soften the blow—Eduardo was on the brink of death. Tears poured down her face as she tried to maintain her composure. After doing my best to console her, I assured the rest of the family that someone would be out shortly to update them when Eduardo was more stable.

---

* Dopamine also increases heart rate and cardiac muscle contractility. Although doctors classify drugs as vasopressors and inotropes, many of these drugs have mixed effects.

Back in the ICU, everything was unraveling. Deb and Jenny scrambled to hang IV bags of fluids and medications as Eduardo's life support monitors chimed dissonantly. He lay near comatose, his blood pressure plunging dangerously again. Across the room, Alex reported the escalating disaster: Eduardo's organ systems were failing one by one. The dopamine had failed to raise his blood pressure, and his CVP had climbed to 12 mmHg, suggesting his tank was full. Alex had ordered a second vasopressor drug—norepinephrine—while Jenny moved quickly to start the infusion.

I was afraid we were losing Eduardo, so I paged the on-call critical care fellow, Mark, now in his final year of ICU fellowship.

"I'm on my way," Mark said.

In the meantime, he recommended maximizing vasopressor support and administering a dose of the steroid hydrocortisone. Though the use of steroids in sepsis was still an ongoing debate, he explained that the latest evidence suggested a potential benefit—especially for a patient as critically ill as Eduardo.

We followed Mark's suggestions to the letter, but it didn't matter. Despite being on maximum doses of two vasopressors, Eduardo's blood pressure refused to rise. Meanwhile, his respiratory system was failing, forcing Sandra to increase the ventilator support to hazardous levels, risking direct injury to his lungs. Eduardo's skin showed a bluish-red lace-like pattern known as livedo reticularis, an ominous sign that his microcirculation was collapsing—and his intravenous lines began oozing blood, a sign that his clotting system had shut down.

Jenny hung the hydrocortisone. I asked her to start a third vasopressor. There was nothing left to do.

Mark arrived shortly after. He shook his head as I delivered my bleak report. Without a pause, he grabbed the portable ultrasound, performing a bedside exam to rule out other potential causes of shock, such as a heart attack or pulmonary embolism.

"It's just bad septic shock," he said, resigned.

Despite filling Eduardo's tank, maxing out multiple vasopressors, and infusing steroids, his blood pressure was abysmally low, barely capable of sustaining life.

All we could do now was watch, wait, and hope.

Eduardo's heart finally gave out at 6:00 a.m., just as the day team began trickling in. His heart monitor displayed a lethal arrhythmia: ventricular fibrillation.*

A team of nurses rushed to his bedside, initiating chest compressions, while Mark and I moved swiftly through the ACLS protocol.

We shocked his heart once, twice, three times. Nothing changed. We repeated the cycle again and again. I kept time—ten minutes, then fourteen, then twenty. As we passed the thirty-minute mark, his heart's tracing weakened, fading into a faint agonal rhythm—then flat.

"It's time to call it," Mark said, exhaling.

I stared at him, disbelieving. I was exhausted and reeling from the emotional roller coaster of the long night at Eduardo's bedside.

I pushed back at first, almost reflexively, clinging to the hope that Eduardo could pull through, that we could somehow save him.

Mark gently patted my shoulder, a silent acknowledgment that it was over.

Alex's face turned red, his eyes filling with tears. I wanted to scream. But I snapped back to reality—I had to keep it together for Alex's sake.

Mark pronounced Eduardo, and we met with his family. We explained what had happened and offered what little comfort we could. Afterward, we had no time to process it—we had to rejoin rounds. When we'd finished, Mark sent Alex and me home for the day.

As I headed out, I returned to Eduardo's room one last time to say goodbye to his family.

Only Anita and Marta were left. They thanked me for taking care of Eduardo. I didn't know what to say.

Instead, I hugged them both and whispered, "I'm sorry."

Before I left, Marta put her hands on Eduardo's face, kissed his forehead several times, and softly said, "Goodbye, *mi hijo*."

---

* Studies later showed an increased risk of ventricular arrhythmias like ventricular fibrillation with dopamine, and it is no longer recommended as a first-line agent in septic shock.

Part II

The Rips

HUNTINGTON BEACH, CALIFORNIA

JUNE 19, 2000

DURING THE SUMMER OF 2000, while visiting family in Southern California, I spent an afternoon at Huntington Beach. With just a few weeks of freedom before starting medical school, I figured what better way to spend it than at one of the world's most iconic surf breaks?

It was a sunny, picturesque day, with a mild breeze carving gentle ripples in the sand. As I stood on the shoreline, the shimmering water beckoned me. I saw myself in a movie scene, running toward the ocean and diving headfirst into the waves.

I was on the verge of becoming a doctor. I had my whole life ahead of me.

With that, I gathered my courage, sprinted into the shore break, and plunged into the water.

The cold water hit my face like a freight train as I torpedoed through the depths, emerging somewhere beyond the break. For a while, I just swam, lost in the moment.

Then, as I began treading water, I glanced back at the shore and spotted a lifeguard truck parked near the guard tower. A lifeguard stood beside it, looking through binoculars, waving to get my attention.

"Great. I'm in trouble."

Reluctantly, I began swimming to shore.

But something wasn't right. Although I was swimming forward, the beach was moving farther away. I swam harder but got pulled into deeper, more chaotic waters that tossed me up and down as the shoreline disappeared. Waves crashed into my face, forcing salt water into my lungs as I began to choke. It became difficult to breathe. My legs cramped. I struggled to keep my head above water.

I was in trouble. I knew it.

A sense of doom fell over me.

I'm going to die.

This is how I die.

———

Toward the end of the 1990s, US hospitals were experiencing higher patient volumes, overcrowded conditions, and increasing delays in medical care. Hospital throughput slowed down as medical wards, particularly ICUs, became regularly congested with sick patients. This bottleneck extended to the emergency room, the hospital's largest entry point for sepsis patients.

Meanwhile, by 1996, the number of uninsured Americans had exceeded forty-one million—many of them suffering from chronic medical diseases. Without access to regular primary care, medications, and preventive healthcare, these less fortunate individuals often sought late-stage medical care in emergency departments, which were now serving as society's medical safety net.[1]

This health inequality was a burden all Americans would carry in some way. Rising premiums often shifted costs associated with the emergency care of uninsured patients onto those with healthcare coverage.*[2] Moreover, whether insured or not, all Americans faced one particularly detrimental consequence of overloaded emergency departments: decreased quality and timeliness of medical care.

By 2000, US emergency departments were seeing 114 million visits per year, while many large centers were regularly operating over capacity, diverting patients to other hospitals. Emergency waiting rooms were often overrun with sick patients, who were sometimes forced to experience wait times as long as

---

* The Emergency Medical Treatment and Active Labor Act (EMTALA), enacted in 1986, requires hospitals participating in Medicare to provide an initial medical screening examination to anyone seeking emergency care, regardless of insurance status or ability to pay. If an emergency medical condition is identified, the hospital must either stabilize the patient or transfer them to another facility capable of meeting their needs.

eight to twelve hours. Patients spilled out of rooms and lined hallways, while those already admitted, like Eduardo, were often "boarded" in the emergency room for hours, sometimes days. One nationwide survey of ninety emergency departments revealed that 73 percent were boarding at least two admitted patients on a typical Monday.*[3]

By the mid-2000s, we were beginning to see the effects of these systemic issues. Studies showed that the longer patients stayed in the emergency department, the higher their mortality. One report revealed that patients who were boarded for more than six hours were 35 percent more likely to die during hospitalization compared to those boarded for less than six hours. This translated to one unnecessary death for every twenty-two boarded patients.[4]

Emergency departments were designed for high-frequency rapid stabilization of sick patients, not for continuous care of those already admitted.[5] Crowded emergency rooms simply weren't the ideal setting for practicing the moment-to-moment, bedside critical care espoused decades earlier by those like Edward Frank. Patients like this needed to be in controlled environments, with dedicated and undistracted staff who could respond quickly to their ever-changing conditions.

The healthcare advisory and research arm of the National Academy of Sciences, known at the time as the Institute of Medicine, described this dysfunction in a jaw-dropping 2007 report, *Hospital-Based Emergency Care: At the Breaking Point*. It summarized the dismal state of emergency departments across the nation and provided a raw portrayal of the US healthcare system as seen through the window of emergency care.[6]

It also gave a prescient warning: the overloaded state of emergency rooms meant that this crucial front line of the healthcare system was ill-prepared for potential large-scale disaster scenarios, such as viral pandemics, natural disasters, or acts of terrorism.[7]

By the early 2000s, over two-thirds of sepsis admissions were occurring in the emergency department, and the numbers were climbing.[8] As ERs were now regularly overwhelmed by patients of all kinds, those with sepsis faced significant treatment delays, increasing their risk of deterioration and death.

Sepsis was now thoroughly entangled with the healthcare system. It wasn't just about how a medical team treated a *particular* sepsis patient. It also related

---

* Many US emergency rooms still operate under these conditions today.

to how many of these patients were being shuffled through the system and, most notably, how they made their way through a busy and complicated emergency room. After that, it involved making sure what needed to be done—important processes like lifesaving antibiotic and fluid administration—could be accomplished quickly.

Additionally, once sepsis patients were admitted to the hospital, there was still wide variation in how quickly their blood pressures were stabilized, with patients often remaining hypotensive for hours.[9] In one 1998 study, patients who progressed to septic shock in the hospital ward could expect, on average, to wait for over five hours before receiving stabilizing treatment with vasopressor drugs—over ten times longer than it would take in the ICU. Even more concerning was a trend toward significantly higher death rates in this patient group, with close to 70 percent dying by the end of their hospital stay.[10] All this meant that there was a great need for a systematic process to quickly identify and treat these patients *before* they could deteriorate.

At the same time, hospitals themselves were their own incubators for deadly diseases. By the early 2000s, the US Centers for Disease Control and Prevention (CDC) estimated that 1.7 million patients were suffering from hospital-acquired infections each year, including *C. difficile* infections, catheter-associated urinary tract infections, central line–associated bloodstream infections, surgical site infections, and ventilator-associated pneumonia—many of which were preventable.[11] This is not to mention an array of other potential hospital-related complications, including blood clots, patient falls, and medication errors.

All of this fueled a lasting meme in hospital culture: "Hospitals are dangerous places."

I first heard it from one of my senior residents, who was trying to convince a patient that he was ready for discharge. I remember her exact words: "Oh, you don't want to stay here too long. A lot of bad things can happen in the hospital."

She wasn't wrong. But over time, this notion became more troubling. Why was it that, as hospital staff, when we brought a patient into our world, we were accepting such an abysmal status quo for their safety? How had the healthcare system's front line become an ocean of danger for the patients it was meant to save?

———

An intangible hollowness arrived in those final moments as I realized my life was about to end. Images of my loved ones flashed before me, followed by a crushing sense of shame—the agonizing feeling that I had let them all down as I felt my connection to the world fade.

Just as I had lost hope, I saw a figure cutting through the water, heading straight for me—a lifeguard!

One must have dove in after me while the other had been watching from shore! And not a moment too soon. My legs were giving out, and I was fighting for each breath.

"Hey! How's it going?" The lifeguard's voice rang out, energetic and unexpectedly cheery.

"I'm getting pretty tired," I mumbled.

"All right, I'm gonna wrap this tube around your body. Just hold on, okay?"

I managed to fit the rescue tube around my waist, and she started towing me back to shore. I could hear her grunting, struggling to drag my dead weight through the water. After a few minutes, the shoreline grew closer. Then, suddenly, a wave of embarrassment hit me.

"I think I can stand up at this point," I said.

"Okay, take it slow," she responded.

Relief set in as my feet touched the sandy bottom. Then I saw them—a crowd gathered near the lifeguard tower. Mortified, I kept my eyes down. But it didn't matter. I was alive. And I was on solid ground.

"How are you feeling?" she asked.

"Good. Thank you," I replied.

We walked toward Lifeguard Tower 8. Across the way, the lifeguard who had first spotted me stood watching.

I waved and yelled, "Thank you!"

He smiled, waved back, then got into his truck and drove off.

"Was that a riptide?" I asked.

"Yeah, the rips are bad right now. We've been pulling people out all week."

"I'm Parsa, by the way."

"Emily."

"Thanks for helping me."

"No problem!"

I owed her more gratitude, but she went about her business as if it had been just another day at the office. We parted ways.

As I walked back to my car, I felt dazed. I took one last look out at the ocean. It felt unreal, like the closing scene of a dramatic made-for-TV movie. I kneeled, sifted through the sand, and captured a small seashell. Back at the car, I pulled a pencil from the glovebox and carefully wrote: "EMILY '00."

———

I've shared this story countless times in my years as a quality improvement leader—a powerful example of a well-coordinated system that saved my life. In my work, we strive to build similar systems in hospitals and emergency rooms.

What struck me most about my experience at Huntington Beach was that the lifeguards knew I was in trouble before I did. The moment they saw me drifting too close to a rip current, they tried to warn me. When that didn't work, they wasted no time—they initiated a rescue immediately. I may have been helplessly caught in the rip, but Emily was already on her way to save me.

The lifeguards' response was proactive and well-executed—exactly the kind of response we should hope for in any emergency. One might expect a similar level of performance on the healthcare front line.

Yet, for most of the twentieth century and into the twenty-first century, medical professionals often fell short in addressing deadly conditions like sepsis. We didn't always think ahead. We reacted late, only really paying attention when the situation was critical.

I can still remember many nights during residency, rushing to a code blue, only to realize there was no hope—the patient's death was foregone. I can also recall long nights in the ICU, battling sepsis long after it had already taken hold of patients like Eduardo.

Even in the modern age, the healthcare front line remained mired by overcrowding, noisy emergency rooms, and elusive syndromes, like sepsis, creeping in and seizing control. By the time we'd recognized something was going terribly wrong, it was often too late.

In *Outlive*, Dr. Peter Attia writes, "Medicine's biggest failing is in attempting to treat conditions at the wrong end of the timescale—after they are entrenched—rather than before they take root."[12]

In the early 2000s, there was no better example of this than sepsis. Until the turn of the century, most medical professionals lacked a reliable system to identify and treat sepsis early. As a result, we were often on the defensive, playing catch-up.

In 1964, members of California's Surf Lifesaving Association of America established what is now the United States Lifesaving Association (USLA).[13] Their mission? To shift the premise of lifeguarding toward prevention while introducing a national standard for reliable lifeguarding practices and procedures.[14] It was a rethinking of the long-honored profession, born out of the realization that, though sometimes thrilling, dramatic rescues of swimmers already drowning or in distress were often unsuccessful.

Drowning happens quickly and quietly. Once a swimmer is distressed, rescuers have only seconds to reach them. Worse, the body's natural reaction to aquatic distress, the instinctive drowning response, can render a victim incapable of doing anything except keeping their head and mouth above water.[15] This makes early intervention critical—lifeguards must spot danger before it escalates.

According to Justin McHenry, a superintendent and aquatic specialist with California State Parks whom I interviewed in the fall of 2022, my Huntington Beach experience was "a pretty typical rescue scenario."[16] Over the past sixty years, lifeguarding has shifted from high-volume rescues toward a more proactive approach. Despite the romanticization of death-defying rescues—the stuff of cinema and *Baywatch* episodes—modern lifeguarding primarily involves prevention.[17] For every one of the ten thousand water rescues California lifeguards perform each year, they log over 100 *preventive* actions.[18] That's over one million preventive actions annually, ranging from something as simple as educating beachgoers about rip currents to pulling a high-risk swimmer like me out of the water before distress sets in.

As Lt. Jim McCrady of Fort Lauderdale, Florida, stated in a 2017 interview for *Slate Magazine*, "A good lifeguard is a dry lifeguard."[19]

Prevention and early intervention.

Sixty years ago, these two pillars revolutionized lifeguarding. Instead of wrestling the juggernaut of a full-blown instinctive drowning response, leaders of this renaissance learned to intervene before it amplified beyond control.

In short, it became glamorous for lifeguards to be unglamorous.

As for the outcome of this change?

The USLA now estimates that having a certified lifeguard on duty reduces the chance of fatal drowning to a staggering one in eighteen million.[20]

Sometimes powerful acts of heroism don't look like heroism at all.*[21]

———

The dawn of the twenty-first century brought similar transformations in the sepsis world, hospital culture, and the medical profession. This included one of the most significant international public health initiatives in history—the Surviving Sepsis Campaign (SSC)—which finally brought sepsis to the mainstream medical consciousness. Additionally, a pair of clinical trials sent shockwaves through the medical world in just two years, promising a new era in sepsis therapy.[22] All of this occurred against the background of a jaw-dropping exposé of the flawed underbelly of the US medical system, kick-starting the modern quality improvement and patient safety movements.[23] The convergence of these events shaped one of the most revolutionary periods in sepsis history.

But the rumblings of a US healthcare quality and safety revolution could be felt as early as the late 1990s. In 1996, the Institute of Medicine organized the National Roundtable on Healthcare Quality, a series of meetings involving key healthcare representatives from the public and private sectors to examine the rapidly changing landscape of modern US healthcare.[24] That same year, President Bill Clinton signed Executive Order 13017, establishing the President's Advisory Commission on Consumer Protection and Quality in the Health Care Industry. Independent reviews produced by these two bodies quickly elevated healthcare quality and safety to a national priority.

A run of groundbreaking publications and governmental actions ensued. If you were following the news around November 29, 1999, you likely heard about the bombshell report from the Institute of Medicine titled *To Err Is Human: Building a Safer Health System*. It exposed a stunning truth: medical errors were a leading cause of death, killing upward of a hundred thousand people each year in US hospitals.[25]

The report concluded that medical errors weren't simply the result of individual mistakes, but of systemic failures. It also introduced a radical concept: medical errors were inevitable, and it was flawed to "rely on individuals not

---

*   I was introduced to the concept of *redefining* heroism in healthcare in the writings of physician-author Atul Gawande, who touches on the subject throughout his writing, most notably in the book *The Checklist Manifesto*.

to make errors rather than assume they will."[*][26]

To Err Is Human depicted the healthcare front line as a collection of imperfect parts struggling to work in harmony. It underscored the need to anticipate errors and prevent adverse events from escalating into catastrophes. At its core, it was about building better systems—ones that supported healthcare professionals by making it "hard for people to do the wrong thing and easy for people to do the right thing."[27]

In 2001, the Institute of Medicine released a follow-up report, *Crossing the Quality Chasm: A New Health System for the 21st Century*. It highlighted the divergence between the ideal modern standard of care and the actual care delivered on the front lines of American healthcare.[28] The report called for urgent improvements in health information technology, payment systems, and the medical workforce.[†][29]

An independent study published around the same time by the RAND Corporation also showed that, when it came to the most common conditions treated by doctors, Americans received the standard of care only about half the time.[30]

To address gaps in healthcare quality, the President's Advisory Commission proposed the formation of the National Forum for Health Care Quality Measurement and Reporting, or the National Quality Forum (NQF). Launched in the fall of 1999, the NQF was a public–private partnership aimed at uniting stakeholders across government, industry, and the clinical community. Its mission was to identify quality improvement goals and chart a strategy for measuring and reporting healthcare quality nationally.[‡][31]

The NQF used a rigorous "Consensus Development Process" to develop and maintain key national healthcare quality measures.[32] In later years, through

---

[*]　There are nuances to understanding the report's conclusions. For one, the study was an extrapolation that used data from a handful of health systems to *estimate* the national figures. In addition, the original figure for the number of deaths was a range of forty-four thousand to ninety-eight thousand—a pretty wide margin. The report also oversimplifies the entropy and chaos permeating hospital care. The immense amounts of data, communications, decisions, treatments, and interactions that go into even a single patient's hospital stay can virtually guarantee that no matter what we do, something can and will always go wrong.

[†]　It also identified a collection of fifteen high-priority medical conditions, such as heart attacks and strokes, for which focused attention and improvement programs were direly needed.

[‡]　There was a general sentiment at the time against government regulation and control of the healthcare sector. Thus, the NQF also served as an open assembly for public and private entities to collaborate on national healthcare initiatives. Its funding sources included a combination of member dues and public and private grants from the US Department of Health and Human Services and the Robert Wood Johnson Foundation.

a collaboration with the Centers for Medicare and Medicaid Services (CMS) known as the Measure Applications Partnership, these endorsed quality measures would be fed to CMS for consideration.*[33]

As its opening act, the NQF released a pivotal report in 2002 titled *Serious Reportable Events in Healthcare,* which outlined twenty-eight life-threatening, preventable healthcare-associated adverse events, laying the groundwork for one of the most robust national patient safety and quality improvement reporting systems in history. While several states had already implemented mandatory reporting programs for adverse events, most of these systems focused on individual providers. *To Err Is Human* highlighted a critical flaw with this strategy: medical errors were severely underreported as many healthcare professionals feared repercussions or legal liability. To address this, the IOM recommended implementing voluntary and confidential reporting systems.[34]

In response, US lawmakers passed legislation promoting wider adoption of error-reporting systems. By 2003, the US CDC had begun developing guidelines for state-level public reporting of healthcare-associated infections, and by 2005, had launched the National Healthcare Safety Network, a nationwide system to track and monitor such infections. This sparked a grassroots movement across multiple states, leading to expanded public reporting of healthcare-associated infections. State lawmakers also enacted regulations to protect patient safety data and shield healthcare professionals who reported adverse events from legal or public retaliation.[35]

In 2005, the Patient Safety and Quality Improvement Act led to the formation of public and private patient safety organizations to collect and analyze patient safety data nationwide while safeguarding provider confidentiality. The Agency for Healthcare Research and Quality (AHRQ) subsequently created the Network of Patient Safety Databases (NPSD), aggregating large pools of deidentified patient safety data for analysis.†[36] That same year, the Deficit Reduction Act authorized CMS to reduce payments to hospitals when preventable hospital-acquired complications—such as catheter-associated infections—occurred,

---

* Ultimate approval of measures rested with CMS. However, endorsement by the NQF carried significant weight.

† The AHRQ was established in 1989 as the Agency for Health Care Policy and Research, based on a predecessor agency, the National Center for Health Services Research. It supports research and quality improvement of healthcare organizations and delivery systems. According to one of its past directors, Robert Valdez, AHRQ's mission is to improve healthcare. (See reference 36.)

a policy implemented in 2008. Collectively, these initiatives set the stage for robust reporting and prevention systems that now underpin hospital patient-safety programs across the nation.[37]

In December 2004, the Institute for Healthcare Improvement (IHI), a leading nonprofit healthcare organization, launched one of the most ambitious hospital safety initiatives in history: the 100,000 Lives Campaign. The campaign's lofty goal was to prevent one hundred thousand unnecessary deaths in US hospitals over an eighteen-month period.[38] To achieve this, it mobilized thousands of hospitals and healthcare associations nationwide, creating a collaborative network to rapidly share ideas, evidence-based best practices, and safety initiatives.

Founded in 1991, the IHI was led by Donald Berwick, a Harvard-trained pediatrician and health policy innovator. Its mission was to redesign the healthcare system by reducing errors, eliminating waste, minimizing care delays, and addressing unsustainable costs. Its strategy was to merge industrial engineering—the work of pioneers such as W. Edwards Deming—with clinical medicine and healthcare operations.[39]

By integrating evidence-based medicine with the science of process and systems, the campaign targeted key drivers of preventable hospital deaths: heart attacks, medication errors, catheter-associated infections, surgical site infections, and ventilator-associated pneumonia.*[40]

It also introduced the concept of a bundle—a set of three to five evidence-based practices shown to improve outcomes when performed consistently. Introduced in 2001, bundles offered structure and reliability when confronting complex hospital problems. For example, the "central line bundle" consisted of five simple steps when placing an invasive central venous catheter that ensured proper hygiene and line insertion and maintenance. When practiced reliably, this approach significantly reduced the risk of central line infections.[41]

The IHI also introduced rapid response teams: hospital teams trained to intervene at the earliest signs of clinical deterioration.[42] Rather than waiting

---

* In the case of medication errors, this work involved promoting medication reconciliation: systematically reviewing patients' medication lists before, during, and after their hospital stay to look for errors and omissions. In the case of surgical site infections, it involved implementing checklists to reliably deliver measures, such as precise doses of pre-operative antibiotics at the right time to prevent infection.

for patients like Eduardo to experience a full-blown code blue, rapid response teams were activated at the first sign of trouble, allowing them to implement critical supportive measures such as fluid resuscitation to stabilize a patient before the situation worsened. In some cases, this meant quickly transferring the patient to the intensive care unit for closer monitoring.[*][43]

The campaign concluded on June 14, 2006, with around 3,100 hospitals enrolled—three-quarters of all US hospitals at the time, and over a thousand more than originally projected. The results were remarkable: 122,000 prevented hospital deaths in eighteen months.[†][44]

———

By the time *To Err Is Human* was making waves and the 100,000 Lives Campaign was in full swing, the seeds of a revolution had already been sown within the sepsis community. Following the 1991 Sepsis 1 definition conference, experts and drug developers recognized that sepsis was complex enough to warrant a dedicated group of specialists—one that could refine its intricate definitions and develop treatment guidelines for the broader medical community. At the time, the academic landscape was relatively barren when it came to expert sepsis guidelines, leaving much of this work to be conducted internally by pharmaceutical companies as they developed and tested new treatments through clinical trials.[45]

In the early 1990s, Roger Bone's path crossed with aspirin maker Bayer while the company was testing a new cytokine inhibitor to treat septic shock. Discussions with Bone and other experts convinced Bayer to sponsor the formation of an international medical society of sepsis experts to provide peer-to-peer education to physicians. By 1996, Bone and colleagues had convened an international panel of ten experts, forming the International Sepsis Forum (ISF), the first organization of its kind. The ISF was officially launched in 1997

---

[*] There has been debate around the effectiveness of rapid response teams. If you ask most doctors and nurses, rapid response teams are invaluable, and studies have demonstrated that they have significantly reduced the number of cardiopulmonary arrests or "code blue" calls outside the ICU. However, these studies have failed to demonstrate a robust mortality benefit. This may relate to many factors and shouldn't discourage us from continuing to utilize and refine what is a self-evident process of earlier intervention in critically ill patients.

[†] This figure is based on an extrapolation derived from audited data from more than three thousand participating hospitals and a case-mix or risk-adjustment of the raw mortality data.

at the International Symposium on Intensive Care and Emergency Medicine (ISICEM) in Brussels, Belgium.* Tragically, Bone passed away from cancer at fifty-six, just before the forum's debut.[46]

Before he died, Bone outlined a bold vision for sepsis care in an op-ed published in 1995. He urged researchers to stop "tilting at windmills" in what he believed was a quixotic search for "imaginary magic bullets" or advanced sepsis therapies. Instead, he encouraged physicians to utilize the SIRS framework to identify sepsis patients as early as possible, initiate rapid treatment using protocols and rigorous standards, and leverage risk prediction tools, like the APACHE score, to better identify subgroups of sepsis patients who might benefit from newer therapeutic approaches.[47]

For its first major initiative, the ISF developed a comprehensive set of clinical guidelines to educate doctors worldwide on best practices for sepsis care. ISF members believed that a unified, widespread effort was essential to raising awareness and improving recognition of the syndrome across the medical community.[48]

"This was not running clinical trials. This was working on educating people on sepsis," as the ISF's executive director, Elaine Rinicker, recounts.[49]

Research showed that certain hospitals consistently following treatment standards and protocols achieved better outcomes. This suggested that the widespread adoption of such protocols could help reduce unwanted variation in sepsis care and, by extension, save countless lives worldwide.[50]

In 1997, Bayer's cytokine inhibitor was found to be ineffective, leading the company to abandon the drug. However, instead of dissolving its investment, Bayer donated its remaining funds to the ISF to support the development of treatment guidelines. Other drug developers soon followed, and when the ISF guidelines meeting convened in 1999, nine pharmaceutical companies had agreed to sponsor the organization.[51]

In 2001, the ISF published its landmark "Guidelines for the Management of Severe Sepsis and Septic Shock," the first comprehensive set of treatment recommendations and best practices for sepsis in history.[52]

That same year, a second International Sepsis Definitions Conference,

---

*   The ISICEM is a large annual international educational conference for intensive care and emergency medicine health professionals hosted by the Departments of Intensive Care and Emergency Medicine of Erasme University Hospital, Université Libre de Bruxelles, and the Belgian Society of Intensive Care Medicine.

known as Sepsis 2, was held in Washington, DC, led by Dr. Mitchell Levy, a prominent sepsis researcher from Brown University, and Dr. Graham Ramsay, president of the European Society of Intensive Care Medicine (ESICM). The work culminated in the publication of a consensus report in 2003, further refining sepsis definitions.

By then, the SIRS concept—defining sepsis as the systemic inflammatory response to infection—had gained traction in the academic and research community. However, many frontline doctors still struggled to define the syndrome. A 2003 survey involving one thousand frontline medical professionals showed that only 20 percent of intensivists and 5 percent of all other physicians used SIRS when diagnosing sepsis. Many clinicians believed that SIRS and other sepsis findings were too nonspecific and could be confused with other conditions. Meanwhile, more than two-thirds of doctors felt that there was still no clear definition for sepsis at all.[53]

While the Sepsis 2 task force recognized that the SIRS framework was useful for enrolling patients in clinical trials, they also acknowledged its limitations as a bedside diagnostic tool. For one, many other conditions could cause a patient to meet SIRS criteria, mimicking sepsis and leading to false alarms if used as a standalone test. Additionally, some of the individual criteria—such as an elevated pulse or respiratory rate—were widely regarded by clinicians as normal or *expected* physiologic responses to infection rather than clear indicators of sepsis. As a result, the task force questioned whether SIRS was too nonspecific to reliably diagnose sepsis in real-world clinical settings.[54]

Ultimately, the task force concluded that while SIRS could be helpful in identifying patients at risk for sepsis, the syndrome was too complex and heterogeneous to be reduced to a few abnormal criteria. Because no single test or biological marker could pinpoint when a normal physiologic reaction escalated into sepsis, the task force opted against redefining the condition, leaving the question for future research.[55]

———

On April 30, 2002, the community of Palm Harbor, Florida, was devastated when twenty-three-year-old Erin Flatley died from sepsis following what should have been a routine hemorrhoid surgery. Despite several visits to the emergency room, Erin was admitted only after her condition had worsened.

Once in the hospital, her health deteriorated rapidly under the nose of her healthcare team. Her doctors had overlooked the diagnosis until she was in septic shock—but by then, it was too late.[56]

In the wake of her death, her father, Carl, struggled to make sense of what had happened, growing increasingly frustrated when trying to get answers from Erin's doctors. He ultimately filed a lawsuit against the hospital and several doctors involved with his daughter's care. A series of depositions further convinced Flatley that Erin's death had been preventable.[57]

After that, Flatley immersed himself in research. Like many others, he had never heard of sepsis—and he was shocked to discover that, by the early 2000s, it had become one of the leading causes of death in the US, claiming over 200,000 American lives each year.[58] Yet despite its staggering death toll, there seemed to be no coordinated effort by hospital systems or government agencies to address it.

Frustrated, Flatley pushed for action.

"I went to the CDC, I went to NIH, I went to halls of Congress, I went to the state of Florida with the governor. I had knocked on all these doors, saying, 'What's going on? Who's taking care of this?' No one was doing anything. CDC wasn't even keeping track of it."[59]

A light went off. He realized the desperate need for sepsis advocacy. Flatley established a foundation in Erin's name and began building a nationwide network to bring sepsis awareness to the forefront of public consciousness.[60]

———

In the years following the ISF's formation, its members grew increasingly convinced that sepsis diagnoses were still being missed or dangerously delayed worldwide. A pervasive lack of sepsis awareness was leading to countless preventable deaths like Erin Flatley's. They also lamented that most frontline doctors weren't following guidelines or standardized processes when treating septic shock patients like Eduardo.[61] Outside of academic circles, many physicians were unaware of the sepsis framework, and most hospitals lacked organized systems to rapidly identify and treat sepsis patients. Worse still, expert guidelines weren't yet widely available to help inform frontline doctors about the best treatment options. For many doctors, sepsis was still flying under the radar.

In the early 2000s, Mitchell Levy, Graham Ramsay, and Phillip Dellinger (one of the founding members of the ISF) began discussing the need for a global sepsis public health initiative—the Surviving Sepsis Campaign.[62]

In 2002, they pitched the concept to three major critical care societies: the ISF, the ESICM, and the Society of Critical Care Medicine. The campaign outlined a comprehensive action plan to improve early diagnosis and treatment while providing education and leadership support to doctors worldwide. The pitch was a resounding success, and all three societies embraced the initiative.[63]

On October 2, 2002—six months after Erin Flatley's tragic death and a decade before Rory Staunton's—the Surviving Sepsis Campaign made its world debut during the 15th Annual Congress of the ESICM in Barcelona, Spain.

Now known as the Barcelona Declaration, this moment marked the first major public recognition that sepsis was a leading cause of death worldwide. The unveiling included a bold, global call for action: to reduce sepsis mortality by 25 percent within five years.[64]

The battle lines were now drawn. With this, we arrive at the modern sepsis era.

CHAPTER ELEVEN

Bending the World

Pure pragmatism can't imagine a bold future.
Pure idealism can't get anything done.
It is the delicate blend of both that drives innovation.

—SIMON SINEK[1]

HENRY FORD HOSPITAL IS A sprawling medical center in midtown Detroit, Michigan. Since opening its doors in 1915, it has served a diverse urban population while evolving into a nationally recognized hub for cutting-edge translational research—a place where scientific discoveries move quickly from bench to bedside.*

In the late 1990s, one of its researchers, a physician named Emanuel Rivers, saw a crucial opportunity to transform sepsis care. Rivers had spent many long nights studying patient charts, looking for patterns that could unlock the secret to reversing septic shock. But he eventually realized that the truth wasn't buried in clinical data; it was displayed across the healthcare system itself—in its processes, blind spots, and inefficiencies.

For Rivers, sepsis didn't begin when a patient arrived at the ICU. Instead, it started in the emergency room—the earliest and most crucial point to intervene. Yet systemic challenges, such as overcrowding, frequently led to dangerous treatment delays, exposing sepsis patients to a high risk of death.[2]

---

* Though not a public safety-net hospital, Henry Ford Hospital plays a vital role in delivering care to many underserved communities in Detroit.

His solution was a protocol, a step-by-step recipe for treating sepsis patients quickly and decisively in the emergency room. In keeping with R. Adams Cowley's golden hour concept in traumatic shock, Rivers's method brought the same level of urgency to the treatment of sepsis. His protocol used objective criteria to quickly identify patients in the emergency room and then treat them using William Shoemaker's decades-old practice of goal-directed therapy, which entailed using sophisticated instruments and techniques to optimize oxygen delivery to vital organs. He named this new protocol early goal-directed therapy (EGDT).[3]

Between 1997 and 2000, Rivers led a clinical trial of 263 septic shock patients in a nine-bed "sepsis unit" attached to the emergency department at Henry Ford Hospital to test the new protocol. After identifying and enrolling eligible patients using SIRS criteria, investigators conducted extensive bloodwork, administered intravenous fluids for resuscitation, and infused broad-spectrum antibiotics. Patients were then randomly assigned to a control group, which received standard septic shock treatment, or an experimental group, which underwent EGDT.[4]

Standard septic shock care at that time involved many of the principles developed by Edward Frank in the 1960s: continuous monitoring of arterial and venous blood pressures and administration of intravenous fluids and vasopressors to maintain organ perfusion.*

EGDT added the step of continuously monitoring oxygen delivery to vital organs and a structured protocol to quickly restore adequate perfusion.

During severe shock, blood flow to the organs falls to dangerously low levels, leading to a sharp drop in oxygen delivery. In response, oxygen-starved organs extract as much oxygen as possible from circulating hemoglobin, the blood's oxygen-delivery molecule.† This leaves venous blood significantly depleted of oxygen by the time it returns to the heart, resulting in a lower venous oxygen saturation level (measured as mixed venous oxygen saturation).

---

* Organ perfusion was monitored by measuring surrogate blood markers, such as lactate, and organ function parameters, such as urine output (in the case of the kidneys) or mental status (in the case of the brain). Doctors followed this standard of care for both groups, which also included the administration of fluids and vasopressors to maintain a MAP of 65 mmHg or higher (or systolic pressure of 90 or higher) and a central venous pressure of 8 to 12 mmHg to keep the "tank" full.

† Hemoglobin, the oxygen-carrying protein in the blood, resides within red blood cells. Each hemoglobin molecule can bind up to four oxygen molecules, allowing red blood cells to transport oxygen from the lungs to the body's tissues.

Rivers hoped to reverse this process by enhancing oxygen delivery to organs. As the organs received more oxygen, their demand for extracting it would lessen, leaving more of it in the venous blood and thereby increasing mixed venous oxygen saturation. This measurable change could allow clinicians to fine-tune the treatment in real time.

This was the crux of EGDT: using red blood cell transfusions and an inotropic heart-stimulating drug called dobutamine to rapidly increase cardiac output and optimize oxygen delivery to a specific therapeutic target, providing a precise, measurable strategy for reversing the effects of septic shock.

Funding for the study was scarce, however. As Rivers later recalled, "There was no money coming from anywhere."

Ultimately, most of the financial support came from the Henry Ford Health Systems Fund for Research.

"It was a grassroots effort," Rivers said, "from nurses to medical and even high school students. We used a little bit of everybody. We were quite proud of it."[5]

To continuously monitor mixed venous oxygen saturation, Rivers needed a specialized catheter equipped with a built-in sensor. This led to a partnership with medical technology company Edwards Lifesciences, which designed an instrument for the study: the Edwards catheter.[6]

The trial's results were striking. By the end, the mortality rate in the experimental group was reduced by *one-third* compared to the control group, from 46.5 to 30.5 percent. Put another way, the Rivers protocol saved one additional life for every six patients treated.[7]

EGDT quickly captured the medical community's attention by offering a structured, scientifically precise approach to treating septic shock—what Rivers called a "standard operating procedure" for sepsis.[8] In the process, it heightened the urgency of sepsis to that of a trauma alert or heart attack, establishing a process to swiftly identify patients in the emergency room, initiate an intensive treatment pathway, and optimize oxygen delivery to vital organs.

Yet some experts in the medical community criticized the study's methodology. One concern was that the initial treatment team was unblinded to the randomization assignment, meaning they could have unintentionally influenced outcomes by paying closer attention to patients in the treatment group, potentially skewing the results in favor of EGDT. Skeptics also argued that because the protocol combined multiple interventions, it was difficult to pinpoint which factor was responsible for the improved outcomes.[9] Perhaps the most important critique, however, was that it was a *single*-center study, making it more susceptible to bias and random error while limiting its generalizability or applicability to other patients worldwide.*

Skepticism aside, by the early 2000s, experts had become grim about sepsis care. Too many patients like Eduardo were dying of septic shock, and sepsis research seemed to be lagging far behind advances in other fields, such as heart disease and cancer. The EGDT trial offered a breakthrough, a signal that we could make a difference in this syndrome.[10] And, at its core, the approach just made sense. How could you go wrong rapidly treating sepsis patients using a goal-directed strategy of improving oxygen delivery to their organs?

Ultimately, considering the strength of Rivers's results, the reasonable quality of the trial, and an urgent desire to help septic shock patients like Eduardo, the EGDT protocol became a crucial inflection point in the modern sepsis saga.[11]

———

The same year EGDT made its debut, an advanced new drug emerged, transforming the sepsis landscape. It also ushered in one of the most controversial chapters in recent sepsis history.

By the 1970s and 1980s, researchers had uncovered the critical role of the blood coagulation system in sepsis.† They found that inflammatory cytokines, such as interleukin-1, and immune system–triggering pathogen-associated molecular patterns (PAMPs), like bacterial endotoxin, could activate a cascade of clotting proteins, leading to the uncontrolled formation of fibrin clots and microthrombi in the microcirculation, impairing blood flow and depriving vital organs of oxygen and nutrients. As a result, drug developers began searching for therapeutic targets within the coagulation system to halt this runaway process. By the 1990s, they had identified a promising candidate: a molecule known as activated protein C (APC).

APC is crucial in regulating the blood coagulation system. Under normal physiological conditions, it acts as a natural anticoagulant by inactivating certain

---

* Generalizability relates to how similar a study's patients are to patients in the real world. The more generalizable the study patients, the more likely one can expect comparable results in the real world.

† See chapter six for a discussion of the blood coagulation system in sepsis.

clotting factors, thereby helping to prevent excessive thrombus formation and inappropriate clotting. A deficiency in protein C, the precursor to APC, can increase the risk of serious thrombotic events, such as deep venous thrombosis (DVT) and pulmonary embolism.[12] Conversely, as we will see, excessive levels of therapeutic APC can lead to an increased risk of bleeding.

By the 1990s, it had become clear that inflammatory cytokines could suppress the formation of APC from its precursor molecule, protein C.*[13] This disruption was tipping the balance toward excessive clotting in the microcirculation. As a result, some sepsis patients developed widespread microvascular thrombosis, which impaired perfusion to vital organs and contributed to multiorgan failure. To counteract this process, researchers thought to synthesize APC directly and administer it as a potential sepsis treatment.[14]

During this period, drug manufacturer Eli Lilly developed a synthetic form of APC called drotrecogin alfa. Branded as Xigris, the drug was produced using recombinant DNA technology, in which genetically engineered human lab cells were programmed to manufacture large quantities of the target protein. Lilly maintained these modified cells in a master cell bank, from which entire cell lines could be cloned and cultivated for large-scale drug production.[15]

In 1998, Lilly sponsored a massive clinical trial called PROWESS, enrolling 1,690 sepsis patients across 164 centers in eleven countries to test Xigris's efficacy in reducing mortality.† Investigators identified sepsis patients using the 1992 Sepsis 1 definition and enrolled them in the study within the first twenty-four hours of meeting sepsis criteria, provided they had at least one dysfunctional organ system.[16]

The trial had all the hallmarks of high-quality research. It was a multicenter study that enrolled a diverse patient population across multiple countries, enhancing its generalizability. It was randomized, ensuring that potential confounding factors were distributed evenly between the treatment and control groups. It was also double-blind, meaning that neither patients nor investigators knew who was receiving the drug, minimizing the risk of bias in both care and outcome assessment.[17]

---

*   Inflammatory cytokines like TNF-α and IL-1β can impair endothelial function by reducing the expression of thrombomodulin and endothelial protein C receptor (EPCR), which, in turn, reduces the conversion of protein C to APC.

†   Clinical trials are often referred to by their acronyms. In this case, PROWESS stands for Recombinant Human Activated Protein C Worldwide Evaluation in Severe Sepsis.

Much like the EGDT trial, the results were remarkable. After two years, the mortality rate in the Xigris group was 24.7 percent compared to 30.8 percent in the control group, an absolute mortality reduction of 6.1 percentage points. In practical terms, this meant that among the 850 patients who received Xigris, approximately 52 additional lives were saved than would have been expected with standard care. The results were so good that Lilly halted the trial early and submitted the drug for FDA approval in the fall of 2000.[*][18]

But several issues emerged during the FDA's review—conducted principally at a public meeting of the agency's Anti-Infective Drugs Advisory Committee (AIDAC) on October 16, 2001.[†] Midway through the trial, Lilly had significantly revised the study protocol, adjusting the enrollment criteria to exclude patients with more severe chronic medical conditions. One can imagine this was done to shift patient selection toward those more likely to benefit from Xigris and *less* likely to die from unrelated causes.[‡][19] Additionally, in August 1999, Lilly had introduced a new master cell bank to manufacture Xigris, effectively creating a new batch of the recombinant protein—right in the midst of the study itself.[20]

In reality, it's not uncommon to amend a study protocol after a trial is underway. Such amendments are often necessary to improve recruitment, address unforeseen challenges, or incorporate new medical knowledge. However, protocol modifications can also influence study outcomes, intentionally or unintentionally, making it essential to evaluate their potential impact on the trial's validity and interpretation.[21]

A review of PROWESS data before and after the protocol changes revealed a substantial improvement in the drug's apparent efficacy—and it wasn't subtle. Before the amendments, Xigris showed no statistically significant benefit at all, whereas afterward, the drug showed an apparent 30 percent relative reduction in mortality—from 31 to 22 percent.[22]

Something had clearly changed, producing dramatically better results. But was it the drug? The patient selection? Chance? There was no way to know for sure.[23]

---

[*]   Patients in the experimental group also had lower levels of the inflammatory cytokine interleukin-6 and decreased concentrations of a byproduct of excessive blood clotting, known as the D-dimer.

[†]   The Anti-Infective Drugs Advisory Committee is now known as the Antimicrobial Drugs Advisory Committee.

[‡]   Interestingly, Lilly also eliminated protein C deficiency status—whether study participants had a measured deficiency in protein C—as a primary variable for the analysis. The full implication of this decision will become more apparent in later chapters.

This posed a major challenge for FDA reviewers, who had to weigh the drug's benefits against its risks and side effects. And with Xigris, those risks were no trifling matter. Due to its anticoagulant mechanism of action, the drug carried a risk of life-threatening bleeding. In the treatment group, 3.5 percent of patients—one out of every twenty-eight treated—experienced a severe bleeding episode. Over the course of the trial, four patients died from hemorrhagic complications.[24]

When it came time to recommend the drug for approval, the advisory committee was deadlocked—ten voting in favor and ten opposed. Some in the medical community were surprised that it was even that close, arguing that the drug should have been rejected outright due to the significant uncertainties that had surfaced.[25]

At the same time, sepsis was a growing public health crisis, and if the results were valid, Xigris had the potential to save thousands of lives. Despite lingering doubts about its efficacy, supporters argued that the drug met acceptable safety standards and offered a possible real-world benefit too compelling to ignore.[26]

The ensuing commotion within the agency was palpable—a flurry of follow-up analyses, internal deliberations, and debate attempting to reconcile the conflicting results from the study's protocol changes. The agency teamed up with Lilly to conduct a meticulous analysis of the updated Xigris product, manufactured from the new master cell bank, and found no discernible structural differences compared to the original. Still, some experts cautioned that subtle, undetectable changes in the recombinant protein could not be ruled out, leaving open the possibility that manufacturing differences may have influenced the results.[27]

Further review of the trial's updated exclusion criteria added an interesting twist. At first glance, one would have expected the changes to exclude patients less likely to benefit from Xigris and more likely to die from other causes. But that's not what the data showed. A review of the final dataset revealed that patients with a higher burden of preexisting conditions appeared to benefit the *most* from Xigris—not the other way around.[28]

The agency conducted a secondary analysis of the trial, examining patient subgroups. It showed that while the overall mortality rate improved significantly after the protocol amendments, consistent survival benefits were observed primarily in the *sickest* patients—those with APACHE II scores greater than 25. These findings suggested that Xigris's efficacy may have been limited to a narrower segment of the sepsis population than originally anticipated.[29]

This was somewhat consistent with where the science was heading at that time. Recall from chapter seven that the challenge of sepsis heterogeneity had plagued trials throughout the 1980s and 1990s. In several of those studies, more sophisticated follow-up analyses suggested that narrowing the focus to the sickest patients might have yielded better outcomes.[30] Now, with Xigris, there was emerging evidence that this pattern was repeating itself.

After considerable review, the FDA opposed its evenly-divided advisory committee and approved Xigris—with strict limitations. To balance its risks and benefits, the drug was authorized only for the most critically ill sepsis patients—those with APACHE scores above 25 *or* two or more failing organ systems—in other words, patients with "severe" sepsis.[31]

It was a seemingly innocuous technicality at the time, yet it would soon fundamentally reshape how frontline doctors diagnosed the syndrome.

Meanwhile, the same data indicated no clear benefit for lower-risk sepsis patients. As a result, the agency required Lilly to conduct a follow-up study to reevaluate the drug's efficacy in this lower-risk population—those with APACHE scores below 25.[32]

Some experts within the agency criticized this move, noting that PROW-ESS had not been explicitly designed or powered to test subgroups. While the post hoc analysis suggested a benefit among the sickest patients, it was far from proven science.[33]

FDA leaders acknowledged these limitations but ultimately stood firm. Jay P. Siegel, director of the agency's Office of Therapeutics Research and Review later defended the decision, writing, "the data currently available for activated protein C strongly support the conclusion that the use of this drug as labeled will save many lives."*[34]

With that, Xigris was officially ready for prime time.

---

*　On October 22, 2001, four of the ten dissenting members of the panel wrote a letter to Dr. Siegel expressing deep reservations about the decision, writing, "Despite many attempts over the last two decades, no drug in this field [sepsis] has reproducibly improved mortality. All agents have failed when tested in a second confirmatory trial. Accordingly, a drug that we know to be toxic should not be released without confirming that it does, in fact, prolong lives . . ."

As the medical community buzzed with the promise of Xigris and EGDT, the Surviving Sepsis Campaign (SSC) entered its guideline development phase, assembling experts from around the world to codify sepsis best practices into an international standard of care.

With the precision of the EGDT protocol—demonstrating its remarkable ability to rescue patients from septic shock—and Xigris, offering the potential to save thousands of lives through a simple intravenous infusion, it was no surprise that these two innovations became key components of the SSC's opening salvo against sepsis.*

The SSC needed clear guidelines with sharp definitions to improve doctors' ability to rapidly identify sepsis patients and determine when and how to use these advanced therapies. Decades of research had exposed critical gaps in the quality of care across modern healthcare systems. Medical experts now needed to bridge those gaps by issuing guidelines and establishing a standard of care.

At the same time, evidence showed that guidelines alone weren't sufficient to improve outcomes. They just didn't work without carefully crafted rollouts to promote and socialize them among healthcare providers. At the turn of the century, nearly two thousand medical "best practice" guidelines were cataloged in the National Guidelines Clearinghouse. Yet evidence of their impact on patient care was inconsistent.[35]

To create a sea change, the SSC needed more than just a set of guidelines. They needed a strategic, well-coordinated plan to disseminate new information to the front line—educational programs for doctors and nurses, performance measurement strategies, and a system for publicly reporting results.[36]

As Mitchell Levy stated in 2002, "Advances in critical care have been among some of the most dramatic in medicine, but we are well aware that a comprehensive program of education and action by policymakers and the medical community could significantly reduce the number of deaths caused by sepsis each year."[37]

This endeavor would also require substantial financial backing—something the SSC lacked. By 2004, funding for the US government's premier patient safety research agency, the AHRQ, had been diverted to information technology

---

* The Xigris treatment protocol involved a continuous intravenous infusion of the drug over ninety-six hours.

research. While this shift ultimately enhanced health systems' efficiency in billing and service accounting, it did little to improve the quality of medical care. As a result, organizations like the SSC faced the difficult challenge of seeking alternative funding sources.[38]

So when Eli Lilly approached the SSC's executive leadership team to sponsor the campaign and its guidelines, Levy and his colleagues seized the opportunity. They recognized that without significant funding, the SSC might never get off the ground.[39] Lilly ultimately provided 94 percent of the financial backing—over 500,000 euros—through unrestricted educational grants. This funding helped launch a global sepsis awareness campaign, starting with the Barcelona Declaration, and provided crucial logistical support for developing its guidelines.[*][40]

On March 3, 2004, the SSC published a groundbreaking set of international sepsis guidelines, titled "Surviving Sepsis Campaign Guidelines for the Management of Severe Sepsis and Septic Shock." It was a monumental collaboration involving forty-four critical care and infectious disease experts representing eleven international medical organizations.[41] Using the International Sepsis Forum's 2001 guidelines as a roadmap, the SSC issued forty-six distinct sepsis treatment recommendations backed by the latest medical evidence from clinical trials.[42]

The guidelines' central theme was urgency—treating sepsis as swiftly as heart attacks and strokes. Additionally, recommendations for lifesaving therapies, including prompt antibiotic administration, intravenous fluids, and vasopressors to maintain blood pressure and organ perfusion, were spread throughout the publication. At the forefront of its advanced treatment protocols were EGDT and Xigris.[43]

The guidelines also served as a comprehensive resource for ICU care, encapsulating decades of advancements in critical care medicine. This included recommendations on mechanical ventilation for conditions like acute respiratory distress syndrome (ARDS) and best practices for patient nutrition, blood glucose management, and advanced care planning.[†][44]

---

[*] The remaining funding was provided by Edwards Lifesciences, maker of the Edwards catheter, which was used to measure venous oxygen saturation during EGDT, and another sepsis medical device manufacturer, Baxter BioScience.

[†] In 2000, the landmark ARDSNet study was published in *The New England Journal of Medicine*. It represented a massive paradigm shift in the management of acute respiratory distress syndrome, using a specific protocol for ventilator management. Some experts have cited

Meanwhile, the campaign set out to establish an international quality improvement program to help hospitals quickly implement its new recommendations.[45] History had shown that the medical front line was often slow to adopt new evidence. Notably, the Institute of Medicine had recently estimated that it took an average of *seventeen years* for newly discovered therapies to become standard practice.[46]

But sepsis was a public health emergency, and lifesaving interventions were now available. The SSC knew it needed to translate its guidelines into real-world change—quickly. So, its leaders turned to the prestigious Institute for Healthcare Improvement (IHI) in Boston. Its recent innovative work using quality-of-care bundles had already improved hospital performance and patient outcomes in conditions such as heart attacks and hospital-acquired infections.[47]

———

On a crisp Boston morning in the spring of 2004, just as the SSC's new guidelines were reverberating, a young critical care physician named Sean Townsend anxiously paced the halls of Mass General Hospital. Townsend's ICU fellowship required a research project, but the sterile world of the laboratory held little appeal. He had heard rumors about the IHI, and that morning, on a whim, or perhaps by fate, he took a brisk walk through the city's historic streets to the IHI's headquarters near the Old State House.[48]

When Townsend arrived, he introduced himself at the front desk and boldly requested a meeting with the institute's director, Donald Berwick. His request stirred a quiet commotion, and after hours of being shuffled around the office, he found himself seated across from Dr. Carol Haraden, one of the institute's senior vice presidents. At the time, Haraden was leading the IHI's Critical Care Collaborative, an ICU-focused quality improvement initiative that included the pioneering use of bundles to prevent central line infections.[49]

Like many physicians of his time, Townsend had little understanding of what "quality improvement" entailed. Yet as he listened, he was captivated by its basic premise: building a better healthcare system. Haraden, meanwhile, saw his potential and immediately recruited him to her team. Before long, Townsend was at the forefront of the IHI's most ambitious initiatives, including

this study as one of the most important advancements in critical care in the twenty-first century.

the 100,000 Lives Campaign.[50]

Shortly afterward, Levy and members of the SSC approached the institute, wanting to translate their newly published guidelines into hospital quality improvement bundles. The two formed a strategic partnership, and Haraden entrusted Townsend to assist the SSC in developing bundles for sepsis care.[51]

Over the next year, Townsend collaborated closely with SSC leaders to establish two crucial sepsis bundles: a six-hour sepsis *resuscitation* bundle and a twenty-four-hour sepsis *management* bundle, both crafted based on recommendations from the 2004 SSC guidelines outlining the key components of high-quality sepsis care. (See Table 11.1.)[52]

Their objective was simple but powerful: to distill the guidelines as "change bundles" that could drive improvements in patient care. By forging connections with hospitals worldwide, the campaign aimed to standardize high-quality sepsis treatment and establish a global benchmark for sepsis management.[53]

6-hour Resuscitation Bundle	24-hour Management Bundle
Measure blood lactate	Administer low-dose steroids
Obtain blood cultures before antibiotic infusion	Administer Xigris
Administer broad-spectrum antibiotics within 3 hours in the ED and 1 hour in the hospital	Maintain blood glucose between 70 and 150 mg/dL
If hypotension and/or lactate ≥ 4 mmol/L, administer fluid bolus and vasopressors if no response to fluid bolus	Maintain median inspiratory plateau pressure < 30 cm H_2O in mechanical ventilation
If septic shock and/or lactate ≥ 4 mmol/L, perform EGDT protocol	

Table 11.1: 2005 Surviving Sepsis Campaign sepsis management bundles.[54]

"You can't improve what you don't measure." This longstanding mantra of management theory and quality improvement science had become a guiding principle for both the IHI and the SSC.[55] Quantifying change was almost as crucial as effecting it. Townsend emerged as a key architect of the SSC's data-gathering and -collection strategy.[56]

As the campaign rolled out, it commissioned a state-of-the-art database with a user-friendly graphical interface designed to streamline sepsis patient screening, facilitate data collection, and provide real-time feedback to frontline providers through improvement reports. The system was deployed in hospitals worldwide, fostering back-and-forth data exchange.[57]

Performance was measured in two ways: "process" and "outcome." Process referred to the reliability with which hospitals accomplished care interventions, specifically, how consistently they completed the sepsis treatment bundles for each patient. Outcome, on the other hand, was the ultimate measure of success: the likelihood of survival for sepsis patients. Bundle performance was evaluated as "all or nothing," meaning that to "pass," care teams had to complete every element within a bundle for each patient. Partial compliance wasn't enough when lives were on the line.

Like the 100,000 Lives Campaign, the SSC propelled its effort through a series of domestic and international learning and performance improvement collaboratives from 2005 to 2012. In the US, nearly sixty hospitals participated from coast to coast. Similar initiatives took root in England, Spain, Brazil, and other countries, forming a global network to improve sepsis care.[58] These networks were essential for gathering crucial real-world data on bundle efficacy.

Despite its noble ambitions, the SSC faced controversy from the outset. Some critics argued that the five-year 25 percent mortality reduction goal was overly ambitious. Others took issue with its "prescriptive methodology," believing that a one-size-fits-all approach was ill-suited for a complex and heterogeneous condition like sepsis. Moreover, it infringed upon physician expertise and autonomy in treating individual patients, threatening the long-standing principle that critical care happens at the bedside.[59]

Another major concern stemmed from the syndrome's nebulous and ill-defined nature. Defining the bundle start time, or "time zero," seemed arbitrary without a precise way to determine when a patient officially became septic. This created challenges in both practice and performance measurement.

Some physicians also criticized the bundles' all-or-nothing nature, believing it could encourage overtreatment simply to meet protocol standards while making it more difficult to pass cases where clinical judgment dictated a different course of action.[60]

SSC proponents considered the broader context. To them, bundles "were essential to drive improvement and resourcing for frontline physicians for whom the SSC resonated."[61] The SSC was focused on strengthening individual centers willing to adopt the guidelines and improving average performance incrementally—not achieving universal bundle adoption.

And with sepsis, changing the absolute mortality figures by even a few percentage points could multiply into thousands, if not millions, of lives saved worldwide.[62]

But the most contentious debate surrounding the campaign involved its ties to the pharmaceutical industry, particularly Eli Lilly, due to one of the SSC's more controversial guideline recommendations: Xigris. Scrutiny mounted over what some pointed out was a significant conflict of interest, as the key financial backer of the SSC guidelines was now seeing its prized sepsis drug listed as a critical sepsis therapy—supported, no less, by a "strong" recommendation. This is not to mention that the most game-changing element of the guidelines, EGDT, required a specialized monitoring device, the Edwards catheter, which was manufactured by Edwards Lifesciences, another major SSC sponsor.

On October 19, 2006, three senior physician researchers from the National Institutes of Health published a sharply critical opinion piece in *The New England Journal of Medicine*. It alleged that the SSC guidelines were part of a coordinated marketing strategy by Eli Lilly's public relations firm, Belsito & Co., to promote Xigris.[63] Its lead author, Peter Eichacker, was one of the original FDA panelists who had reviewed the drug in 2001 and voted against its approval. Since then, he and his group had published multiple opinion pieces raising concerns about the drug's efficacy and safety.[64]

The report's most serious assertion was that the SSC itself was an extension of Belsito's strategy to promote and sell Xigris. This suspicion deepened when it came to light that in 2003, the campaign had hired Belsito to manage its media relations.*[65] According to the authors, Lilly sought to boost Xigris sales by raising sepsis awareness and embedding the drug into the official sepsis guidelines.[66] They argued that the drug had received an unusually strong recommendation in the guidelines, despite the irregularities that surfaced during the PROWESS trial. They also pointed out that several members of the SSC guidelines panel had financial ties to Lilly, serving as paid consultants and speakers.[67] In a follow-up letter, they suggested that these experts may have been strategically positioned as "local champions and thought leaders" to advance Lilly's interests.[68] Eichacker and his colleagues went on to suggest that Belsito

---

*   To support their claims, Eichacker and his colleagues cited an online marketing communication by Belsito—which has since been removed—as well as a 2003 investigative report published by *The Wall Street Journal*.

and Lilly were exploiting medicine's emerging resource utilization crisis as part of a broader marketing strategy: framing Xigris rationing in hospitals as an ethical dilemma to drive demand.*[69]

Adding to the vitriol, in 2004, the prestigious Infectious Diseases Society of America (IDSA) declined to endorse the SSC guidelines, citing concerns over the quality of evidence and conflicts of interest surrounding Xigris. When asked for comment, the IDSA's guidelines panel chair, Dr. Naomi O'Grady, said, "Let me choose my words carefully. This guideline really, I believe, was designed to promote a product."[70]

The records show that Eli Lilly marketed Xigris aggressively, which might be an understatement. It was the kind of high-profile promotional blitz you would expect from a Hollywood film release, complete with swanky hotel parties and Xigris-emblazoned key cards.[71]

Perhaps this was to be expected. After all, Xigris was Eli Lilly's crown jewel: a miracle drug promising to save thousands, if not tens of thousands, of lives in its first year alone. It culminated a two-decade development project, costing hundreds of millions of dollars. The stakes were high, as were the expectations: projected revenues of a billion dollars a year or more.[72]

Lilly may also have been under enormous financial pressure at the time as its flagship antidepressant, Prozac, was set to lose patent protection. Competitors would soon begin selling generic versions of the drug, threatening a multibillion-dollar revenue stream. In this context, Xigris might have represented not only a promising medical breakthrough, but also a financial imperative.[73]

By the spring of 2002, Xigris sales were falling far short of expectations—only one hundred million dollars, a fraction of the blockbuster revenue Lilly had projected. Facing mounting pressure, the company overhauled its external public relations strategy, firing its existing PR firm and putting out new bids for Xigris.[74] Ultimately, the winning bid didn't come from a large powerhouse but a small boutique firm in Manhattan: Belsito & Co., run by Marybeth Belsito. Her pitch? Simple: "It was unethical not to use the drug."[75]

Belsito framed Xigris's poor sales as a consequence of hospital rationing, attributing it to cost concerns rather than skepticism about the drug itself. This narrative fed into a broader debate around the growing crisis of ICU

---

* When asked to comment on these implications and the fact that Lilly and the SSC were sharing the same public relations firm, a spokeswoman for Lilly, Judy Kay Moore, insisted that there was no master plan and that it was all a mere coincidence.

rationing and resource utilization in the twenty-first century.

That same year, a survey of 620 physician members of the Society of Critical Care Medicine, conducted by Mitchell Levy himself, revealed that 55 percent of ICU doctors reported having to sometimes ration medications due to limited supply, cost constraints, or institutional restrictions. What's more, the most widely rationed drug in the study was Xigris.[76]

Part of this related to its hefty price tag—sixty-eight hundred dollars per treatment—but supply issues and lingering doubts about its efficacy also played a role. In an interview with *The Wall Street Journal*, Dr. Levy explained that his motivation for the survey stemmed from concerns that Xigris was being used inconsistently within his own hospital network, Lifespan Health Systems Corp.[77]

Belsito and Lilly reached out to Levy with a proposal: lead a study specifically on Xigris rationing. However, Levy managed to persuade them to fund a broader investigation into ICU rationing. Lilly agreed and awarded Levy a 1.8 million dollar grant to establish a consortium of medical experts and bioethicists: the Values, Ethics & Rationing in Critical Care (VERICC) Task Force. Its goal was to examine the complex issue of rationing in intensive care and develop ethical guidelines for physicians.[78] Levy later remarked, "It was an opportunity to study something that would never otherwise get funding."[79]

Meanwhile, Lilly recruited patient advocates and physician speakers to champion Xigris. Among them was Nevada State Senator Sandra Tiffany, who had personally received the drug during a near-fatal bout of septic shock in March 2002. Tiffany later lobbied US Secretary of Health and Human Services Tommy Thompson, successfully persuading him to grant Xigris "new technology" status. This designation led to a special federal dispensation, reimbursing hospitals for 50 percent of the drug's cost.[80]

The drug manufacturer also played an indirect role in shaping how sepsis was documented and billed at the national level.[81] On November 2, 2001, shortly after the FDA had approved Xigris for patients with "severe sepsis," Dr. Peter Morris—a leading critical care researcher and paid consultant for Eli Lilly—successfully petitioned the CDC's ICD-9-CM Coordination and Maintenance Committee to add the diagnosis codes "severe sepsis" and "systemic inflammatory response syndrome (SIRS)" to the ICD-9-CM, the official US catalog of medical billing codes.[82]

Some critics believed the introduction of new diagnostic codes was part of a broader effort to increase Xigris use—encouraging hospitals to report more "severe" sepsis cases, thereby aligning with the FDA's approved indication for using the drug. Around the same time, Lilly encouraged state legislators to pass laws mandating sepsis case reporting to public health agencies, a move that could have also expanded the eligible patient pool for Xigris.[83]

SSC leaders like Phil Dellinger pushed back against assertions that the SSC was anything other than a critical public health initiative. He emphasized that Xigris was merely a small component of the campaign's broader mission to improve recognition and treatment of a syndrome that was claiming the lives of countless individuals worldwide.[84] While he acknowledged concerns regarding potential conflicts of interest related to industry funding and the financial ties of some experts, he maintained that the SSC had upheld transparency by publicly disclosing all industry affiliations while barring industry representatives from participating in the guideline development process.[85] Additionally, sponsors had been blinded from the guideline recommendations until they'd undergone peer review by the medical community and been formally accepted for publication.[86] The process operated independently of industry influence, and the evidence-grading system adhered to the standards used at that time.[87]

To unpack this, it's important to recognize that before the International Sepsis Forum and the SSC, much of the innovation in sepsis treatment—and some influence over evolving definitions—came from pharmaceutical-sponsored research and clinical trials. These efforts frequently involved collaboration with leading sepsis experts and researchers, who served as company advisors and consultants.

Since the dawn of modern medicine, the pharmaceutical industry and the medical research community have been interwoven in a complex web of collaboration, innovation, and, at times, controversy. This partnership has yielded tremendous advancements: penicillin, vaccines, and countless other lifesaving therapies. Yet it has also tested, and at times breached, the boundaries of medical ethics.

David Blumenthal captured this paradox in an eloquent 2002 health policy report in *The New England Journal of Medicine*, writing, "On display are the power, social contributions, and occasional venality of a very profitable industry whose products contribute in important ways to the health and longevity of the American people but that at times employs methods that are deeply troubling and even criminal."[88]

While Belsito's involvement complicated perceptions of the SSC, the campaign's core principles and foundational work had been established for decades before the PR firm entered the picture. The push for standardized definitions, early recognition, and structured treatment protocols was not a product of corporate marketing but the culmination of years of academic research and clinical experience.

There was also the issue of pragmatism in the face of a global imperative like sepsis. Most funding for guidelines and drug development came from the pharmaceutical industry at the time, as government and independent research funding were often insufficient.

Dr. Levy acknowledged this reality in a 2006 interview, stating, "In an ideal world, where there was enough NIH funding for purity, it would be great not to have to use industry funding."[89]

Levy's focus remained on the patients.[90] Reflecting on his experience in 2022, he remarked, "One of the things I learned early on in working with the Surviving Sepsis Campaign is that academics are much more interested in arguing minutiae than doing the right thing for patients."[91]

It was also hard to ignore the reported efficacy of these therapies. The potential benefits of EGDT were among some of the most substantial in modern medicine, and Xigris, despite its controversy, demonstrated an absolute mortality risk reduction nearly three times greater than that of aspirin for a heart attack.

In the end, ask yourself this: if you had the power to promote a drug like Xigris, knowing it could potentially save thousands of lives each year, what would you do? As Bono famously said, "Idealism allied with pragmatism, with rolling up your sleeves and making the world bend a bit, is very exciting. It's very real. It's very strong."[92]

———

In 2002, Senator Tiffany came across the website Carl Flatley had created to honor his daughter Erin. Moved by a shared mission, the two quickly became friends and collaborated to establish a major sepsis advocacy group: the American Sepsis Alliance. Tiffany's connections to Eli Lilly proved beneficial, as the pharmaceutical company pledged one hundred thousand dollars to help launch the organization.[93]

The Alliance held its inaugural meeting in Chicago in 2003, electing Flatley as its first chairman. Though Lilly later withdrew its funding, other prominent organizations, such as the American Association of Critical Care Nurses and the Paralyzed Veterans of America, joined the Alliance's efforts and helped sustain its mission.*[94]

In 2007, Flatley founded the Sepsis Alliance, which has grown into one of the largest sepsis advocacy groups in the world. Organizations like the Sepsis Alliance introduced a new dimension to the modern sepsis movement, empowering families of victims and survivors to unite around the shared mission of raising sepsis awareness and reducing its death toll. They have since become a powerful megaphone, amplifying the voices of those affected by sepsis and awakening the public to this critical health threat. Through advocacy and outreach, they have also pressured healthcare leaders and policymakers to drive systematic change and innovation in sepsis care.

———

The assertions in Eichacker's report and the media firestorm that followed delivered a severe blow to the SSC, threatening to derail the entire movement. The implications were deeply distressing for its members like Sean Townsend. As he later recalls, "It was a brutal time."[95]

The SSC's leadership responded decisively, terminating all industry sponsorship and stripping the campaign's financial ties to pharmaceutical companies. But this move came at a steep cost—the campaign was left without the resources to update its sepsis guidelines, much less sustain its international hospital improvement efforts.

At first, it seemed as if the SSC wouldn't survive.

Then, one morning, Townsend received a phone call from a grant writer at the Gordon and Betty Moore Foundation.

The voice on the other end simply said, "We'd like to help you continue your work."

Townsend dropped everything and immediately drafted a grant proposal, securing a critical lifeline for the campaign.[96]

As the accusations faded, the SSC regained momentum. While Eichacker's criticisms and the IDSA's rejection had tarnished the campaign's reputation, the

---

*   By the summer of 2005, Mease Dunedin Hospital and the doctors involved in Erin's care had agreed to settle her case. Flatley recalled having "mixed feelings" about the settlement but realized that the financial award would be enough to fund his sepsis advocacy work for years to come.

broader critical care community still recognized the urgent need for change. Meanwhile, a growing patient advocacy movement highlighted the syndrome as a public health crisis. The campaign pressed on, and the controversy surrounding Eli Lilly faded from the limelight. Yet the events left a rift in the medical community. Even years later, as I began my own sepsis quality improvement work, a shadow of cynicism lingered as a faint reminder of the turbulent past.

CHAPTER TWELVE

Surviving Sepsis

PORTLAND, OREGON
FALL, 2009

"LOOKING FOR SEPSIS CHAMPIONS."

The subject line caught my eye as I scrolled through work emails in the fall of 2009. It was from David Schmidt, the critical care director for Kaiser Permanente's Northwest regional healthcare system. He was inviting applicants for the region's first sepsis quality improvement committee, based at Kaiser Sunnyside Medical Center, in Portland, Oregon.

I had just joined the Northwest Permanente medical group as a staff hospitalist and was eager to take on a leadership role. I emailed Dr. Schmidt and arranged to meet with him the following week.

By then, sepsis had become a top priority for Kaiser Permanente. As the largest nonprofit health plan in the US, the organization served nearly nine million patients in eight distinct regions nationwide.[1] Just a year earlier, an analysis of twenty-one hospitals in its flagship region, Northern California, had shown sepsis to be the leading cause of hospital death. Data showed that an average sepsis patient had about a one in four chance of dying by the end of their hospital stay, while a septic shock patient's chances were closer to one in three.[2]

According to Dr. Schmidt, who liked to be called Dave, sepsis was also the number one killer of patients hospitalized at Kaiser Sunnyside Medical Center in Portland. Moreover, research suggested that we could significantly impact those numbers. This meant there was a huge opportunity to save lives. By the meeting's close, I was hooked. I leaned forward and asked, "When can I get started?"

———

After his landmark early goal-directed therapy (EGDT) trial, Emanuel Rivers saw an opportunity to drive similar improvements in other hospitals and healthcare systems. In addition to mentoring sepsis programs nationwide, he and his team at Henry Ford Hospital set their sights on the nation's largest healthcare payer: the Centers for Medicare and Medicaid Services (CMS). By convincing CMS to adopt the sepsis bundles, they hoped to sway most US hospitals to upgrade their sepsis care delivery and, by extension, potentially save tens of thousands of lives.

CMS had a vested interest in the quality of care and services delivered at US hospitals. By 2010, just over 47 million Americans were enrolled in Medicare alone, representing a nearly 150 percent increase compared to 1966.[3] Medicaid enrollment was even larger, at around fifty-four million, over half of whom were children. Medical costs were also skyrocketing, with national health expenditures now approaching 2.4 *trillion* dollars, or just over 16 percent of the US gross domestic product.[4]

Stark revelations from the Institute of Medicine had already revealed an emerging crisis in the quality of care in twenty-first-century US hospitals. In response, CMS had launched the Hospital Quality Alliance in December 2002, a public–private partnership involving multiple governmental and non-governmental healthcare organizations.[5] It aimed to enhance hospital care by measuring and publicly reporting performance on quality metrics for a range of critical medical conditions. The Hospital Inpatient Quality Reporting Program was officially established by the Medicare Modernization Act of 2003 and later expanded by the Deficit Reduction Act of 2005.[6] It required hospitals to report their performance on these measures under the threat of payment penalties. With results publicly displayed on the CMS Hospital Compare database, hos-pital performance became more transparent, helping patients—as healthcare consumers—make more informed decisions about their healthcare services. In 2003, CMS also established pay-for-performance programs, directly linking hospital payments to quality performance metrics to drive improvements.[*] This shift allowed the government to incentivize hospitals to adopt specific quality measures.[†][7] During this time, the National Quality Forum (NQF) developed a partnership with CMS through the Hospital Quality Alliance, becoming its principal feeder for hospital quality measures.[8]

In 2007, Rivers submitted a national sepsis quality measure to the NQF: the "Severe Sepsis and Septic Shock Management Bundle," or NQF #0500. This measure incorporated key Surviving Sepsis Campaign (SSC) bundle elements and required EGDT for all adult septic shock cases. The ultimate objective was to secure its inclusion in CMS's Inpatient Quality Reporting program, effectively ensuring widespread hospital adoption and positioning sepsis at the forefront of medicine's twenty-first-century quality improvement renaissance.[9] Within a year, the NQF had endorsed a portion of #0500 but stopped short of approving the entire measure. Its reviewing committee required more rigorous data and broader expert representation to evaluate some of the measure's more complex components, such as EGDT.[10]

To develop a national quality measure, you need robust baseline and field data to support its design and quality specifications. You also need complex statistical tools to ensure the measure is feasible and reliable and produces valid data. Rivers didn't have all the necessary components, but the SSC did. So, when he approached the SSC for support, Sean Townsend—one of the key architects of its sepsis bundles—was ready to step in. As Townsend later recalls, from that moment on, he and Rivers were "tied at the hip" as they began codeveloping NQF #0500.[‡][11]

---

[*]   Most pay-for-performance programs were not fully formalized until the Affordable Care Act of 2010.

[†]   Standardization and monitoring of hospital quality work began a century earlier when an American orthopedic surgeon named Ernest Codman devised the idea of an "End Result" system for hospitals: following every patient's progress long enough to determine whether or not the treatment was successful. This inspired another American surgeon, Franklin Martin, to establish the American College of Surgeons in 1913, which launched the Hospital Standardization Program in 1918 to establish best practices for hospitals. Later called the Minimum Standards for Hospitals, it was ultimately adopted as the nationwide hospital accreditation process. In 1951, the American College of Surgeons joined several other medical societies to form the Joint Commission on Accreditation, now most commonly referred to as the Joint Commission, currently North America's principal independent nonprofit hospital accreditation organization.

[‡]   This occurred during the 2007–2008 housing and financial crisis, which left many hospital systems unable or unwilling to fund participation in the Institute for Healthcare Improvement's (IHI) national healthcare quality collaboratives. During this time, the IHI lost some

———

In the spring of 2008, quality and safety leaders from Kaiser Permanente Northern California invited Rivers and the Henry Ford team to meet with hospital leaders across their Northern California region. This event spawned a collaboration to overhaul sepsis care delivery nationwide at Kaiser Permanente hospitals. Over a series of visits spanning several years, Rivers and the Henry Ford team trained over two hundred physicians, nurses, pharmacists, respiratory therapists, and laboratory scientists using the latest in evidence-based sepsis care.[12] During this period, Kaiser Permanente integrated Rivers's sepsis treatment bundles into its care protocols, leveraging its extensive resources and state-of-the-art information technology systems to build one of the most advanced sepsis surveillance and treatment programs in the world.

Word travels fast across Kaiser Permanente's various regions. By the time I'd attended my first sepsis committee meeting at Sunnyside Medical Center in the Northwest, Dave Schmidt had already established a mentorship program under Kaiser Permanente's Northern California region. Drawing on Northern California's experience, our committee set to work adapting and implementing a sepsis improvement model in our own hospital.

———

Just a few months earlier, the SSC had also published the second edition of its sepsis guidelines. This time, the campaign had removed all direct industry sponsorship and strengthened its methodology by adopting the more rigorous Grading of Recommendations, Assessment, Development, and Evaluation (GRADE) framework.[13] GRADE is a well-established standard used by medical guideline developers to objectively assess the quality of medical evidence and formulate clear, evidence-based treatment recommendations.[14]

The core framework of the guidelines was unchanged: treat sepsis urgently and rescue patients from septic shock with rapid, goal-directed therapy. However, the SSC strengthened recommendations for rapidly initiating self-evident therapies, such as antibiotics and intravenous fluids. Fluid resuscitation

---

prominence, and the quality improvement and patient safety revival lost momentum, leading to a future loss of perspective among healthcare professionals and medical trainees regarding the origins and importance of major quality improvement initiatives like the SSC.

strategies themselves remained nuanced, with the SSC favoring an incremental approach: administering small amounts of fluid while closely monitoring the patient's response. Recommendations for advanced therapies, like steroids and Xigris, were still moving targets, with the SSC notably downgrading its recommendation for Xigris to a "suggestion," limited to patients with APACHE II scores of 25 or higher.[15]

Skepticism around EGDT persisted. While Rivers maintained that the protocol's effectiveness stemmed from the combined impact of all its components, many experts sought to isolate and evaluate the individual interventions to determine which were truly responsible for the improved outcomes.*[16]

For example, some researchers noted that patients in the EGDT group received, on average, larger volumes of intravenous fluids and more blood transfusions than those in the control group. This raised the possibility that the improved outcomes were driven primarily by rapid and aggressive correction of blood volume deficits, rather than by the entire protocol itself.

EGDT was one of the most important developments in medical history—a paradigm shift in sepsis care. But the protocol's intricacies weren't settled in science, and more data were needed to confirm its efficacy while also establishing its generalizability to other patients and centers across the nation. (This would also be an essential step given that the protocol was being considered as a national measure.)

Other research groups around the world began working to replicate Rivers's findings. In 2006, the US National Institutes of Health (NIH) awarded the University of Pittsburgh Medical Center an 8.4 million dollar grant to conduct a large, multicenter trial designed to validate EGDT. The study, known as ProCESS, aimed to enroll nearly two thousand patients across twenty-four

---

* On August 14, 2008, *The Wall Street Journal* published a story citing concerns about the legitimacy of Rivers's data and conflicts of interest surrounding his relationship with Edwards Lifesciences. The report contended that the EGDT study excluded twenty-five patients— mostly control patients who had survived or EGDT patients who had died—from its final analysis, thus potentially skewing the results in favor of EGDT. The article also referenced numerous payments to Dr. Rivers and Henry Ford Hospital by Edwards Lifesciences in the years following the study. Rivers and Henry Ford Hospital responded on August 19, 2008, noting that the hospital's Internal Inquiry Committee had formally addressed the original complaint. After a reanalysis of data, it confirmed the original EGDT results and found no evidence of wrongdoing. It also confirmed that the EGDT trial had received no funding support from the industry and that Rivers had released his intellectual property rights to Edwards without receiving any royalties.

US centers.*[17]

Patient recruitment for ProCESS was well underway by 2008. Simultaneously, on the other side of the globe, a coalition of medical societies in Australia and New Zealand was launching a similar study: ARISE. A few years after that, researchers in the United Kingdom began recruiting patients for a third EGDT trial called ProMISe. These three large, multicenter studies aimed to determine whether EGDT's benefits could be reproduced in broader, more diverse populations of sepsis patients.

The story of Xigris was also evolving quickly. In 2005, Eli Lilly completed its follow-up trial examining the efficacy of Xigris in lower-risk sepsis patients. The study enrolled 2,640 patients across 516 centers in thirty-four countries, specifically selecting individuals with APACHE scores less than 25 or only one failing organ system. The results showed no mortality benefit for lower-risk patients. Additionally, the trial confirmed a higher risk of severe bleeding in the treatment group, with data showing one additional serious bleeding episode for every fifty-nine patients treated.[18]

At the same time, large patient registries were documenting significantly higher bleeding rates than what had been observed in randomized trials. This implied that, in real-world clinical practice, the risk of severe bleeding with Xigris was much greater, likely because community doctors were less adherent to strict safety protocols compared to those involved in rigorously conducted clinical trials. In response to these reports, the European Medicines Agency (EMA)—Europe's equivalent of the US FDA—conducted a formal review in 2007. The agency concluded that Eli Lilly would have to conduct another follow-up trial to reevaluate the drug's safety and efficacy.†[19]

By the time I was educating providers about the SSC guidelines in the Northwest, much of the early controversies had become a distant memory in the medical community. While some physicians still harbored resistance to the guidelines, the origins of that skepticism were mostly unclear to me. Occasionally, I'd catch a glimpse—a passing remark during a sepsis lecture or a vague reference to "industry sponsorship" in a medical blog or op-ed. However, the growing momentum behind the SSC's initiatives largely eclipsed these lingering doubts.

---

* ProCESS: Protocolized Care for Early Septic Shock.

† Many doctors were hesitant to use Xigris back then, as it was known to be associated with dangerous bleeding complications. As one of my ICU partners recalled recently, "I'd always find a reason not to use it."

And it was for good reason. As the healthcare system gradually reoriented itself around the SSC's powerful narrative about sepsis, the syndrome was finally being recognized as the medical emergency it had always been. Moreover, data indicated that patient outcomes were improving alongside the creation of sepsis programs and the adoption of sepsis bundles.[20]

While it is true that the industry had provided much of the initial impulse and funding for these new guidelines and therapies, something more important was happening here. Sepsis care was evolving beyond commercial interests. This transformation wasn't just about clinical trials and guidelines; it was about a fundamental shift in how the medical community was approaching the syndrome.

———

In 2010, the SSC published a striking report involving 15,022 patients treated at 165 centers worldwide that participated in the campaign's guideline-based performance improvement program between January 2005 and March 2008. The study found that, in the first two years of participation, absolute in-hospital sepsis mortality decreased by 5.4 percentage points.[21] Another way of looking at the data is that an estimated eight hundred *additional* lives were saved during the period.[22] These results represented a major milestone for the campaign—the first large-scale evidence validating its quality improvement efforts.

Other studies were also beginning to establish a link between the timeliness of sepsis bundle elements, such as rapid antibiotic administration, and patient survival. One influential study published in 2006 by Canadian researcher Anand Kumar found a remarkable association between delays in antibiotic therapy and increased mortality in patients with septic shock. According to the analysis, the risk of death rose by 7.6 percent for each *hour* that lifesaving antibiotics were delayed.[23] Although the study was observational and not a randomized clinical trial, its findings quickly captured the attention of the medical community. It remains one of the most widely cited studies in sepsis research, reinforcing the importance of early intervention in sepsis care.

We officially launched our sepsis program in January 2010: the Kaiser Permanente Northwest Regional Sepsis Initiative. Its vision was clear: to create a hospital culture centered on the early recognition and treatment of sepsis patients using bundles. The organization had already formed a strategic partnership with the Institute for Healthcare Improvement (IHI), which meant Dave had immersed himself in the IHI's principles of healthcare quality improvement, learning how to drive systemic change. In the process, he realized that success hinged on assembling the right stakeholders. Not surprising, then, was his team: an eclectic group of physicians, nurses, hospital administrators, laboratory specialists, pharmacists, and data analysts, each of whom brought unique expertise to the table.

We had a core leadership group. It felt like a family. Dave was the father figure, mentor, and leader. Then there was Anne, our "mother" and project manager—a brilliant and cheerful quality analyst who crunched the numbers with precision. Dave called her "the heart and soul of our program." Then came Briar and me, the young physician champions—Dave's protégés. Briar was a charismatic ER doctor, her sharp intellect tempered by a dry, effortless wit. I brought a passion for medical evidence and an obsession with PowerPoint. We were a tight-knit unit, tracking progress, refining strategy, and troubleshooting challenges.

The meetings were nearly uncountable, mapping out process and workflow, fine-tuning every leverage point in a sepsis patient's journey through the hospital. For instance, to ensure that frontline teams consistently checked blood lactate levels on every sepsis patient, we embedded the test into the physician computerized order sets, implemented new nursing triage protocols, and enabled nurses to order the test themselves automatically. We tried to make it easy to do the right thing. Then we reinforced these changes with electronic alerts, paper flyers, and email reminders.*

Many hours went into educating frontline clinicians on the new definition of sepsis. Data from the SSC showed us that these updated definitions were helping identify sepsis patients sooner, leading to faster treatment and improved

---

* We also embedded antibiotic guidance directly into physician order sets with the most up-to-date antibiotic recommendations for the treatment of common sepsis-causing infections such as pneumonia or cellulitis.

outcomes. Projections suggested that millions of previously overlooked sepsis patients were now being diagnosed each year worldwide.[24] Sepsis was no longer a shadowy figure lurking in the dark corners of hospitals. It was becoming a prominent condition, standing alongside heart attacks, strokes, and trauma.

———

As more sepsis diagnoses surged in the early 2010s, data from Kaiser Northern California revealed a disconcerting trend: an astonishing number of sepsis patients were dying without ever developing shock. Before the 2000s, these cases often went unrecognized and unclassified by frontline providers. But with the adoption of new sepsis definitions, more doctors were identifying these non-shock sepsis patients. We began referring to them as the "intermediate-risk" sepsis population—a group whose average mortality risk hovered around 10 percent, lower than that of septic shock patients, whose risk was closer to 30 percent in our system.[25]

As a term, however, "intermediate" was misleading. In reality, a 10 percent mortality rate is exceptionally high by medical standards. To put this into perspective, around that time, only 3 to 4 percent of heart attack patients died in our hospitals. But beyond the individual risk, there was a greater concern: due to their sheer number, intermediate-risk sepsis patients were accounting for most sepsis-related deaths in many hospitals.

Small percentages multiply into large numbers when applied across broad patient populations. Data from Kaiser Permanente Northern California showed that *two-thirds* of their sepsis deaths involved patients who never progressed to shock. At Sunnyside Medical Center in Portland, our data showed that, by 2010, intermediate-risk sepsis patients outnumbered those with septic shock three to one, and they accounted for just over *half* of all sepsis deaths.

It was a sobering and powerful revelation, demanding an evolution in our understanding of sepsis and our systems for detecting it. Before our eyes, this once-familiar syndrome was revealing itself to be far more complex, nuanced, and, at times, elusive. This only reinforced the need to develop an objective, systematic approach to its identification—one capable of catching sepsis in all its forms. We not only had to strengthen our front line to identify and treat critically ill septic shock patients quickly; we also had to reconfigure our entire system to better detect and manage the newly recognized population of *intermediate*-risk sepsis patients.

But how had these intermediate patients gone undetected for so long? Wouldn't they have simply gotten sicker and then been diagnosed with sepsis later in their illness? While it's true that a significant fraction of sepsis patients progressed to the more advanced stage of their illness—septic shock—emerging data revealed an important distinction: not *all* sepsis patients followed that predictable trajectory; many were dying in other ways.

Take Tom from chapter four as an example. While he undoubtedly had sepsis, he never progressed to septic shock. Instead, his condition deteriorated due to worsening respiratory failure from acute respiratory distress syndrome (ARDS). In similar fashion, many intermediate-risk sepsis patients were dying from severe organ dysfunction without ever developing shock—whether respiratory failure, kidney failure, or multiple organ system failure. As a result, we were misidentifying many of these cases, failing to recognize that they had been septic all along.

In 2012, a group led by Dr. Gordon Carr from the University of Arizona uncovered an even more troubling pattern while analyzing a vast database of cardiac arrest patients from over 500 hospitals in North America. The study, spanning from 2000 to 2009, identified 4,453 cardiac arrests in patients admitted for pneumonia. Many of these patients had experienced sudden cardiovascular collapse during hospitalization. Moreover, only a third of them had been diagnosed with septic shock before their cardiac arrest.[26]

This challenged the prevailing notion that sepsis patients followed a linear progression: from sepsis to septic shock, then to cardiac death. Instead, the findings suggested that many sepsis patients bypassed septic shock entirely, suffering abrupt cardiovascular collapse without warning. The study also hinted that just beneath the stable facade of "normal" blood pressure lurked a chaotic mess of microvascular and organ dysfunction—a hidden storm within the body. In some cases, this reaction was so severe that it led to sudden cardiac death.[27]

When examining the long-term outcomes of sepsis survivors, the picture became even more complicated. In life-threatening conditions like sepsis, research has historically focused primarily on survival, usually within the hospital or up to thirty days after admission. However, as early as the 1990s, researchers discovered that even when patients survived their initial sepsis hospitalization, they didn't survive for long.

For example, a 1997 study found that sepsis survivors were twice as likely to die within five years following their hospitalization compared to non-sepsis controls.[28] Similarly, in the original EGDT trial by Rivers and colleagues, in-hospital mortality in the treatment group was reported as 30.5 percent, but rose to 44.3 percent when extended to sixty-day mortality.[29] In the control group, mortality rose from 46.5 percent to 56.9 percent over the same time period.

It seemed as if something was happening to sepsis patients that we weren't quite capturing yet. Survival wasn't merely about making it through the hospital stay. An injured sepsis patient might survive only to die within a few weeks or months. The long-term consequences of the syndrome were just as devastating. This meant we needed a broader, longer-term view when it came to recovery and post-sepsis care.

This brings us to morbidity, which is the general state of living unhealthily or the experience of having a disease and its accompanying detriments. Morbidity includes factors such as kidney damage, limb loss, brain injuries, bedsores, and loss of muscle mass, among others. Traditionally, discussions around sepsis have prioritized survival, often overlooking survivor*ship*. Yet sepsis inflicts profound collateral damage, leaving many survivors in a state of chronic illness and diminished quality of life.

In 2010, Dr. Theodore Iwashyna and his team from the University of Michigan published a stark report on sepsis survivorship. Their study examined 1,194 sepsis patients from 1998 to 2006 and found that sepsis survivors were three times more likely to develop cognitive impairment, such as dementia, and 1.5 times more likely to develop significant physical disability after their initial hospitalization. The authors acknowledged that the study was observational, meaning that it couldn't definitively *prove* that sepsis directly caused this morbidity. However, even after statistically adjusting the data to account for other factors, a strong association between sepsis and long-term morbidity remained.[30]

Iwashyna's report exposed a chilling new reality about sepsis, one that physician researcher Derek Angus from the University of Pittsburgh characterized as a "hidden public health disaster" in an editorial accompanying the study.[31] Just as one example, the data projected an additional twenty thousand new dementia diagnoses annually from sepsis alone, with each diagnosis requiring up to forty hours a week of additional caregiver support.[32]

Angus also underscored the need to better understand the pathophysiology of sepsis. He encouraged researchers to develop laboratory disease models that could more effectively study sepsis morbidity rather than just survival. He went on to suggest that systems could be implemented both before and after hospitalization to focus on the rehabilitation of sepsis patients, minimizing potential collateral damage. Angus even suggested that it might be time to replace traditional short-term mortality outcome measurements with longer-term survival data and functional outcomes, as the former were too blunt to adequately capture the devastation caused by this syndrome.[33]

As for the extent to which this was purely correlation, no one knew for sure. Sepsis patients are often quite sick at baseline, which means they typically have shorter life spans compared to healthier individuals. Since all the data were observational, untangling sepsis from the confounding variables proved challenging. Even the most advanced statistical tools couldn't prove causation. What we could say for sure was that more was happening beneath the surface. This morbidity sometimes led us to question whether treating certain patients would genuinely alter their outcomes. However, for the majority, it made a strong case that we needed to enhance the treatment process itself.

———

For as long as there have been hospitals, nurses have served as their lifeblood. They are its primary caregivers, its watchful eyes and ears, and often the first responders in a crisis. In the emergency room, they are frontline decision-makers, rapidly assessing patients, recognizing early warning signs, and initiating crucial interventions. They draw blood, conduct essential tests, administer lifesaving antibiotics and intravenous fluids, and ensure that treatment begins without delay. Their vigilance and expertise form the backbone of patient care and the foundation of every hospital.

They are also the cornerstone of any sepsis program.

As an emergency physician, Briar understood this better than anyone, often reminding us, "Nothing happens without nurses."

As a result, we spent countless hours collaborating with nurse managers and educators—disseminating sepsis education, conducting hospital-wide sepsis "road shows" to raise awareness, and recruiting local nursing champions to advocate for best practices. In the end, they became one of the strongest forces behind our quality improvement efforts. When it came to saving lives, nurses were always on board.

Physicians were a different story. Briar used to joke that leading doctors was "like herding cats." Each had their own opinion or interpretation of the science and an unwillingness to surrender autonomy. Dr. Gordon Rubenfeld from the University of Toronto described them as "great chefs"—self-proclaimed masters of their craft who balked at the idea of being replaced by protocols or recipes.[34] Many doctors, myself included, had already developed deeply ingrained mental shortcuts, or heuristics—rules of thumb shaped by experience that enabled us to navigate the fast-paced, high-stakes world of frontline medicine. But these same heuristics made change difficult. Before learning new practices, we had to unlearn stubborn old habits.

This meant supplementing our clinical gestalt with a more objective framework. By the early 2010s, the definition of sepsis had firmly evolved into the model illustrated in Figure 12.1. Yet, for most frontline physicians, this was still a relatively new concept. Many still associated sepsis with a visibly *toxic-* appearing patient or a late-stage shock scenario. This outdated mindset needed an overhaul to shift focus more upstream and in line with the modern sepsis concept: the body's systemic response to infection.

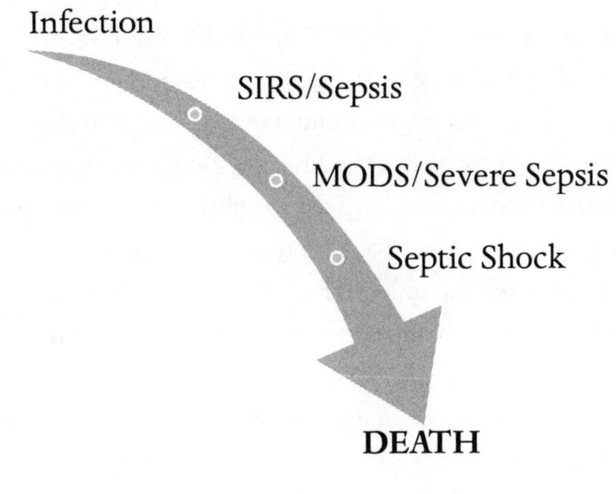

Figure 12.1: The sepsis concept we were working with around 2010.

But one of the problems with the sepsis definition at that time was that many doctors viewed signs like fever and tachycardia as the body's *expected* response to infection—not evidence of sepsis. As a result, there was broad skepticism toward the SIRS criteria, which were seen as too nonspecific to reliably identify the syndrome. In 2008, while attending an administrative meeting as a junior faculty member at the University of New Mexico School of Medicine, I sat in awe as one of the department chiefs lambasted the SSC for incorporating SIRS into the definition of sepsis.

To his credit, many sepsis patients diagnosed this way were not as ill as the more classically defined patients of the past—many didn't have sepsis at all. For instance, a young twenty-five-year-old woman with a mild viral illness could have easily been diagnosed with "sepsis" based solely on having a fever and a rapid heart rate. Initiating an aggressive sepsis bundle for such a patient could lead to harm from excessive intravenous fluids or unnecessary antibiotic therapy.

Even more concerning, many *non*infectious conditions—such as heart attacks, strokes, pulmonary emboli, and pancreatitis—could also generate abnormal SIRS criteria. In such cases, thinking a patient had sepsis could lead a physician to overlook another serious diagnosis or condition. In fact, these pitfalls were already apparent to members of the 2001 Sepsis 2 Definitions Conference, who cautioned against relying too heavily on the SIRS framework due to its limited specificity.[35]

But despite its limitations, the SIRS-based definition brought some clarity to a concept that had long been vague and imprecise. Sepsis had always been a syndrome without a single defining test—its signs and symptoms were nonspecific, and diagnosis often relied heavily on clinical intuition. The new definitions offered a way to standardize recognition. In the words of Dr. Levy, they were bringing "structure" to something that had been too "nebulous" for years.[36] Instead of relying on gestalt to decide that a patient "looks septic," clinicians could now point to objective criteria: an infection plus two abnormal SIRS markers. This structure allowed for earlier identification and intervention. While it may have led to some degree of overdiagnosis, many sepsis leaders saw this as an acceptable trade-off if it meant saving more lives.

———

Beyond just early identification, improving sepsis outcomes demanded rapid treatment and consistent delivery of sepsis bundles. However, the challenge lay buried in a mountain of detail. Implementing the bundles was a monumental task, with varying degrees of complexity depending on whether the patient was in septic shock or classified as intermediate risk.

Septic shock is rarely subtle.* Patients are critically ill, usually experiencing extremely low blood pressure, lethargy, and multi-organ dysfunction. Identifying these patients wasn't the hard part—it was completing EGDT efficiently.

Along with the prompt administration of antibiotics and fluids, the protocol required the rapid insertion of a central line—a delicate procedure that could take thirty minutes to an hour. This was followed by the initial measurement of central venous pressure and venous oxygen saturation to guide further resuscitation. From there, EGDT called for precise titration of vasopressors, blood transfusions, and fluids to achieve targets for central venous pressure, mean arterial pressure, and mixed venous oxygen saturation. This intensive, hands-on process added significant pressure to emergency physicians and nurses who were already juggling multiple crises.

To support the emergency room during a septic shock admission, we adapted a concept already proven effective for expediting treatment in other urgent conditions, such as heart attacks and strokes: the sepsis alert.

Once the ER team had identified a patient in septic shock, they would trigger the alert, activating a dedicated septic shock response team. This included the ICU charge nurse and a rapid response nurse, both trained in setting up the necessary monitoring equipment and rapidly completing the sepsis bundle measures.

As for intermediate-risk sepsis patients, they were more challenging to identify but had less complicated treatment bundles. Their clinical signs and symptoms were often vague and nonspecific. Questions persisted regarding just how sick they really were. However, once the ER doctor recognized a patient with intermediate sepsis, it was a simpler matter of administering antibiotics and fluids promptly while also checking blood cultures and lactate levels.

Meanwhile, we were already facilitating early blood culture collection and lactate testing by adding a SIRS screening process to the nursing triage workflow. Since triage is where a nurse first evaluates patients, it was also the perfect

---

* The one exception is the so-called "cryptic" septic shock patient—a patient with normal blood pressure but blood lactate level greater than 4 mmol/Liter, signifying severe microvascular shock. Such patients can sometimes languish right under the radar.

location to perform the SIRS screen.*

During this time, something interesting was emerging from Kaiser Permanente Northern California. Data from its registry indicated that if doctors obtained a *repeat* lactate a few hours after initial treatment, they could gain valuable insights into a sepsis patient's condition and prognosis.

This made perfect sense. Lactate serves as a marker for underlying sepsis-induced organ dysfunction and metabolic dysregulation. A *decreasing* lactate level can indicate that the initial treatment measures—fluids and antibiotics—are working and that the sepsis-induced dysfunction is improving. In fact, data from Northern California revealed that if the lactate improved by at least 10 percent within the first few hours, a patient's risk of death decreased by half.†[37] With such compelling evidence, by mid 2012, we had embedded a lactate clearance process into our sepsis bundles.‡

———

Morbidity and mortality data were intellectually compelling but sometimes too abstract. Beyond the statistics and clinical outcomes lay the deeply personal stories of survivors, victims, and families forever changed by the syndrome. Thanks to the efforts of a growing movement of sepsis advocacy groups, like the Sepsis Alliance, these stories were coming to light. By connecting frontline providers to this syndrome's human and emotional toll, we could cultivate a stronger sense of connection and responsibility to patients and their families.[38]

———

In the early spring of 2012, Dave, Briar, and I met to discuss the state of the program and plan our strategy for the upcoming year. Our sepsis initiative

---

* Triage nurses were encouraged to automatically draw blood cultures and lactate tests on any patients with a suspected infection and positive SIRS criteria; thus, by the time the physician saw a patient, they often already had the lactate result as well as a notification from the nurse that the patient was SIRS-positive.

† Debate persists today regarding the clinical utility of checking repeat blood lactates in sepsis.

‡ Our rapid response nurses kept constant watch on intermediate-risk sepsis patients, regularly rounding on them, ensuring they had repeat lactates checked, and following their progress until they were deemed stable.

had become fully operational, and the data presented an impressive picture.

For one, we were identifying more cases. Between 2009 and 2011, the average number of sepsis diagnoses at Sunnyside Medical Center had more than doubled, rising from 54 cases per month to 122. Much of this was driven by improved processes, particularly more frequent blood lactate testing, which helped detect sepsis earlier and more reliably.

Beyond that, outcomes had improved. Our overall sepsis mortality rate had dropped by more than half, from 12 percent down to just 5 percent.

But perhaps most importantly, we had fostered a cultural shift in the hospital. Sepsis was now on everyone's radar. The question "Could it be sepsis?" became second nature—a simple yet lifesaving reflection among doctors and nurses as they assessed their patients.

Challenges remained. With its many moving parts and overlapping roles, EGDT had become a major burden on the emergency department. Simply inserting a central line in a busy ER was hard enough, but with EGDT, nurses had to assemble the measurement apparatus, calibrate the instruments, and start taking readings.

The equipment itself was also cumbersome. Device cables tangled, key components went missing, and the protocol's logistical complexity led to frustration. Other emergency departments experienced similar barriers.[39]

I often wondered whether we would have been better served by a dedicated sepsis ward, much like the one in the original EGDT study. Our rapid response team was a blessing, stepping in during sepsis alerts to support the emergency room staff. Yet even with their help, we struggled to get it right each time.

Additionally, a growing number of ICU doctors began opposing the rigidity of EGDT. Some believed that not every patient needed such aggressive measures, while others wanted more flexibility in deciding when to follow the protocol. As we enforced adherence to the bundles, we encountered credibility problems.

Briar and I heard similar concerns from some ER and hospitalist physicians. There was a growing sentiment that we were overdiagnosing sepsis. While the large-scale numbers were hard to ignore, the bundles sometimes pushed doctors out of their comfort zones.

Dave, who was always pragmatic, recalls at one point leveling with the ICU doctors: "We're giving up some autonomy, and we're going to have to accept some overtreatment as the price to pay so that we don't undertreat others.

Let's agree to do this together."[40]

It was a delicate balance: ensuring that sepsis patients received timely, life-saving care without alienating the clinicians responsible for that care.

At the meeting's close, Dave left us with a piece of wisdom I still hold on to: "In medicine, we sometimes need to do something right over and over again, sometimes even a hundred times, to save one person's life. That's why we're doing this. So we don't leave anyone behind."

Reliability was everything. We were building a better system—one that could genuinely safeguard our patients. One that would ensure no one fell through the cracks.

CHAPTER THIRTEEN

Rory's Lessons

THE ANNALS OF SEPSIS TRAGEDY are filled with victims whose stories hold the weight of the world. Our timeline now brings us back to Rory Staunton, whose account I shared in the prologue and who has become one of modern history's most publicized and transformative sepsis figures. Some experts consider his death a "never event"—an appalling outcome involving so many missteps that it should never have occurred. Yet, while documented breakdowns in care took place, his tragedy does more to unmask wider systemic issues and entrenched biases that have plagued medical professionals in their struggle against this syndrome. In this light, Rory teaches us many lessons and can help us chart a better path forward. His account illustrates the complexity of sepsis in our society and healthcare system today and serves as a devastating postmortem on how our most vulnerable patients can slip through our fingers.

In this chapter, I'll revisit Rory's story and reflect on moments when events might have unfolded differently.

———

On Wednesday, March 28, 2012, Rory Staunton scraped his elbow during gym class. The wound was covered without being cleaned—an apparently minor oversight that may have opened the door to the infection that would later claim his life.[1] Prevention remains our most powerful tool against sepsis, yet this basic tenet still eludes us. Something as simple as prompt wound care or proper hygiene can often make the difference between life and death.

By the following morning, Rory had a high fever, was vomiting, and complained of severe leg pain. He was clearly sick. In the pediatrician's office, he had a fever of 102°F, a heart rate of 140 beats per minute, and rapid breathing. Clinical gestalt aside, you might recognize three out of four SIRS criteria, suggesting a serious infection and possibly sepsis. However, sepsis wasn't considered at this point. As for the mottled rash on his skin? A subtle but ominous sign of poor blood flow: livedo reticularis.[2]

One of the earliest links in the lifeguarding chain of survival is recognizing distress. This grants lifeguards time to intervene before the instinctive drowning response overwhelms a potential victim. Seconds spell the difference between life and death, so lifeguards take a systematic approach when scanning the water for distressed swimmers.

With sepsis, half the battle is promptly recognizing that a patient is in trouble. In many cases, this begins in the outpatient setting—at home, school, a doctor's office, or an urgent care clinic. Recent studies estimate that anywhere from a third to half of all sepsis patients have had an outpatient encounter with the healthcare system in the week before they were hospitalized.[3] Although it's unclear from the data whether a significant portion of these encounters represent missed opportunities, the findings underscore the need to broaden sepsis awareness into the outpatient setting.[4] Had sepsis been suspected at Rory's first visit to the pediatrician's office, prompt intervention might have changed the course of events.

In the years leading up to Rory's death, the Surviving Sepsis Campaign (SSC) had slowly spread its influence to hospitals worldwide, but it wasn't moving fast enough, and it faced constant skepticism and resistance from healthcare leaders and frontline doctors.

In the end, this expanding sphere of vigilance fell just shy of converging with the plight of a twelve-year-old boy.

———

By 2012, data from the SSC showed that with each incremental improvement in bundle compliance, hospitals demonstrated higher sepsis survival rates. More importantly, nearly all the survival benefits were attributed to the six-hour resuscitation bundle. Thus, the most critical factors were the rapid administration of antibiotics and restoration of blood perfusion with fluids and supportive care.[5]

An examination of 29,470 sepsis patients treated between 2005 and 2012 showed that each 10 percent increase in bundle success produced a 3 to 5 percent improvement in hospital sepsis mortality.[6] It was an impressive finding, even more pronounced in high-performing hospitals—those participating in the SSC's program for at least three years and displaying particularly impressive bundle compliance.

Some in the medical community remained skeptical. They weren't convinced the improved mortality was solely due to sepsis bundle compliance.[7] Since the study data were observational and not derived from randomized clinical trials, there were too many potential confounding variables to prove causation between the bundles and improved outcomes.

Recall from chapter seven that one of the key advancements in medical science was randomization: the ability to study the effect of a single intervention and test its impact on a group of patients. The problem with observational studies? You can't truly randomize; thus, you are unable to isolate a single intervention in question—in this case, sepsis bundle compliance—making it difficult to be sure it's the sole variable responsible for the result.

It could have been that the superior mortality outcomes were due to an overall improvement in critical care medicine throughout the study's period.

As Dave Schmidt explains, "The story of critical care has been that of a whole lot of little things improving over time."[8]

Over many years, doctors became more skilled at managing the complex needs of critically ill patients, including those with sepsis. This is not to mention that the SSC coincided with other large quality improvement initiatives, like the 100,000 Lives Campaign. Perhaps it was the cumulative effect of all these system-level improvements that drove the observed gains in sepsis outcomes, not the sepsis bundles alone.[*][9]

Further illustrating this point, investigators analyzing ICU data from Australia and New Zealand between 2000 and 2012 found that sepsis mortality was effectively cut in half. However, they also saw a similar decline in mortality among non-septic ICU patients during the same period. This parallel improvement suggested that the observed mortality benefits were likely driven by overall changes in critical care practice, rather than by changes in sepsis management alone.[10]

---

[*]　While the campaign embedded many of these evolving standards of care in the SSC treatment guidelines, they didn't include them all in the bundles.

Epidemiologists also suggested that the SIRS definitional framework was skewing overall mortality data by helping doctors identify "healthier" sepsis patients, creating an apples-to-oranges comparison problem in studies.[11] Many of these newly diagnosed sepsis patients, like the intermediate-risk patients from chapter twelve, had less severe manifestations of the syndrome and were less likely to die in the first place, regardless of the intervention. Thus, their addition to the overall pool of sepsis patients likely decreased or diluted the overall mortality average.

This phenomenon is sometimes referred to as the "Will Rogers effect," owing to a famous joke Rogers made in the 1930s about migration during the Great Depression: "When the Okies left Oklahoma and moved to California, they raised the average intelligence in both states."[12]

Anticipating these concerns, the SSC used sophisticated statistical tools to adjust for differences in illness severity. It used a severity of illness modifier—the sepsis severity score—which allowed researchers to risk-adjust mortality estimates, ensuring that comparisons before and after bundle implementation involved patients with similar baseline illness levels—in other words, comparing apples to apples.[13]

To disentangle the confounding problem, they examined how long centers participated in the SSC's program. They found that hospitals with longer participation tended to show greater improvements in mortality. Looked at another way, the sepsis bundles appeared to have a *dose-response* effect: more exposure to the program resulted in better outcomes. This temporal association strengthened the case that bundle performance may have played a causal role in improving survival.[14]

Large healthcare systems, such as Kaiser Permanente, used similar risk-adjustment approaches to evaluate sepsis outcomes—specifically by tracking the mortality ratio (observed mortality divided by expected mortality). This standardized mortality ratio accounted for how severely ill patients were at the time of presentation.* Using this analysis, researchers found that the average sepsis mortality ratio declined significantly across Kaiser Permanente hospitals in Northern California from 2009 to 2012. The consistency of this risk-adjusted improvement suggested that the effect was likely real—reflecting genuine gains in sepsis care rather than a statistical artifact or dilution from

---

* See chapter eight for a discussion of the mortality ratio.

changing the case mix.[*][15]

Sepsis treatment bundle trials also presented ethical and logistical difficulties. By the early 2000s, the necessity of initial treatments such as antibiotics, fluids, and vasopressors had become so self-evident that withholding them from patients during a study was considered unethical.

In clinical research, the concept of equipoise holds that a randomized clinical trial is ethically permissible only when there is genuine uncertainty about which treatment is superior. If a physician has knowledge that one option is clearly better, such as administering antibiotics for sepsis rather than withholding them, the ethical obligation is straightforward: she must offer the proven therapy.[†][16] In time-sensitive conditions like sepsis, however, this ethical clarity can pose logistical challenges. Because early treatment is critical, researchers often struggle to enroll and randomize patients quickly enough to meet both scientific rigor and clinical urgency, complicating experimental design and implementation.[‡][17]

Beyond the ethical and logistical challenges, sepsis also posed a substantial public health threat. To maximize the potential for saving lives, hospitals needed to adopt systemwide strategies quickly. In this context, waiting for definitive randomized clinical trial data was often impractical.

Ultimately, while the SSC brought much-needed structure to the sepsis concept and raised awareness in hospitals around the world, the complexity of *measuring* the true impact of its bundles ensured that doctors would debate the data for years to come. It also meant that reliable sepsis systems would take even longer to spread across the healthcare landscape.

---

[*]   Even more striking was a sharp drop in observed mortality from 30 percent to just under 20 percent in septic shock patients, which, for the most part, had about the same expected mortality.

[†]   The equipoise argument gets tricky when you think about *time* to antibiotics. Some might say early antibiotics are also self-evident, but the devil is in the details. If the antibiotics are poorly selected, it could be catastrophic.

[‡]   A waiver of consent is required for clinical trials examining the earliest stages of sepsis treatment. In such trials, patients are enrolled before formal consent is obtained. The rules and specifications around such a process are rigorous, and it is rare for institutional review boards (IRBs) to grant such waivers.

———

The Stauntons brought Rory to the emergency room at NYU Langone Pediatric on Thursday, March 29, at 7:14 p.m., where his initial vital signs included a pulse of 143, respirations of 20, temperature of 100°F (just shy of the fever cutoff), and normal blood pressure.[18]

Although the Stauntons didn't know it at the time, the nurses checked Rory for sepsis using a clinical screening tool that was part of the Greater New York Hospital Association's Stop Sepsis Collaborative, a multi-hospital quality improvement project aimed at improving sepsis recognition and care. But because Stop Sepsis required at least three out of eight abnormal clinical signs to trigger a positive screen, it didn't flag Rory as abnormal, as he had only two signs at the time.*[19] An hour later, his blood tests showed a white blood cell count of 14,700, which meant that he had now met *three* out of four abnormal SIRS criteria.[20] However, because he'd already been screened on arrival, he never tested positive for sepsis.†

Sepsis algorithms and alert systems are powerful tools, but without attention to detail and fine-tuning, they don't always work. They might even create a false sense of security. Perhaps the most agonizing part of this tragedy is that, like many Greater New York hospitals at the time, NYU Langone Pediatric *had* a sepsis screening process in place; it had simply failed.

Screening tests shouldn't replace clinical gumption but *supplement* it. High-quality sepsis care entails well-trained staff, a robust sepsis culture, and a practice environment that allows unimpeded clinical judgment. Yet bringing all these pieces together in every hospital can be challenging.

When the emergency medicine physician assessed Rory, she diagnosed him with viral gastroenteritis ("stomach flu"). There had been a report of a recent outbreak in the community, and Rory's pediatrician had made the same diagnosis. Orlaith now believes that the emergency medicine physician may

---

* Stop Sepsis criteria: suspected infection, temperature greater than 100.4°F, pulse greater than 90, respirations greater than 20, altered mental status, oxygen saturation less than 90 percent, systolic blood pressure less than 90, and suspected or known to be immunocompromised.

† Orlaith doesn't believe these laboratory results were seen by the emergency room treatment team, and they certainly were not communicated to her and Ciaran while Rory was being discharged. Furthermore, Orlaith reports that Rory's pediatrician indicated that she would call ahead to the emergency department to notify them about Rory's condition, but this never happened.

have committed a medical error known as *premature closure*, where a clinician draws a conclusion too early in a patient's workup, remaining closed-minded to other possibilities.*[21]

At 9:14 p.m., the emergency physician signed Rory's discharge order, writing, "Patient improved" in the chart. The records show that ten minutes later, he spiked another fever of 102°F while his heart and respiratory rates remained severely elevated. This meant that he was now firmly meeting the hospital's Stop Sepsis screening criteria as well as all four SIRS criteria. But by then, the physician had made her decision, and the discharge was already in process.[22] While viral gastroenteritis could have caused such abnormal vital signs, it's uncertain if sepsis was also considered a possibility at this point.

Based on reporting by *The New York Times* in 2012, the emergency room printed additional results from Rory's blood tests three hours later. These results showed that over half of his white blood cells were immature bands.[23] Recall from chapter eight that this can be a sign of a catastrophic bacterial infection. Unfortunately, Rory had already been discharged, and there was no effort to call the Stauntons back to the emergency room.[24] According to Jim Dwyer's *New York Times* article, NYU Langone wouldn't say if the doctors treating Rory at that time had seen the report.[25]

———

Back at Kaiser Permanente Northwest, I used to call the emergency room "ground zero." The ER was a crucial front line. Most of our sepsis patients came through its front doors, either as ambulance patients or walk-ins, making it imperative to understand the challenges of practicing medicine in that environment.

In the ER, sepsis lurks under the radar, not always presenting obvious signs of infection or shock. Complicating matters is that emergency rooms are often flooded with very sick *non*-septic patients, many displaying fevers, tachycardia, and high white blood cell counts. This is especially problematic during flu seasons or viral outbreaks, which bring droves of young, healthy patients with abnormal vital signs, creating an exceptionally distracting environment. Here, singling out a sepsis patient amid a flurry of viral illness

---

* If the ER physician had also been aware of Rory's pediatrician's assessment, it may have biased or anchored her to the initial diagnosis of gastroenteritis.

becomes a game of *Where's Waldo*—especially when it comes to children. Adding to the chaos is the cacophony of interruptions, alerts, and crises that typifies the daily ER experience.

By the late 2000s, hospitals like Kaiser Sunnyside Medical Center and NYU Langone began using screening tests to scan wards and emergency rooms for potential sepsis patients.[26] These are tests that aim to catch a disease or syndrome before it inflicts too much harm by testing those who haven't been diagnosed yet.

A good screening test should cast a wide enough net to avoid missing any potential cases while also detecting the condition early in its course. A classic example is a mammogram.

Such tests are a good idea—in principle. But they can be mired in problems, making it difficult to interpret their results. These tests are imperfect and can generate false positive or negative results, leading to unnecessary treatment or missed diagnoses. In addition, factors like the patients themselves, the setting where the test is conducted, and the baseline prevalence or "commonness" of a condition influence the accuracy of the results.

Altogether, these issues make sepsis screening an incredibly nuanced process that can easily go awry.

In 2008, during my residency at the University of New Mexico Hospital, we implemented a sweeping sepsis screening program. Nurses were instructed to screen all their patients regularly for SIRS. Minutes after the initiative went live, physicians were inundated with hundreds of notifications as numerous hospitalized patients tested positive for SIRS, regardless of their underlying conditions. Many didn't have infections. Their SIRS criteria resulted from serious non-sepsis conditions, making it difficult to identify which patients really needed attention. Unsurprisingly, the initiative collapsed within days.

Researchers use the terms "sensitivity" and "specificity" to describe medical tests. Sensitivity indicates the likelihood that a person with a condition will test positive. The higher the sensitivity, the more likely the test is to detect the condition, resulting in fewer false negatives. In contrast, specificity represents the likelihood that someone without the condition will test negative, with higher specificity leading to a lower chance of false positives. A highly sensitive test can catch most cases of a disease, but if its specificity is low, it may also generate false alarms by flagging healthy individuals.

In other words, if you cast a wide net, you're more likely to catch the fish you want, but you'll also haul in a lot of other things you don't want, which you'll then have to sift through. The University of New Mexico Hospital's SIRS screening process was behaving like a wide net—while it was catching a lot of sepsis patients, it was also generating too many false alarms and, in the process, creating a "Boy Who Cried Wolf" scenario. So, the physicians might have received ten false alarms for every true sepsis alert. Within just a few days, a "sepsis alert" was more likely to prompt an eye roll than a rapid response.

The issue of false alarms is not easy to solve. A specific syndrome's baseline prevalence greatly affects the chances of false positives when screening. A positive screen is more likely to be accurate if the syndrome is prevalent in a specific environment. However, if it's not that prevalent, a positive screen is more likely to be false. Put another way, it's easier to find a needle in a haystack if the haystack contains a hundred needles. As for the average prevalence of sepsis in a typical emergency room, it's only between 1 and 2 percent. *Why so low?* you may be wondering. The explanation is that while sepsis is indeed common, emergency rooms are filled with patients who have a wide range of other conditions, diluting the overall proportion of sepsis cases.

At Kaiser Permanente Northwest, we overcame these challenges by using a two-step screening process. We began with a *sensitive* test, SIRS, to identify as many potential sepsis patients as possible. However, we instructed nurses and doctors to apply the SIRS screening test only on patients who either *had* an infection or were *suspected* of having one. This helped us avoid drawing too many noninfected patients into the process.* Next, we had physicians follow up each positive SIRS test with a second, *risk-assessment* step, designed to identify patients with evidence of organ dysfunction—in other words, "sicker" patients, who were in greater need of urgent attention. As it turned out, one lab test fit the bill perfectly for this second step.

Between 2003 and 2004, Dr. Nathan Shapiro led a group at Beth Israel Deaconess Medical Center in Boston, Massachusetts, examining the relationship between blood lactate levels and sepsis mortality. It studied 1,278 patients diagnosed with infections in the emergency room over one year, measured their blood lactate levels, and followed them to see what happened. It revealed that as lactate levels increased, the risk of death also rose. His group used this data to stratify patients into low-, intermediate-, and high-risk groups based on lactate results. (See Figure 13.1.)[27] A few years later, another group from the

---

* We instructed providers to ask themselves two questions: Is your patient infected? If so, do they meet the SIRS criteria?

University of Pennsylvania found that the same association between lactate and death was independent of other factors, such as shock or other measures of organ dysfunction.[28]

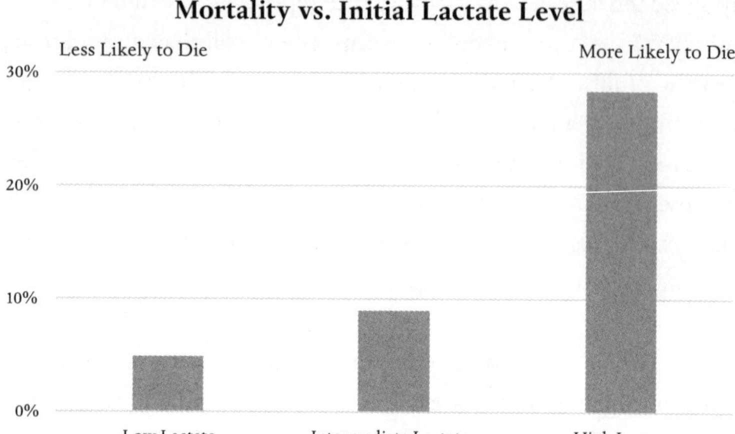

Figure 13.1: Initial lactate level in the emergency room and risk of death by day three in the hospital.[29]

You may recall from chapter eight that SIRS helped identify sepsis patients but failed to provide much information about *how sick* a particular patient was. However, applying a second step—the APACHE risk score—to the same group of SIRS-positive patients instantly reshuffled them across a spectrum of severity, from low to high risk. Similarly, adding a simple lactate test to our screening process dramatically improved our ability to spot sepsis patients.

This approach created a kind of sepsis *two-step*. For any patient with suspected or confirmed infection, we first applied the SIRS criteria, and if it was positive, we then checked their lactate level. An elevated lactate not only supported the diagnosis of sepsis but also signaled the need for immediate treatment. This second step improved the specificity of our screening process, helping us focus on patients with early signs of organ dysfunction—those who were sicker and more likely to benefit from urgent intervention.

By the 2010s, the blood lactate test had become one of the most essential innovations in sepsis recognition. When used correctly, it identified the earliest signs of sepsis-induced organ dysfunction, even in patients who didn't obviously "look septic." This improved our ability to recognize sepsis patients quickly and treat them rapidly, leading to better outcomes. In fact, a 2012 internal study at Kaiser Permanente Northern California showed that the simple act of checking lactate levels improved a patient's likelihood of survival by almost 4 percent, translating to one additional life saved for every twenty-five lactates tested.[30] This simple test was transforming our entire system when it came to sepsis survival.*

One of the great challenges with sepsis is that no single test or process can diagnose it. It's a heterogeneous syndrome caused by various infections, manifesting in numerous ways. Unless you specifically run tests to look for organ dysfunction, it's often difficult to know precisely when the body's immune response has switched from normal to abnormal. All this is to say that a relatively "normal" physiological reaction to infection, such as fever, can quickly and covertly escalate into an avalanche of immune dysregulation and organ dysfunction.[31] This can happen right under the noses of busy doctors and nurses, who are already engaged in caring for patients in the demanding and chaotic environment of emergency rooms and hospital wards.

As the former chief of emergency medicine at Kaiser Permanente Northwest, Dr. Eric Roth, used to say, "Sepsis is sneaky."[32]

———

After returning from the emergency room, the Stauntons had a false sense of security. No one had mentioned sepsis at any point before Rory's discharge. As he lay in a deep sleep, they took comfort in his rest, unaware that his life was slipping away with each passing hour.

By Friday morning, Rory was clearly deteriorating. He had lost his appetite, was extremely lethargic, and was experiencing severe weakness. Having held out for just over a day, it seemed now that his body was finally shutting down. After a tense exchange with his pediatrician, the Stauntons decided to return to the emergency room.

---

* We provided electronic decision support to help clinicians remember to order the test. We programmed our electronic health system to produce a pop-up alert reminding the provider to order the lactate whenever they were ordering blood cultures. Within two years, we saw the percentage of lactates ordered on suspected sepsis patients increase from 25 to 99 percent, and our ability to detect sepsis improved by a factor of three.

Pediatric sepsis is a challenging problem. Affecting around twenty-five million children and resulting in three million deaths each year worldwide, sepsis wages its harshest war on the youngest and most vulnerable members of our population.[33] Some of this relates to host factors. With underdeveloped immune systems, infants and young children are at high risk for developing sepsis. In other cases, it stems from a lack of access to clean water, vaccines, and healthcare in low- and middle-income countries, with diarrheal diseases leading in terms of sepsis-related childhood mortality.[34]

Detecting sepsis in children is especially difficult. According to pediatric sepsis expert Scott Weiss from Nemours Children's Hospital in Delaware, "Children, and particularly young children, often have a harder time relaying their symptoms, so it can be challenging to understand exactly what a child is experiencing early on in the course of illness." What may seem relatively nonspecific, such as fever, abdominal pain, or irritability, could represent "red flags that someone is on the path of developing sepsis."[35] In Rory's case, stomach symptoms and leg pain appeared nonspecific, yet they indicated a severe infection. Parents and healthcare workers should remain vigilant when caring for a sick child and always consider sepsis as a possibility.

Making matters worse, the signs of sepsis manifest differently depending on the child, making it especially perilous for frontline doctors. Based on age alone, children can vary considerably in terms of the normal ranges for vital signs. Moreover, it's not uncommon for healthy kids without sepsis to display abnormal vital signs, such as fever and tachycardia.* This makes standard sepsis screening tests less effective at differentiating an actual sepsis patient from a relatively healthy child with a few abnormal vital signs. In fact, this led the first expert panel on pediatric sepsis, the International Pediatric Sepsis Consensus Conference (IPSCC), which convened in 2005, to develop modified SIRS criteria for diagnosing sepsis in children.†[36]

Children with sepsis can also maintain normal blood pressure until very late in their course, leading to an illusion of stability. By the time a child develops

---

* Compounding matters, most infected children never develop sepsis, which makes for an even larger haystack to sift through while you're looking for that one child who has it.

† The 2005 IPSCC pediatric sepsis definition requires at least one SIRS criterion to be an abnormal temperature or white blood cell count while also using age-specific SIRS criteria.

septic shock, they're often much sicker than an adult would be at the same point in their illness, making for an especially dire situation.

All this is to say that designing an appropriate screening test for pediatric patients is no easy task. Sepsis develops on a continuum, starting with an uncomplicated infection. Doctors need a method to quickly determine whether a child has sepsis, but the difficulty lies in establishing the appropriate cutoff point for the test. As Weiss explains, "The challenge is trying to dichotomize something that's otherwise a continuous spectrum."[37] For instance, what happens to a patient like Rory, who missed the cutoff by one vital sign?

Much of it comes down to the specific screening process and the general culture built around it. Weiss describes the system he used while working at the Children's Hospital of Philadelphia (CHOP). His team began by examining baseline data for their emergency room, which showed that physician clinical judgment alone had poor sensitivity for detecting sepsis in children. As a result, doctors were missing about 17 percent of pediatric sepsis diagnoses in the emergency room.[38] They needed a process that could catch most children with sepsis without overwhelming the system with false positive alerts.

Weiss and his team developed a two-step computerized electronic sepsis screening process using criteria established by the American Academy of Pediatrics. The first step involved generating an automated alert for nurses based on sensitive criteria, such as a simple elevation in a child's age-adjusted heart rate. This alert would prompt the nurse to input additional information: whether they were concerned about infection and other specific indicators of organ dysfunction and reduced perfusion. The computer then conducted a second screening test. If this new information triggered a positive screen, it would launch a system-wide electronic sepsis alert (ESA). That would prompt the care team to conduct a sepsis huddle: a focused meeting to discuss the patient in question. Following the huddle, the team would classify patients into green, yellow, and red risk zones based on their likelihood of sepsis and estimated risk of death.[39]

They also implemented another interesting strategy: instructing clinicians to activate a sepsis huddle whenever they had concerns that a child might have sepsis, even in cases where the sepsis screening alert *didn't* trigger. They referred to these instances as "clinician-identified" sepsis. This approach encouraged doctors and nurses to think critically and rely on their clinical judgment when the computer system fell short. It was a crucial step, as the ESA couldn't catch every case on its own. In fact, of the 326 children ultimately diagnosed with sepsis, the ESA missed 45 of them. However, emergency room clinicians were able to identify and catch 43 of those missed cases.[40]

When he and his team studied the total effect of the ESA between June 2013 and May 2015, they found that the overall percentage of missed sepsis cases had dropped sharply from 17 to 4 percent. This meant that, over an average year, twenty-five *additional* children with sepsis were identified in the emergency room. More importantly, when they combined the effect of the ESA *and* clinician-identified sepsis cases, they improved the overall sensitivity of their emergency room's sepsis detection to 99 percent.[41]

As for the issue of false positives, by tuning the process this way, the positive predictive value, or hit rate for the system, was about 25 percent, meaning that one out of every four alerts was real.[42] That may not seem very effective, but when you're looking for a needle in a haystack, it's pretty good if it only takes four attempts to find the needle.

———

On arrival back at the emergency room Friday evening, Rory was clearly in septic shock, obviously recognizable by the staff, who responded swiftly. But by then, as had been the case with so many other sepsis victims before him, it was too late. We had already passed the point where we could have changed his outcome. Despite all their advanced technology and training, the staff at NYU Langone could not overcome the firestorm of immune dysregulation that was now raining upon Rory's entire system. In just a few hours, he needed to be put on life support, and at that point, his chance of survival sat on a razor's edge. One can only wonder how greater sepsis awareness might have placed Rory on someone's radar early enough to have steered him away from disaster.

———

The early 2010s saw increased awareness of sepsis and expanding global quality improvement programs. The syndrome was finally on the radar of many clinicians in hospitals and emergency rooms. However, sepsis leaders continued to face a general lack of urgency and difficulty in balancing over- and under-diagnosing cases. With more data accumulating each year, our understanding evolved quickly and sometimes dramatically. This was a positive development, allowing us to gain real-time knowledge. However, it also unintentionally undermined confidence in the core guidelines while empowering skeptics of the SSC and fostering a pervasive nihilism toward sepsis bundles.

In the fall of 2011, Eli Lilly shocked the medical world once again when it withdrew Xigris from the market. As promised, the pharmaceutical company had been conducting a long-awaited post-marketing follow-up study of its flagship drug, known as PROWESS-SHOCK. This time, Xigris failed to demonstrate any survival benefit in septic shock patients, leading Lilly to abandon the drug.[43] It also left many wondering how Xigris had gone from miracle drug to complete dud in only ten years.

There's certainly reason to suspect methodological flaws in the earlier studies. The irregularities that arose during the FDA's review suggest as much. Lilly's aggressive marketing tactics didn't help either, overpromising the drug's benefits and damaging the company's credibility.[44]

However, closer examination also reveals something more fundamental, which ties Xigris back to chapter seven's clinical trials conundrum and the issue of heterogeneity.

"Part of the problem was that a lot of the pharma companies would develop a molecule and then test it on all sepsis patients," explains Dr. Mitchell Levy. "There's enormous heterogeneity in the septic population. You could have a twenty-year-old post motor vehicle accident who develops infection and sepsis and an eighty-five-year-old with chronic lung disease and diabetes. Those are just different populations . . . the idea that we could find a single therapeutic agent that could allow us to treat all septic patients was the downfall of a lot of these trials."[45]

We now understand that Xigris's mechanism of action—targeting abnormal coagulation through activated protein C—may have been too narrowly focused for the diverse population of patients with septic shock. In retrospect, only about 40 percent of patients enrolled in PROWESS SHOCK had significantly reduced protein C activity, the very abnormality the drug was designed to treat.[46]

Much to the understandable frustration of pharmaceutical executives evaluating the profitability of drug development, the future of advanced sepsis therapeutics seemed to lie increasingly within the evolving field of precision medicine.[47]

Unfortunately, this shift has had the unintended consequence of discouraging further investment in sepsis drug development. Precision therapies are generally less lucrative as they target a smaller patient population, limiting overall market potential compared to widely prescribed blockbuster drugs. This is not to mention that, after incurring billions of dollars in losses, many pharmaceutical companies had grown wary of investing in advanced sepsis therapeutics.[48]

Experts like Levy have since learned from these lessons and are now beginning to redesign clinical trials to account for all the different sepsis fingerprints. Finding better ways to identify patients likely to respond to special therapies like Xigris may ultimately solve the sepsis clinical trials conundrum.

Something else might have been at play to explain the disparate trial results: Medicine is a story of gradual progress. The rise of the SSC and other quality improvement initiatives in the early twenty-first century led to substantial improvements in sepsis care across hospitals worldwide. In other words, the *baseline* had changed. Over the course of just a decade, "usual care" improved so significantly that it may have stolen Xigris's thunder.[49] By the time PROWESS-SHOCK was conducted, patients enrolled in the study just weren't as sick as those in the original PROWESS trial. Comparing the baseline mortality of the control groups reveals the stark difference: 31 percent in 2001 compared to 24 percent ten years later.*[50]

PROWESS-SHOCK's rigorous methodology also made patient recruitment a slow and challenging process. Because enrollment required patients to remain in septic shock despite initial fluid resuscitation and vasopressor support, many had already received essential elements of early sepsis care, such as antibiotics and fluid resuscitation, before randomization.[51]

As physician-author Judy Stone explains, "Advances in supportive care during the enrollment period resulted in enough improvement in the patients' conditions to wipe out any evident difference between the active study drug and placebo groups."†[52]

Ultimately, the Xigris saga serves as a cautionary tale about the complexities of medical research—how the urgent desire to save lives, combined with flawed methodologies, can sometimes lead well-intentioned researchers to draw incorrect conclusions about a drug's effectiveness.[53] It also underscores

---

* Another observational trial published in 2012 showed that any benefit of Xigris was only seen in subgroups of patients where there had been significant delays in antibiotic treatment.

† All PROWESS-SHOCK participants received the recommended intravenous fluid bolus, and 84 percent received appropriate antibiotics within three hours.

the limitations of viewing sepsis as a single disease with a one-size-fits-all treatment. Finally, it reminds us of the relentless march of time and the power of medical progress—how, in just a decade, a once-promising therapy can be diminished, outpaced, or even rendered obsolete.

————

By 2012, the SSC had issued a third edition of its sepsis guidelines, including a revision of the previous six- and twenty-four-hour bundles to a new three- and six-hour *resuscitation*-focused bundle, incorporating the latest developments in the changing landscape of evidence-based sepsis practice. As expected, Xigris was no longer a bundle element. Meanwhile, a repeat lactate measurement was now included in the initial six-hour bundle. (See Table 13.1.) Most importantly, the bundles were now entirely focused on early recognition and rapid treatment, firmly emphasized as the foundation of sepsis care.

3-Hour Bundle	6-Hour Bundle
Measure lactate level	Start vasopressor (for septic shock)
Obtain blood cultures	Start EGDT (for septic shock or lactate ≥ 4 mmol/L *aka* cryptic shock)
Administer broad-spectrum antibiotics	Remeasure lactate level
Administer 30 mL/kg fluid bolus for hypotension or lactate ≥ 4 mmol/L	

Table 13.1: 2012 Surviving Sepsis Campaign Bundles.[54]

By then, more doctors and nurses were thinking about sepsis, but we still lacked the critical mass necessary for a sea change. Most healthcare professionals still didn't take the syndrome as seriously as other emergencies, like heart attacks and strokes.

Meanwhile, resistance was growing in the academic community against the SSC guidelines and bundles. Many doctors were concerned that the sepsis threat was exaggerated. The idea that SIRS was an early stage of sepsis didn't resonate well with the medical community. Many believed SIRS was leading to overdiagnosis and often resulted in the overtreatment of patients with fluids and antibiotics.

All of this contributed to persistent and worrisome inertia.

———

As was often the case with sepsis diagnosis around the turn of the twenty-first century, all the pieces of the puzzle finally came together days into Rory's hospitalization—when his blood cultures returned positive for *Streptococcus pyogenes*, and he was in fulminant shock. But by then, the sepsis response had amplified out of control and was no longer within anyone's ability to stop it. It quickly dismantled his organ systems, leaving him trapped in a death spiral, ultimately leading to a series of cardiac arrests as his heart finally gave out.

I first encountered Rory's tragic story in the summer of 2012. In retrospect, it's clear that all the information about a dangerous bacterial infection was there early in his illness. But his doctors and nurses didn't recognize it in time. It vexes the mind to imagine all the moments when Rory's course could have shifted toward a different outcome.

What made it all the more demoralizing was the syndrome's ability to remain obscure—even within a system designed to catch it. Combined with the rising complexity of modern healthcare, it created the perfect storm. Rory languished, unseen, right under the noses of his healthcare providers.

Beyond that were deeper failures: communication, partnership, responsibility. Rory was a five-alarm fire that no one seemed to notice until it was too late. In a case like this, who was responsible for warning the Staunton family of the danger? How were we supposed to monitor him once he'd left the hospital? Who was ultimately accountable for sounding the alarm?

Rory's death was a sentinel event not only for NYU Langone or even New York State's broader medical community, but for the entire sepsis movement. Although the groundbreaking work of the SSC and many others had catalyzed a revolution in sepsis awareness, Rory Staunton's story was a critical inflection point. The growing pressure from an unacceptable status quo had finally hit a tipping point, and it was about to pave the way for a series of decisive public and governmental actions that would reshape the sepsis landscape forever.

CHAPTER FOURTEEN

Regulations and Regression

*Hundreds of thousands of Americans contract sepsis infections each year—
so we must take bold steps to prevent these needless illnesses and deaths.*

—US SENATOR TOM HARKIN, September 13, 2013[1]

AFTER RORY'S DEATH, AN UNSPEAKABLE grief fell upon the Stauntons.
For Orlaith, it was as if a voice in her life had gone silent. His empty bed and
his vacant chair at the table were haunting reminders of a life stolen. No one
could fathom how an infection had taken Rory so suddenly and cruelly.

Word of his tragedy quickly spread, sending shockwaves throughout Sunnyside Gardens and Greater New York. Friends, neighbors, and even strangers
reached out in sorrow and support. It seemed as though everyone had heard
about it.

News reached New York Senator Charles Schumer, who had met Rory
several times, once at an Irish–American immigration meeting in Queens and
another time at a St. Patrick's Day parade in Brooklyn. Schumer immediately
called Ciaran to express his deep condolences and offer his support.

"This is my cell number. Whatever you need going forward, please call me."[2]

When the Stauntons turned to the hospital for answers, they were told that
Rory had died from sepsis. It was an unnerving clue in an otherwise tragic
mystery—the first time they had ever heard the term. No one had mentioned
sepsis while Rory was hospitalized.[3]

Orlaith and Ciaran pored over the medical literature, consuming every word with an insatiable thirst for understanding. But with knowledge came dismay. Like Carl Flatley a decade before them, they uncovered a devastating truth: Sepsis wasn't rare. It wasn't some medical anomaly. It was none of those things. It was a leading cause of death in children worldwide. Worse still, Rory had shown the telltale signs of sepsis early on—clear, undeniable warnings. Yet the people entrusted with his care had failed to recognize them until it was too late.[4]

They visited the US CDC website and found no information about sepsis. Nothing. It wasn't even listed under the CDC's "Health Topics A-Z" index. Orlaith was furious—at the world, at the doctors, and at the medical institutions. How could something so common and deadly receive so little attention from the CDC? It seemed that neither the medical profession nor public health agencies were paying enough attention to this common and deadly syndrome.[5]

It was time to take matters into their own hands. The Stauntons contacted Jim Dwyer of *The New York Times*, which published Rory's harrowing account, "An Infection, Unnoticed, Turns Unstoppable," on July 11, 2012. It quickly went viral, becoming one of the most shared stories in the newspaper's history.[6]

Shortly afterward, a glimmer of hope. The Stauntons received a letter from a woman in Florida named Cara Byington, whose son Nate had recently been diagnosed with sepsis. Nate had been complaining of ear pain. Byington took him to see his pediatrician, who diagnosed him with a minor ear infection and prescribed topical antibiotics. After Nate's condition worsened at home, Byington's sister, who had read about Rory's tragedy two days earlier, asked if it could be sepsis. Byington rushed her son back to the emergency room, where he was diagnosed with early sepsis from a severe bacterial infection of the mastoid sinus—mastoiditis. Byington later remarked, "The ER doctor told me that we were probably down to hours before he was in serious trouble."[7] There was no doubt in her mind: Nate would have died if not for the Stauntons' advocacy. After overhearing the news, Rory's sister Kathleen said, "Isn't it a pity that nobody did that for Rory?"[8]

Driven by a blend of anger and altruism, the Stauntons turned their focus to the government. They became relentless advocates for sepsis awareness, pushing for action at both the state and local levels, engaging with leaders like Congressman Joe Crowley of Queens and State Assembly members. They leveraged virtually every opportunity to push sepsis onto Governor Andrew Cuomo's agenda.

But nothing came easy—it required unbelievable persistence, working around the clock, fighting for each meeting with the governor's top advisors.[9]

Ultimately, it paid off. Their efforts led to a series of conversations at the highest levels of state government, eventually bringing sepsis to the attention of State Health Commissioner Nirav Shah.

Shah was struck by the tragic loss of a child in a New York hospital—an outcome that felt both shocking and personal. As a practicing physician at Bellevue Hospital, affiliated with NYU Langone, he had worked alongside highly trained, conscientious providers in one of the country's premier medical centers. Yet, in Rory's case, they had completely missed the mark. It was hard to believe.[10]

He dug deeper and uncovered an unsettling reality: Sepsis was claiming an alarming number of lives in New York each year, yet it had received little attention from the state's health department. And while the Surviving Sepsis Campaign (SSC) had been active for over a decade, there was still considerable variation in sepsis care across the state's hospitals. Sepsis mortality ranged from 15 to 36 percent—a huge disparity—depending largely on where patients received care and, more importantly, whether those hospitals had robust sepsis programs.[11] It also incurred billions in hospital costs annually in New York alone. What's more, the data were inconsistent, not always aligning with a particular hospital's overall quality of care or reputation. So, on top of everything, there were issues with the reliability of the data too. Health officials were essentially flying blind when it came to tracking the syndrome.[12]

Shah needed a large-scale quality improvement initiative, and he had just the person in mind to lead it: his chief medical officer, a charismatic and thoughtful physician named Foster Gesten. Gesten had spent years conducting public health and quality improvement initiatives throughout the state. During that time, he had forged strong relationships with stakeholders from powerful trade groups, such as the Greater New York Hospital Association, while establishing the infrastructure for large-scale health initiatives. Shah saw him as the kind of leader who brought people to the table and convinced them to do the right thing.[13]

Gesten was in. The two proceeded to tap their professional contacts, including members of the academic sepsis community and local and national healthcare leaders. Shah had heard of Kaiser Permanente's success in reducing sepsis mortality by 60 percent in its hospitals. He reached out to its CEO, George Halvorson, who explained the essentials of good sepsis care: "It's not rocket science. It's about systems thinking, team-based care, checklists, paying attention to the problem, and measuring what matters."[14] Meanwhile, Gesten approached New York's largest healthcare provider, Northwell Health, a trailblazer for sepsis care under the leadership of its CEO, Michael Dowling, and researcher Kevin Tracey, director of Northwell's Feinstein Institute for Medical Research.[15]

Sepsis was Tracey's life mission—and it was deeply personal, sparked by the devastating loss of an eleven-month-old patient named Janice decades earlier. Janice had succumbed to complications related to septic shock following a severe burn injury. In 2005, Tracey helped make sepsis a top priority across Northwell's hospitals, aligning its research and clinical teams around the common goal of improving patient outcomes. Four years later, the organization formed a task force dedicated to increasing sepsis awareness among healthcare providers and the public while enhancing its systems for rapidly recognizing and treating it.[16]

In 2010, Northwell hosted a historic international symposium, drawing top scientists, experts, advocates, and policymakers from countries worldwide, including those from the International Sepsis Forum, Sepsis Alliance, and the World Federation of Societies of Intensive and Critical Care Medicine. This collaboration ultimately formed a large international sepsis advocacy group: the Global Sepsis Alliance. A year later, Northwell developed a strategic partnership with the Institute for Healthcare Improvement and became a statewide leader in sepsis bundle performance and outcomes.[17]

Next, Shah asked Orlaith and Ciaran to share their story.

Nobody should lose sight of why this work has to be done, he thought.[18]

The Stauntons had already teamed up with two of Northwell's top sepsis leaders, Drs. Martin Doerfler and John D'Angelo, to raise public awareness of the syndrome. By the fall of 2012, the group had formed the Rory Staunton Foundation, later becoming End Sepsis.[19]

On October 26, 2012, the state's most influential hospital leaders gathered at the New York Academy of Medicine for the Invitational Sepsis Symposium, marking the launch of the New York State Sepsis Initiative. The meeting took place in the Academy Library, a space reminiscent of Hogwarts, with lofty mahogany bookshelves and creaking wood floors, making it the perfect backdrop for such a historic endeavor.[20] Among the invited speakers were leading sepsis researchers, Northwell Health and Kaiser Permanente representatives, members of the two major New York hospital trade associations, the Greater New York Hospital Association and the Healthcare Association of New York State, and the Staunton family.[21]

In his closing remarks, Shah emphasized the devastating toll that sepsis had taken on the Stauntons: 25 percent of their family lost in a matter of days.[22] A preventable tragedy.*[23] What's more, it wasn't an isolated incident—it was happening every day in hospitals around the state.

At first, many hospitals resisted. They said there were too many discrepancies in the data and too much disagreement on which patients to include in the analysis. It was 2013—a full decade after the SSC's inception—yet the medical community was still deeply divided over how to define sepsis. Additional factors, such as patients' baseline comorbidities and hospital acuity levels, complicated the mortality statistics.† People disagreed over the extent of the problem; some were reluctant to accept there *was* a problem. Moreover, there was limited bandwidth for another unfunded initiative.

"These were good people trying to do the right thing, but many of them had a lot to juggle at once," Shah recounts. "While the Stauntons' tragedy was compelling, adding sepsis to their plates was a difficult ask."

Some of them said plainly, "We just can't do it."[24]

Medicine is rooted in morality and science, yet its daily operations are dictated by economics. At the end of the day, Shah and Gesten needed a strong business case. Fortunately, this wouldn't be difficult; by then, sepsis had become the most expensive hospital condition in the United States. To persuade hospital administrators to allocate the necessary resources and to strengthen sepsis programs, they reframed the issue:

Sepsis is not only a leading cause of death but also a major driver of hospital costs and utilization.[25]

---

*   The Stauntons ultimately sued NYU Langone, and while the details of the lawsuit remain confidential, afterward the large health system updated its procedures to include new checklists, better tuning of its sepsis screening tests, and a mandatory process for signing off on test results and vital signs, while also briefing parents on important lab tests before discharge. That same year, Ciaran also teamed up with a leading patient safety researcher from Brigham and Women's Hospital, Dr. Gordon Schiff, to lead a discussion on Rory's case at the Fifth International Conference on Diagnostic Error in Medicine, hosted by Johns Hopkins School of Medicine.

†   The acuity of a hospital refers to how sick the patients are. Some centers, particularly academic hospitals and referral centers, may see higher-complexity patients, which may skew their mortality data.

The next step was securing buy-in. Early in the initiative, Gesten leveraged existing relationships with stakeholders across the state to create a collaborative advisory group, providing hospital leaders with a private forum for candid discussions. He embraced a "big tent" approach, bringing in a diverse mix of quality directors, clinicians, epidemiologists, data experts, and hospital executives.[26] As Shah put it, "There was no such thing as too many stakeholders."[27] This helped shape a "bedside to policy" approach, ensuring that regulations were grounded in the realities of frontline medical care. Together, they addressed critical questions like, "What are the data? What do they show? And what do we need to do about it?"[28]

On January 29, 2013, New York became the first state to pass a sepsis mandate known as Rory's Regulations. It required every hospital in the state to adopt evidence-based protocols for rapidly identifying and treating sepsis.[29] The core framework was based on the SSC bundles and mandated hospitals to adhere to three- and six-hour treatment bundles. However, hospitals were granted significant latitude in their screening processes and methods for identifying sepsis cases.[30] The mandate also called for a separate pediatric sepsis bundle requiring antibiotics, intravenous fluids, and blood cultures within one hour of identification.[*][31]

Orlaith remembers a bittersweet realization: they couldn't save Rory's life, but there were still others they could save.[32]

———

Meanwhile, in the battle for public recognition, sepsis had fallen far short of virtually every other deadly medical condition. By the early 2010s, nearly two-thirds of Americans had never heard of sepsis.[33] This meant it had a major public relations problem and was missing the same brand recognition of other deadly conditions like cancer and heart disease.

This bias also lurked within the medical profession, which housed deeply ingrained misperceptions about sepsis and the need for early detection. As in the early 2000s, many doctors still took a passive stance when diagnosing the syndrome, likely contributing to delays in recognition and treatment on the front line.[34]

---

[*] The data were kept private for the first few years to avoid negative public attention while fostering better partnerships among health systems.

Additionally, public health agencies, like the US CDC, were reluctant to adopt the SSC's definition of sepsis. The health agency, heavily comprised of infectious disease specialists and epidemiologists, resisted the broader sepsis framework. It categorized infectious diseases as distinct syndromes, like pneumonia or meningitis, though sepsis often accompanied them and, in many cases, was the ultimate cause of death.

Orlaith and Ciaran aimed to persuade the CDC to change its approach to sepsis and take on a greater role in education and prevention. After months of lobbying and pressure from Senator Schumer's office, Congressman Crowley, and others, the Stauntons secured a meeting with the CDC's director, Tom Frieden, at the agency's headquarters in Atlanta, Georgia, in January 2014.

At first, the CDC headquarters felt cold and unwelcoming. While sitting in the lobby, Frieden's staff handed the Stauntons a packet of health information—materials on heart disease, dietary fat, and salt intake. It contained no mention of sepsis.

"Not one page. Not one piece of paper in this office or in this massive secure building about sepsis," Ciaran grumbled.

Throughout the meeting with Frieden, Orlaith couldn't shake the dismissiveness in their tone. *How dare you come in here?* she imagined them thinking.[35]

At that moment, they both realized how steep the climb would be. Even after convincing Frieden to acknowledge sepsis on the CDC website, it took six months to make it happen. Even then, the agency classified sepsis as a hospital-acquired condition—only correcting it after intense pressure from the Stauntons.[36]

———

Months before Rory's Regulations were released, a national sepsis mandate was also taking shape at the National Quality Forum (NQF) in Washington, DC. During the summer of 2012, Drs. Rivers and Townsend resubmitted a proposal for measure #0500—the three- and six-hour bundle for adult sepsis patients originally developed by Rivers in 2007.

Measure #0500 was aligned with the SSC guidelines, and its core component for septic shock management, early goal-directed therapy (EGDT), promised to cut mortality rates by a third, saving one additional life for every six treated. However, in its first go-round at the NQF, EGDT was removed from the measure for a lack of supporting evidence.

To be established—along with EGDT—as a national standard for sepsis care, the measure needed a strong endorsement from the NQF, the primary source of quality measures for the Centers for Medicare and Medicaid Services (CMS) at the time.

Thanks to Townsend and the SSC, the proposal was now packed with extensive data supporting the protocol.*[37]

According to CMS, national quality measures should address crucial public health issues and be feasible, scientifically acceptable, and easy to use. A CMS-endorsed measure must be backed by strong and credible evidence, be tested for reliability and validity, and foster meaningful improvements in healthcare delivery. Its benefits must also outweigh any potential burdens of measuring and reporting it.[38]

The NQF needed to rigorously evaluate #0500 using its Consensus Development Process, a six-step method for assessing and endorsing quality measures. The process involved assembling a steering committee, conducting both private and public meetings to review the data, and allowing open periods for public commentary.[39] As a public–private partnership, the NQF represented a diverse array of stakeholders: health insurers, patient advocacy groups, medical societies, drug and device manufacturers, hospital trade associations, and public health agencies.[40]

But beneath the NQF's carefully structured process was a storm of heated debate, politics, disagreements, and compromise. Measure #0500 was unlike any other national quality measure—it sought to define and standardize one of the most elusive syndromes in medical history.

Experts remained divided on the definition of sepsis and the objective markers that signaled its onset. There was conflict over its most basic assumptions—which patients to count in the denominator, and when exactly the sepsis clock should begin (time zero).

Like the SSC bundles, #0500's time-sensitive nature could place significant pressure on doctors—especially those in the emergency room—to quickly administer antibiotics, fluids, and other potentially lifesaving therapies to patients, often with limited information about the diagnoses.

---

*   To focus the attention of providers on the *sickest* sepsis patients, Rivers and Townsend added an additional qualifier: patients had to either have *severe* sepsis or septic shock to qualify for the treatment bundles.

Furthermore, while EGDT appeared to be highly effective, experts disagreed about the quality of the data supporting it. This is not to mention that it was an intricate procedure, requiring an invasive central venous catheter and a coordinated team of doctors and nurses to carry it out. Beyond that, the necessary equipment was expensive and difficult to store and maintain, posing a significant hurdle for hospitals with limited resources.[41]

One of the most contentious debates surrounding the measure revolved around when to establish time zero. Rivers and Townsend wanted to start the sepsis clock when a patient arrived at the emergency room, or "triage time," as it represented a clear reference point that everyone could agree on.[42] This approach would also encourage hospitals to enhance their initial screening processes to identify sepsis patients as quickly as possible.

However, multiple medical societies pushed back, arguing that, unlike other emergency conditions such as heart attacks and strokes, pinpointing the exact moment a patient developed sepsis was far more complex. No single symptom, sign, or test could definitively diagnose it.[43]

Mitchell Levy elaborates on this: "I think one of the biggest challenges with sepsis is that it's a syndrome, unlike heart disease. For example, if somebody comes in and they're grabbing their chest and they say they're having chest pain, there are a number of very objective markers that will enable you to say, 'Oh, this person is having a heart attack.' [This is] not true for sepsis. And so, unfortunately, what we're left with is the suspicion of sepsis."[44]

Identifying sepsis required more detective work than other conditions, making triage an imperfect starting point for time zero. This would result in a measure that was challenging and at times impossible to meet. It also risked pressuring providers to hastily administer treatments, such as fluids and antibiotics, driven more by compliance than clinical judgment.

In the end, Rivers and Townsend compromised, crafting a set of coded specifications to identify the earliest moment a frontline provider could reasonably diagnose sepsis. The result was a system within a system, one that required the convergence of three critical events: (1) documented evidence or suspicion of infection, (2) at least two out of four SIRS criteria, and (3) the presence of organ dysfunction and/or shock. When all three elements aligned, this moment was designated as the "severe sepsis presentation time," or time zero.

Reflecting on the decision, Townsend later commented, "What we ended up with was a very complex way of doing it. I'm not in love with it. But I've never been able to find a really solid substitute for this. You have to start measuring your efforts at some point."[45]

Another area of sharp dispute centered on intravenous fluids. By 2012, the SSC had shifted its recommendation to a standardized, weight-based intravenous fluid bolus of 30 milliliters per kilogram for patients with hypotension or septic shock. This replaced the more cautious, incremental fluid resuscitation strategy from previous guideline editions and was now embedded as a mandatory therapy in Measure #0500.

While the use of fluid therapy to raise blood pressure in sepsis had been recognized as early as the nineteenth century, doctors soon discovered its limitations. In patients with compromised cardiac function, fluid therapy often failed to raise their blood pressure and could even worsen heart failure. In others, the effects were short-lived, as injured blood vessels allowed fluid to leak into surrounding tissues, diminishing their intended impact.[46]

Larger volumes could also bring harmful effects, such as the extravasation (leakage) of fluid through permeable blood capillaries into organs—most damagingly in the lungs, where it could fill the alveolar air sacs with fluid (aka "fluid overload"), resulting in respiratory compromise.[47]

Decades earlier, these inherent challenges had prompted Edward Frank to champion a practice of "moderation" when it came to administering intravenous fluids during shock. This evolved into the modern practice of judiciously titrating fluids—a "half-liter bolus" here or a "liter bolus" there, looking for a response, and then reassessing. Using this Goldilocks approach, physicians could incrementally arrive at just the right amount of fluid.[48]

In 1991, Joseph Carcillo, a pediatric intensivist at the University of Pittsburgh Medical Center, published a study in the *Journal of the American Medical Association* challenging the prevailing approach of incremental fluid resuscitation. His research demonstrated that pediatric sepsis patients who received larger fluid boluses—above 40 milliliters per kilogram of body weight—within the first hour had significantly lower mortality rates than those resuscitated incrementally.* Interestingly, despite the initial difference in bolus size, the *total* volume of fluids administered by the six-hour mark was nearly identical in both groups. This suggested that the key factor in improving survival was not the amount of fluid given but rather the speed of delivery. Further analysis revealed that

---

*   In pediatrics, weight-based fluid dosing is common practice to account for dramatic differences in age and body size.

patients in the incremental group had lower blood pressures at the six-hour mark, linking their lower survival rates to prolonged hypotension—another example of the golden hour concept.[*][49]

Carcillo championed this approach at medical society meetings, sparking widespread discussion and eventually influencing the treatment of adult sepsis patients as well.[50] Over time, with further refinement, the practice of rapidly administering larger boluses—30 milliliters per kilogram of body weight (roughly two to three liters for an average adult)—was formally incorporated into the SSC's bundles.[51]

At the same time, other studies revealed that, in as many as half of sepsis patients, intravenous fluid boluses failed to raise blood pressure; such patients became known as fluid non-responders.[52] In everyday practice, it was tough for doctors to accurately assess how full a sepsis patient's tank was or whether they had a failing heart pump. This meant that while a large fluid bolus could work for one sepsis patient, it might be problematic for another.[†][53] Context mattered. But despite these nuances, Measure #0500 called for the same fluid treatment strategy for every patient, regardless of their baseline physiology. This made many medical professionals uneasy while leaving some apoplectic.[‡][54]

The most controversial issue with #0500 was its EGDT requirement. A debate simmered in academic circles regarding the quality of the data supporting the protocol. The 2012 SSC guidelines panel had determined that the evidence for EGDT was of low quality, yet it still gave it a strong recommendation.[§][55] This flummoxed many experts, who argued that only therapies backed by high-quality evidence should receive such endorsements.[56] Further complicating matters, emerging studies suggested that less-invasive approaches, such as

---

[*] In the late 1980s and early 1990s, the American Heart Association recommended increments of 20 milliliters of intravenous fluid per kilogram of body weight until the normalization of blood pressure for pediatric shock.

[†] By the early 2010s, small clinical trials conducted in Africa showed that, in certain contexts, prescribed or protocolized fluid boluses in the emergency room could even *increase* the risk of death due to dangerous extravasation of fluid into the lungs.

[‡] For example, a 70-kilogram woman with a healthy heart might easily handle a two-liter weight-based fluid bolus, while a 120-kilogram man with congestive heart failure may struggle to tolerate *his* weight-based fluid bolus of 3.6 liters.

[§] This recommendation stemmed from the significant treatment effect observed in Rivers's original 2001 trial and findings from a recent Chinese follow-up RCT published in 2010, indicating a "number needed to treat" of six. Furthermore, large observational studies revealed similar benefits without showing any evidence of harm to patients.

targeting treatment to improve blood lactate levels, were just as effective as EGDT.[57] Meanwhile, several large confirmatory EGDT trials were still ongoing, leaving many wondering whether it had been premature to embed the protocol into a national quality measure.*

EGDT also presented the challenge of central venous catheter placement. At the time, up to 15 percent of patients who received central lines suffered from complications, including blood clots, bloodstream infections, and even collapsed lungs from misplaced needles.†[58] The procedure posed a considerable burden on emergency doctors, particularly in busy urban hospitals, while many smaller hospitals didn't have the resources to perform it consistently and safely.

Those opposing #0500 also raised concerns about potential conflicts of interest involving NQF committee members and the measure's developers. For instance, one of the NQF's steering committee co-chairs was a board member at a prominent medical technology trade association that represented biotech companies, including Edwards Lifesciences, the manufacturer of the specialized catheters used in EGDT.‡[59] As Edwards stood to gain financially from widespread adoption of the protocol, this association raised serious ethical questions.

Additionally, Rivers and Henry Ford Hospital had previously disclosed financial ties to Edwards Lifesciences. While Rivers had forfeited his rights to any intellectual property related to the Edwards catheter and hadn't received any financial compensation from the company since 2009, skepticism remained.[60] Some critics argued that the past association still cast a shadow over the measure.

As the primary developer of #0500, Rivers played a crucial role as both a content and technical expert throughout the NQF endorsement process. Concerns arose that his involvement may have influenced committee members' support for the measure. Critics pointed out that such ties appeared to

---

* A discussion of all the nuances of the guidelines is beyond this book, but suffice it to say that it can be misleading to focus only on the quality of evidence when interpreting guidelines. For example, evidence supporting early antibiotic administration in sepsis is technically *low* quality, as very few randomized controlled trials have examined the issue. However, based on the existing observational evidence and their self-evident basis, early antibiotics are still strongly recommended.

† A recent 2024 review demonstrated a 3 percent risk of significant complications with CVC placement and/or use.

‡ The trade association in question, AdvaMed, actively promotes medical technology companies, such as Edwards Lifesciences, though there is no direct evidence of any intent to influence the NQF proceedings.

contradict the NQF's internal conflicts-of-interest policy, raising questions about the potential for commercial influence in the committee's deliberations. At the least, they believed it weakened the measure's credibility.[61]

According to the NQF's conflict-of-interest policy, committee members must complete disclosure of interest forms, undergo an internal vetting process, and disclose relevant interests during public committee meetings.[62] However, no conflicts of interest were reported during the #0500 review process, and during the public disclosure phase of the meetings, the committee co-chair in question stated on the record, "I don't have any disclosures to make."[63]

Controversy aside, NQF committee members clearly saw sepsis as a public health crisis and recognized the measure's potential to save tens of thousands of lives annually. Moreover, time was of the essence, with one member emphasizing, "Waiting or delaying this could risk lives for minimal gain."[64]

After extensive discussion, public commentary, and multiple rounds of voting, the NQF officially endorsed #0500 on March 6, 2013, paving the way for its adoption by CMS.* Its Consensus Standards Approval Committee (CSAC) approved the entire measure, including EGDT, with the condition that as new evidence emerged, it would form an ad hoc committee to revisit the more contentious issue of EGDT.[65] The decision was immediately appealed by a coalition of medical societies representing frontline professionals and upheld in a subsequent vote by the NQF Board of Directors on June 13, 2013.[66] With that, the measure had moved one step closer to becoming the national standard.

On September 13, 2013, Senator Tom Harkin, then chairman of the Committee on Health, Education, Labor, and Pensions, became the first US lawmaker to acknowledge World Sepsis Day in Washington, DC. The annual event, first launched a year earlier by the Global Sepsis Alliance, was now the pinnacle of a decades-long crusade to increase international awareness of what had become one of the most underappreciated conditions of all time.[67]

---

* There was a vote on August 28, 2012, which was thirteen to four in favor of the measure, followed by a public commentary period. This included concerns from various medical societies regarding the quality of data supporting EGDT and the risk of central line placement in the emergency room. The steering committee met again and voted to endorse the measure, which then went to a larger vote at CSAC, where it was approved by forty-five votes to fourteen, with five abstentions.

Now in its second year, World Sepsis Day 2013 landed during a flurry of activity, quickly following Rory's Regulations earlier that year—much of it driven by Orlaith and Ciaran's intense advocacy. The Stauntons had connections to Senator Harkin, having met him alongside Rory at a White House St. Patrick's Day event the year before.

But that connection hadn't eased their fight. The two had spent the summer pressing Harkin's staff to hold a public sepsis hearing. As Ciaran recalls, "It was painstaking work that Orlaith and I went through to organize those hearings."[68] Every call, every meeting, was a battle.

On September 24, 2013, Harkin led the first-ever US Senate hearing on sepsis, part of a larger session titled "U.S. Efforts to Reduce Healthcare-Associated Infections," organized by CMS and CDC officials.[69] The session's primary focus was on the escalating threat of healthcare-associated infections, which were rapidly reaching unsustainable levels.[70]

Determined to make their presence felt, the Stauntons called on advocates from around the country and organized buses to bring family and friends from New York City to the hearing, which was broadcast live on C-SPAN. Some family members even flew in from Ireland in solidarity.

Amid a shuffle of panel members and discussions, Ciaran was scheduled to testify—the first family member ever to speak before Congress on the topic of sepsis. Yet, as he took his seat, his heart sank as he watched CDC representatives walk out of the chamber. *How could they act so uninterested in this public health crisis?* he thought.

It was a blow, but it didn't shake his resolve. The cause was too important, and too many lives were being lost. Ciaran stood strong and delivered a powerful, gut-wrenching testimony about Rory's death.[71]

Mounting pressure from Harkin and other lawmakers put the US Department of Health and Human Services, which oversaw agencies like CMS and the CDC, in a defensive position. As a result, and in accordance with the new requirements of the Affordable Care Act—signed into law two years earlier by President Barack Obama—it officially designated sepsis as a priority quality measure for its upcoming measurement cycle.[72] This meant that CMS was now in urgent need of a quality measure like NQF #0500.

Meanwhile, the Stauntons continued to press government agencies to take greater responsibility for sepsis, urging them to adopt a more proactive role in national surveillance, education, and treatment guidelines. Orlaith and Ciaran were adamant that all US government health agencies collaborate to address this public health crisis. Their advocacy efforts culminated in the first End Sepsis National Forum on Sepsis in Washington, DC, an event that united prominent politicians, sepsis experts, representatives from federal health agencies, and key advocates. Within a year, they had also established the National Family Council on Sepsis, a network of sepsis survivors and families of victims, representing all fifty states.[73]

———

In the spring of 2014, the academic sepsis world again stirred with the publication of a historic septic shock trial, ProCESS. It was the first of three long-awaited studies to verify the landmark 2001 EGDT trial.[*] By then, EGDT was being championed by many as a standard of care and was soon to be a core component of the national sepsis quality measure. However, many experts remained skeptical that the protocol was superior to an experienced doctor's gumption. In their view, the complexities of managing sepsis patients were best handled on a case-by-case basis, adhering to the adage "critical care happens at the bedside."

ProCESS was conducted at thirty-one US hospitals from March 2008 through May 2013. A total of 1,341 patients were randomized to one of three six-hour treatment arms: Rivers's original EGDT protocol; a second, non-EGDT protocol developed using the latest medical literature and survey data from emergency and intensive-care doctors worldwide; and a third arm consisting of "usual care": physicians treating patients based on their own experience and judgment, without any protocol.[†][74]

So, at the end of the day, ProCESS wasn't just testing EGDT—it was also addressing a broader question: do we need sepsis protocols at all?

The results, published on March 18, 2014, were striking. Investigators found no difference in mortality among the three groups, with an average risk of death of around 20 percent for all groups and a baseline mortality of only 19 percent in the usual care control group.[75] Within a year, results from the

---

[*]   The other two were ARISE and ProMISe.

[†]   The primary outcome was death at sixty days. Patients were recruited into the trial if they had a suspected or confirmed infection, two or more SIRS criteria, and evidence of septic shock.

two other EGDT confirmatory trials, ARISE and ProMISe, were published, showing the same null result.[*][76]

There it was: whether doctors followed EGDT, a different protocol, or no protocol at all, patients fared the same. If you were practicing medicine in 2014, when it came to treating septic shock, a doctor's gumption seemed to be just as effective as any protocol.[†]

What followed was a flurry of articles and blog posts with eye-catching headlines like "The End of Early Goal-Directed Therapy" and "A New Era in Sepsis."[77] In some circles, this fueled a growing narrative that EGDT had been flawed from the beginning and that the SSC had missed the mark.[78] Experts raced to make sense of the results, while critics seized the opportunity to pounce.

How had the sepsis clinical trials conundrum struck again? Were our most recent focusing lenses revealing a more profound truth? Were protocols unnecessary? Was the original EGDT trial flawed? Were the newer trials missing something?

To answer these questions, we must revisit the idea of sepsis as a heterogeneous disorder. Just as it was misguided to think that a single drug like Xigris could effectively treat a diverse group of sepsis patients, it may have been equally flawed to conclude the same for EGDT.

The 2001 EGDT trial was a single-center study, and there may have been something unique about that group of patients that didn't apply to the broader population. This is especially evident when comparing the baseline mortality rates in the studies: 46.5 percent in 2001 versus just 19 percent in 2014.[79] Reflecting on the apples-to-oranges comparison problem from chapter seven, it's clear that these were very different patient populations, potentially at different stages in the progression of sepsis.[‡]

---

[*]   ARISE was conducted at fifty-one centers across Australia and New Zealand and involved 1,600 patients randomized to receive either EGDT or usual care. ProMISe took place in the United Kingdom and involved 1,260 patients across fifty-six hospitals, randomized to receive EGDT versus usual care.

[†]   ARISE investigators prohibited the usual care group from measuring the venous oxygen saturation, which made it impossible to follow the EGDT protocol. There were no such restrictions in ProCESS and ProMISe, but data from the trials show that usual care physicians followed venous oxygen saturation levels only 1 percent and 3.5 percent of the time, respectively.

[‡]   An aspect of EGDT also worth considering is that sepsis involves not only impaired oxygen delivery but also impaired oxygen *extraction* at the tissue level. As a result, mixed venous oxygenation saturation may be a less reliable measure of oxygen delivery in certain contexts.

At this point, one might speculate that the 2001 Rivers patients had simply been sicker, making them more responsive to EGDT. However, this might only be part of the story.

In 2017, a group led by researcher Derek Angus from the University of Pittsburgh conducted a follow-up study called PRISM, which pooled data from the three ProCESS-era trials—a meta-analysis. The aggregate data from the three trials granted Angus increased statistical power to look for subtle differences between subgroups of patients. His group found that EGDT showed no benefit even in the sickest subgroups of sepsis patients.[80] So, while patients in the original trial might have appeared sicker at baseline, it wasn't enough to explain the difference in their outcomes.

But a closer look at the data reveals something else interesting about the patients. The average initial mixed venous oxygen saturation level of Rivers's patients was considerably lower than that of patients in the three ProCESS-era trials—49 percent compared to 71 percent.[81] Applying what we've learned, we can speculate that because their venous blood oxygen saturation was so low at the beginning of the study, Rivers's patients might have been in a more profound state of shock, similar to the trauma patients examined decades earlier by William Shoemaker.*

When might sepsis patients demonstrate such low mixed venous oxygenation levels? One possibility is early on in the emergency room before they have been adequately resuscitated with fluids. Angus explains, "On the front end, totally unresuscitated sepsis resembles classic shock." In such cases, "you can right a lot of wrongs just by fixing the low mixed venous oxygen saturation."[82]

Angus also points out that, before the twenty-first century, sepsis patients often arrived at the ICU in severely compromised states, with profoundly low blood pressure, poor perfusion, and inadequate oxygen delivery.[83] Yet, by the time the ProCESS trial began, early sepsis care had dramatically transformed. Antibiotics and intravenous fluids were being routinely administered as soon as patients arrived at the emergency department, and in some cases, paramedics were already beginning resuscitation en route to the hospital.

Thus, one plausible explanation for the ProCESS results is that *early* sepsis

---

* Recall that during severe shock, there's little if any blood flow to vital organs, which leads to a sharp drop in oxygen delivery. During such a state, oxygen-starved organs will avidly grab or extract as much oxygen as they can from the circulating hemoglobin, resulting in a much *lower* oxygen saturation in the venous blood returning to the heart.

care had advanced so substantially in the decade following EGDT that patients had already received effective resuscitation *before* randomization. This was reflected in their significantly higher mixed venous oxygen saturations at baseline. In other words, their circulatory "tanks" were already full, and their hearts were contracting more effectively. As a result, the once-transformative impact of EGDT was diminished, as many patients no longer required the aggressive interventions that had originally set the protocol apart.

Of course, there is also the possibility that Rivers was dealing with a distinct sepsis phenotype—one characterized by a more classic shock-like state, with impaired cardiac function and low oxygen delivery. Such patients might have been uniquely responsive to EGDT irrespective of their initial emergency room treatment. If so, when future investigators attempted to replicate the protocol across thousands of patients in multiple centers, they may have encountered the problem of averages discussed in chapter seven, when a treatment that benefits a specific subgroup gets diluted when applied to a broader, more heterogeneous population.

What might still exist in the vast PRISM database, as Angus explains, "is a subset of [patients] that might look quite like the Rivers trial, and then another subset of patients in whom the effects were in the reverse direction, and so on average there was no effect."[84] Angus and others are now exploring the possibility of this so-called "heterogeneity of treatment" effect in the same database. In fact, preliminary analysis suggests that "there could be significant heterogeneity, enough to imagine that within PRISM there are several hundred patients who, by the luck of the draw, had they been the only patients we had studied, we would have had a result very similar to the Rivers trial."[85]

Some experts were convinced that the ProCESS trial had validated the SSC's journey to capture the essence of sepsis, turn it into an emergency, and encourage rapid, goal-directed treatment. When Roger Bone first led the Sepsis 1 conference in 1991, the syndrome was a late-stage catastrophe, often killing half or more of those suffering from it. Over two decades, Bone, Rivers, members of the SSC, and many others slowly brought structure to this shapeless entity, allowing doctors and researchers to identify and treat it earlier. Sepsis itself became something more visible, less deadly. In the end, perhaps the real story was that the baseline mortality rate in ProCESS was only *19 percent*. Regardless of the differences between the groups, by 2014, we were obviously doing something right.*

The numbers confirm this. In all three ProCESS-era trials, the median time to sepsis recognition was only 83 minutes. Additionally, 97 percent of patients received an intravenous fluid bolus, and 93 percent received antibiotics within 75 minutes of entering the emergency room.[86] In essence, ProCESS wasn't a rebuke of structured sepsis care—it was a strong endorsement of it.

At the same time, the field of intensive care medicine was steadily advancing. Year after year, incremental improvements refined our ability to treat sepsis *and* other conditions. We improved our skills in managing ventilators, controlling blood glucose, and administering blood transfusions while implementing various hospital-based preventive care measures. I like to think that what we also witnessed during the ProCESS-era trials was the unwavering momentum of medical progress.

Unfortunately, not everyone saw it this way. ProCESS seemed to intensify a nihilism toward structured sepsis care among doctors, and some members of the academic medical community began organizing to dismiss the sepsis bundle concept as an exercise in futility.[87]

Back home in Portland, Dave was worried that we would see backsliding as our broader sepsis efforts began losing momentum. For better or worse, we were now entering the post-ProCESS era of sepsis care.

———

In April 2014, the NQF conducted a scheduled maintenance review of the recently approved measure #0500. As promised, it formed an ad hoc committee to reexamine the measure in light of new ProCESS data. After considerable debate, members voted to remove EGDT.[88] As expected, there were passionate discussions, disputes, and even harsh accusations. In the end? Compromise. The developers agreed to make EGDT optional in exchange for a formalized clinical assessment of a patient's perfusion and blood volume status, documented as a "physician's reassessment examination."†[89]

---

*　This is especially true in the large academic centers participating in these clinical trials. These centers are staffed by highly trained and experienced critical care providers who know the ins and outs of septic shock management.

†　This requirement is a six-hour follow-up reassessment of a patient's perfusion and blood volume status, documented by the clinician. It seemed like a reasonable concession, as there was no evidence that EGDT was ineffective or harmful. It was simply no better than

CMS officially adopted the embattled NQF #0500 as the first national sepsis quality measure in October 2015, naming it "SEP-1." Hospitals across the United States would soon be required to report adherence to the new national sepsis quality bundle. (See Table 14.1.) For many, it was a prodigious development—a national measure that promised greater attention to this deadly condition and more structure around treating it, and perhaps a future marked by a drastically reduced death toll from it.

But SEP-1 faced a shaky launch. The ProCESS trial had undermined confidence in structured sepsis care and protocols. The medical community was divided over the measure, with more academic physicians expressing concern over what they viewed as insufficient data supporting it. There was also animosity over its encroachment on physician autonomy and the potential risks to patients from overtreatment with antibiotics or intravenous fluids.

Resistance also grew among medical societies against the SSC and its expanding influence on sepsis care standards. At the same time, prominent medical bloggers and academic skeptics launched a full-scale campaign against SEP-1 and the SSC guidelines. One prominent group, EMCrit, organized an international petition calling for the retirement of the SSC guidelines, citing concerns about evidence quality, overprescription of antibiotics, and lack of flexibility in bedside care.[90]

This sparked heated debates in the medical literature, to say the least. Some critics argued that the measure was "infantilizing doctors" while others resorted to sensationalized rhetoric, spreading provocative memes, such as "how to drown a patient with 30 mL per kg fluid," stoking fear among frontline doctors about the potential dangers of the standardized fluid bolus for sepsis patients.[91]

Additionally, implementing SEP-1 was far more complicated than initially anticipated. CMS enlisted two private healthcare consultancy groups to transform the intricate measure into a set of rules or specifications for future hospital data abstractors, who would be responsible for collecting and reporting the data. The final specifications manual was a daunting 51 pages long, accompanied by a 393-page supplemental guidebook.[92] This promised a substantial administrative burden for hospitals attempting to meet the measure's requirements.

That said, pressure had been mounting for decades to change the status quo. CMS was now shining a spotlight on sepsis, while SEP-1 embodied what

an experienced doctor's judgment or "usual care," which undoubtedly involved some form of goal-directed therapy.

sepsis experts felt were the most critical aspects of sepsis care: early recognition and treatment.[93]

Required within 3 hours	Required within 6 hours
Draw blood cultures *before* antibiotic administration	Initiate vasopressor therapy if *sustained* hypotension
Draw initial blood lactate	Perform and document organ perfusion/blood volume assessment (invasive central venous pressure and $ScvO_2$ *aka* EGDT optional)
Administer intravenous antibiotics	Repeat blood lactate level if initial lactate elevated
If initial hypotension and/or lactate of 4 mmol/L or higher, administer *prescribed* intravenous fluid bolus	

Table 14.1: The CMS SEP-1 National Sepsis Quality Measure, October 2015.[94]

Back in New York State, data were pouring in from its new sepsis initiative. Between April 1, 2014, and June 30, 2016, 183 hospitals reported data on 91,357 eligible sepsis patients to the State Department of Health. During that period, overall compliance with sepsis bundles increased, and the absolute mortality rate dropped by 4.4 percent, translating to just over 3,200 additional lives saved.[*][95]

A study published in 2017 in *The New England Journal of Medicine* showed that the time to complete the three-hour bundle was directly associated with survival, with longer times resulting in a higher risk of death.[96] In the same period, 54 hospitals reported sepsis cases involving 1,179 children, indicating that the more likely a hospital was to complete the one-hour bundle, the more likely the patient would survive, with a risk-adjusted absolute mortality reduction of 4 percent, translating to one additional life saved for every twenty five-patients treated.[97]

When New York health officials first reviewed their sepsis data in 2014, they were taken aback by the findings. The state performed "average at best"

---

[*]   Compliance increased from 53.4 to 64.7 percent with the three-hour bundle and from 23.9 to 30.8 percent with the six-hour bundle.

in sepsis care.[98] Many hospitals questioned the reliability of the data, skeptical of what they were seeing. As Nirav Shah explains, "When you first look at something, it often looks much worse."[99] But slowly, they began to see change. Despite the complexity of modern healthcare, incremental improvements were possible, and those small victories led to better patient outcomes.

While public health leadership played a crucial role, in the end, as Gesten reflects in a 2024 conversation, "it took a village." He credits the nurses, doctors, and their associations for their willingness to collaborate. "They came to the table in good faith, giving freely of their time and expertise to make changes where they work, for the good of their patients."[100]

As Shah later remembers, "In the end, the story tells itself . . . even the naysayers were glad we did it, and then it was an issue of everyone wanting to take credit for it." In the end, they made a difference. "This kind of improvement can occur in our time, real-time, with quantifiable lives saved. And when you pull it off, wow."[101]

CHAPTER FIFTEEN

Mickey

ON THE BRISK MORNING OF Tuesday, November 7, 2017, Mickey, a sixty-six-year-old man from Portland, Oregon, woke up with a crushing fever, his body wracked with terrible aches and flu-like chills.

For most of his life, Mickey had been the picture of health: a longtime pescatarian with an active lifestyle. But something had shifted. A few months earlier, he had started taking colchicine and allopurinol—medications prescribed for gout—and ever since, an inescapable fatigue had drained his vitality, leaving him a shell of his former self.

By Friday, his fever persisted, often worse at night. Vomiting and diarrhea had left him exhausted. His wife, Claudette, watched over him, anxious and worried. His close friend, a hospital administrator, said, "You need to go to the hospital. Now." Mickey called his primary care provider. The doctor said, "If there's no improvement by morning, go straight to urgent care."

He decided to wait it out. "Let's give it one more day," he said.

That night, Mickey woke up restless and nauseous. He needed to get to the bathroom, so he crawled out of bed and slowly stood up. But something was clearly wrong. A violent chill shook his body to its bones. Each step was a battle as he gripped the walls, inching his way down the hallway.

Then, as he entered the bathroom, he fell into darkness.

The loud crash awoke Claudette. She ran in to find Mickey sprawled on the floor, unconscious. She fell to the ground in a panic and frantically rubbed his chest.

"Mickey! Are you okay?" She screamed.

Seconds later, a gasp, and his eyes opened. Sweat was beading down his skin. "You're burning up," she whispered, wiping his forehead. She tried to help him up, but it was no use. His strength was gone.

Claudette knew there was no time to waste. She grabbed her phone and dialed 911.[1]

———

Two days earlier, across town, I sat anxiously, shuffling through my note cards, preparing to lead my first Kaiser Permanente Northwest regional sepsis meeting. It was a moment I had spent months preparing for—Dave Schmidt had announced his retirement earlier in the year and asked me to take his place as program leader. Now, as I was taking the helm, my body tightened up like a coiled spring. Filling his enormous shoes would be no small feat.

Two thousand seventeen was a tense year for hospital quality improvement. With SEP-1 looming, hospitals were bracing for a major shift. Mandatory reporting for the measure was set to begin in January, with the first public results scheduled for release in July 2018. Sepsis was now in the spotlight—a top priority for hospitals and healthcare systems.

Meanwhile, online discussions among doctors, quality-improvement leaders, and health administrators surged. News briefings flooded the internet, dissecting every component of the measure and debating its potential impact on frontline care delivery.[2] With the chatter came uncertainty. How aggressively would regulators enforce SEP-1? Some called it an outright mandate, while others, including the measure's developers, insisted it was simply an instrument for quality improvement.*

And while the Inpatient Quality Reporting (IQR) program didn't explicitly penalize hospitals or individual physicians for performance, its influence was undeniable. As the nation's largest healthcare payer, CMS set the benchmark for quality measures, easily influencing physician behavior.[3] Thus, even though SEP-1 wasn't technically a "mandate," some worried it could effectively function

---

*   Some also worried that the country's premier hospital accreditation agency, the Joint Commission, could threaten hospital accreditation by enforcing certain SEP-1 performance thresholds, as with other CMS measures. However, this never materialized, as the Joint Commission declined to endorse the measure because it hadn't been sufficiently tested and its specifications were too complex.

as one. Critics also viewed IQR as a stepping stone to the government's Value-Based Purchasing Program, which tied payments to performance. They raised concerns that financial incentives could pressure physicians and health systems to overly comply with the measure.[4]

The ProCESS-era clinical trials only complicated matters, fueling the medical community's skepticism about structured sepsis care and protocols. Dissenters churned out medical blogs, op-eds, and letters opposing what they saw as a deeply flawed measure.[5] Some critics even likened the Surviving Sepsis Campaign (SSC) to the Empire from *Star Wars*, imposing its will on the medical profession.[6]

———

At the same time, revelations from the Third International Consensus Definitions for Sepsis and Septic Shock Task Force, aka Sepsis 3, were echoing in the medical community. The latest iteration of Roger Bone's original 1991 Sepsis 1 task force, Sepsis 3 promised yet again to update the sepsis definition to better match the evolving science.[7]

When Sepsis 1 was released in the 1990s, infectious disease experts worried its main concept—sepsis = SIRS plus infection—failed to match the actual physiology at play. To them, SIRS was an *expected* reaction to severe infection, not an indication of the more abnormal or harmful sepsis response.[8] They believed that using the SIRS definition could lead to a confusing mix of patients with and without sepsis.

In addition, while SIRS helped draw attention to patients with severe infections, it wasn't particularly effective at predicting who was at greatest risk of dying.[9] This weakened the signal-to-noise ratio on the front line, making it difficult for doctors to determine which patients truly needed urgent intervention.*[10] For example, take a young, otherwise healthy woman with a mild viral respiratory infection: an abnormal SIRS score alone didn't provide meaningful insight about her actual risk of death. In some cases, it could even mislead providers into overprescribing antibiotics or administering unnecessary intravenous fluids.

---

* The signal-to-noise ratio is "a measure of the strength of the desired signal relative to background noise (undesired signal)." For example, in a crowded room, the signal-to-noise ratio of a one-on-one conversation may be lower than that of an empty room.

During this time, many doctors felt that sepsis was being overdiagnosed. A meme emerged among frontline physicians: "Is it true sepsis or just 'sepsis?'" Even the 2001 Sepsis 2 Definitions Task Force had acknowledged these limitations, leaving the SIRS concept an open question for future research.[11]

What's more, by 2015, the Sepsis 1 definition had been fully embedded into the vast medical billing system, the ICD-9-CM. With CMS officially adopting this definition, hospitals now had a financial incentive to classify patients with SIRS as having "sepsis" to secure reimbursement for medical services.*

Healthcare systems witnessed a steep rise in sepsis diagnoses, as professional coders—medical documentation experts—helped capture a growing number of infected patients meeting SIRS criteria and labeling them as having sepsis, or more precisely, "sepsis without organ dysfunction." The net result of this was to inflate the number of total sepsis cases—a phenomenon I call "sepflation."

On the positive side, increased sepsis diagnoses meant that healthcare professionals were paying more attention to infected patients in hospitals and emergency rooms. Simply having more eyes on these patients often translated to better care, as clinicians could more quickly recognize early signs of deterioration and respond before patients fell into an unsavable state.

But sepflation also had unintended consequences. Much like the example from the University of New Mexico Hospital in chapter thirteen, it risked paradoxically reducing our overall attention to sepsis by flooding the system with false positives—a "Boy Who Cried Wolf" effect.

Additionally, it muddied the waters by ensuring that the overall pool or denominator of sepsis cases was a clutter of patients with vastly different illness severities. This made it increasingly difficult to discern whether observed declines in sepsis mortality were truly a reflection of better care or merely a statistical "dilution effect"—a classic example of the Will Rogers phenomenon.

One of the primary objectives of the Sepsis 3 Task Force was to draw a clear line between a severe infection and true sepsis. It began with a crucial assumption: while it was essential to recognize and treat severe infection, sepsis was something more—a distinct, life-threatening condition that could not be equated with infection alone.

---

* Medicare Advantage programs use a capitated payment system, where the insurer pays a fixed amount per beneficiary each year based on an individual risk score called the Hierarchical Condition Category (HCC), which factors in a patient's age, demographics, and medical comorbidities. This incentivizes healthcare systems to document high-risk diagnoses like sepsis.

Identifying a severe infection still involved traditional clinical indicators—fever, heart rate, and even SIRS—but these variables fell short in predicting which patients were truly at risk of death. The Sepsis 3 developers were interested in a more decisive and precise framework that could distinguish sepsis from what was now being patchily referred to as "uncomplicated infection" by some but probably more aptly described as "not sepsis."

In other words, Sepsis 3 asked, now that we've identified a severe infection, who is genuinely at risk of dying? Who truly has sepsis?[12]

Over the period of a year, a panel of nineteen of medicine's brightest minds spanning the disciplines of infectious disease, surgery, and critical care, forged a solution. It was an elegant synthesis of modern physiology, biochemistry, and immunology, informed by vast datasets from sepsis clinical trials, basic science, and translational research.

According to Sepsis 3, defining sepsis as "infection plus SIRS" was no longer accurate, as the latter could be seen as an *expected* physiological response to infection—not an abnormal or dysregulated response. In other words, patients needed to show some degree of organ dysfunction to be diagnosed with sepsis. The syndrome was now officially defined as "life-threatening organ dysfunction caused by a dysregulated host response to infection." (See Figure 15.1.)[13] This definition also rendered the term "severe sepsis" redundant since *all* cases of sepsis were, by definition, severe. (See Figure 15.2.) Patients either had an "uncomplicated" infection, sepsis, or septic shock, which was now considered a deadlier subset of sepsis, characterized by "profound circulatory, cellular, and metabolic abnormalities associated with a higher risk of mortality."*[14]

In addition, the task force sought a more objective and universally applicable sepsis definition, ensuring consistency across medical centers and research studies.[15] Even in 2016, sepsis faced a significant measurement problem as researchers struggled to agree on standardized criteria for identifying patients in clinical studies.

---

* It also put the nail in the coffin for the term "septicemia," which had somehow survived the ages despite the assertions of the Sepsis 1 task force twenty-five years earlier.

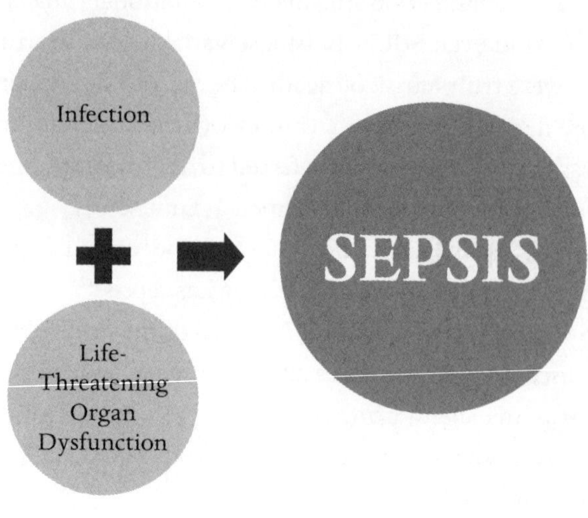

Figure 15.1: The Sepsis 3 (most current) definition of sepsis.

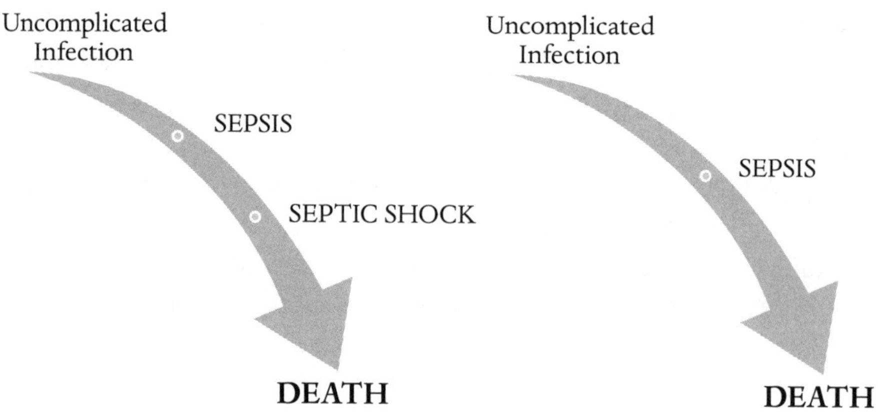

Figure 15.2: The arrow on the left shows the new 2016 sepsis concept—all sepsis is severe, making "severe sepsis" redundant. The arrow on the right reflects the fact that not all sepsis patients progress to septic shock before dying.

To address this, Sepsis 3 introduced the Sequential Organ Failure Assessment (SOFA) score, a method for assessing organ dysfunction and estimating mortality. First developed in the 1990s by Belgian researcher Jean-Louis Vincent, SOFA assigned point values to dysfunction in vital organs, including the kidneys, lungs, and liver. It provided a quantitative framework to categorize patients based on severity, with a score of two points or more signifying sepsis.*[16]

Beyond this, researchers could use SOFA criteria to mine patient databases and identify those who met objective sepsis criteria.[17] Like the APACHE score, it also served as a predictive tool, correlating higher scores with increased mortality risk, thus offering clinicians an idea of the patient's trajectory.†[18]

Despite its sophistication, Sepsis 3 faced significant hurdles in clinical practice. While SOFA was a valuable research tool, it proved impractical for bedside use. Calculating the score required a cumbersome table of organ dysfunction criteria, some of which—such as arterial blood gas measurement—were rarely measured or even available in many hospitals worldwide.[19]

Aside from these logistical challenges, the previous definition of sepsis as infection plus SIRS had been ingrained in medical practice for over a decade, making the transition to a new framework challenging. As a result, many clinicians continued to rely on the older sepsis concept.

Meanwhile, large payers such as CMS failed to adopt the Sepsis 3 framework and continued to use billing codes associated with older definitions, including "severe sepsis" and "SIRS without organ dysfunction."[20] This misalignment between clinical guidelines and administrative coding led to confusion, particularly as SEP-1 required hospitals to identify "severe sepsis" and "septic shock" using outdated criteria.

The result left frontline providers uncertain about how to define sepsis. The growing discord between evolving science, regulatory measures, and reimbursement policies only added to the frustration.

That said, the most problematic aspect of Sepsis 3 was its potential to shift the clinical focus downstream to a point where patients were more significantly compromised. Developed primarily by intensive care specialists, the new definition framed sepsis through the lens of critical illness, often identifying patients who required ICU-level care. In contrast, the earlier

---

*   It also provided specific criteria for septic shock: (1) a need for vasopressors to maintain normal blood pressure *and* (2) a blood lactate value greater than 2 mmol/Liter.

†   For example, a SOFA score of 16 translates to an estimated mortality rate of 50 percent.

definition was designed to flag sepsis *before* organ failure had fully set in, allowing for earlier intervention and the possibility of preventing ICU admission altogether.*[21]

Thus, while the new definition offered greater specificity, it also introduced blind spots, leading to delayed recognition and intervention. There was a real risk of backsliding to an era when the sepsis clock started only once a patient was already caught in an avalanche of immune dysregulation. Ironically, this unsettling implication was embedded within its definition: *"life-threatening organ dysfunction."*†[22]

This emphasis on organ injury may have also overshadowed a more complex underlying process. Dr. Laura Evans, co-chair of the 2021 SSC adult guidelines, explains, "We still don't know what constitutes a dysregulated host response to infection." She goes on to suggest that organ dysfunction alone is "probably not the only way to define it."[23]

There are likely deeper and subtler biochemical markers of an emerging sepsis response—clues that may ultimately prove far more effective in rapidly identifying the syndrome. As Evans says, "I hope we learn how to define earlier what is not a constructive response to infection and that we can change the trajectory of the patient before organ dysfunction occurs."[24]

In the end, confusion reigned. Many large healthcare systems, including Kaiser Permanente and New York State, aligned their sepsis definitions more closely with the SEP-1 national measure rather than with Sepsis 3.[25] This decision was pragmatic: most clinicians were already familiar with the older definitions, and the SEP-1 framework was less likely to miss sepsis patients on the front lines.

To this day, many medical professionals remain uncertain about how to define and diagnose this syndrome.

---

* While SIRS is a physiologic response to an infection, SIRS patients still have an average mortality of around 3 percent.

† A study by Dr. Sarah Sterling from the University of Mississippi Medical Center showed that Sepsis 3 failed to identify 57 percent of patients who met the older criteria for septic shock. These missed patients still had a mortality rate of 14 percent and high organ failure scores. At least half the time, they also needed ICU-level care.

Firefighters and paramedics rushed into Mickey's home. After rapidly assessing his vital signs, they carefully secured him onto a stretcher and carried him downstairs and into an ambulance.

They arrived just after 11:00 p.m. at Kaiser Westside Medical Center in Hillsboro, Oregon. As the resuscitation bay doors swung open, a team of medical staff sprang into action, swiftly gathering biometric data, drawing blood, connecting intravenous lines, and monitoring equipment with almost flawless precision.

At first, Mickey's vital signs were stable: his blood pressure was normal, his heart rate steady, and he had no fever. Though visibly weakened, he remained alert and talkative, recounting the details of his recent illness to Dr. Amy Watts, the emergency medicine physician on duty that night.

His bloodwork revealed an elevated lactate and kidney and liver dysfunction. His blood neutrophil count was nearly zero—a dangerous condition known as neutropenia—leaving him virtually defenseless against microbial attacks. It was a rare but known side effect of both allopurinol and colchicine, which he had been taking for several months.

The picture wasn't entirely clear, but the pattern was familiar: fevers, neutropenia, and organ dysfunction. Sepsis was at the top of a short list of possibilities.

Watts quickly connected the dots.

She ordered blood and urine cultures, a chest X-ray, and two powerful antibiotics to cover an array of possible bacteria.

Minutes later, Mickey's blood pressure plummeted. He began losing consciousness. Alarms rang as the nurses prepared for a crash resuscitation.

"Let's bolus two liters of saline with a pressure bag *stat* and prep for a central line," Watts said decisively.

Years of experience had honed her instincts for treating septic shock. From her time in residency, she was well-versed in early goal-directed therapy (EGDT)—its tactics and philosophy. She knew the importance of promptly restoring perfusion. Time was of the essence.

Mickey's blood pressure transiently improved, and he regained consciousness. Watts patted his shoulder and explained calmly what she would have to do: place a venous catheter in his neck, start vasopressors, and restore blood pressure.

He responded, "Absolutely. Do whatever you need to do."

Years of muscle memory moved her hands swiftly and deliberately as she prepped and draped Mickey's neck to place the central line. Moments later, the line's position was verified by X-ray.

Not long after, Mickey's blood pressure dropped again. A nurse, Desi, infused a vasopressor. With that, his blood pressure stabilized.

———

By late summer 2017, our monthly sepsis meetings had grown significantly, featuring a new group of executives, department heads, nursing leaders, and quality consultants. Many fresh faces attended, while others, like Briar and Anne, had moved on to different roles. That year's meetings were often chaotic, with heated debates about essential processes, workflows, and responsibilities for improving our sepsis bundle performance. Some executives questioned the effectiveness of our existing tactics—everyone seemed to have their own solution.*

SEP-1 had made sepsis the leading quality priority for our hospitals, resulting in more organizational resources and bandwidth. I used this new capital to assemble a team of physicians and nursing leaders from the ER and ICU, quality analysts, medical informaticists, data analysts, laboratory systems experts, and a dedicated project manager. I tried to surround myself with the best experts and engage the right stakeholders. We each had to complement one another. For example, I didn't understand how the emergency room operated, and the ER nursing leadership didn't appreciate the nuances of sepsis or the SEP-1 measure.

On November 8, 2017, I opened my first regional sepsis meeting by sharing Rory Staunton's story. I displayed a data graph from the New York Sepsis Initiative, which showed a dramatic decrease in sepsis deaths from 2014 to 2016. Finally, I presented our internal Kaiser data, indicating that in 2016, we had seen 155 sepsis deaths between our two major Portland hospitals and 2,004 sepsis survivors.

"This is why we're doing this," I stated. The committee members' expressions conveyed everything as a deep reverence settled in the room.

---

* At this time, the national average SEP-1 performance for hospitals was less than 50 percent.

To pull out all the stops, we built a computerized sepsis alert in the emergency room to help ER doctors and nurses identify sepsis patients and deliver the bundle elements. The key was to tune the system with the right sensitivity and specificity to catch as many cases as possible while minimizing false alarms. Our ER doctors were already skilled at diagnosing sepsis. Thus, we didn't need to replace their gumption so much as supplement it.

According to Dr. Derek Angus, "[sepsis] surveillance systems nearly always tell the doctor what they already know."[26]

We haven't yet reached a point where computers can utilize available biometric data, such as vital signs and laboratory tests, to identify sepsis patients any faster than a well-trained, undistracted clinician. Therefore, computer sepsis tools primarily serve a role in decision *support.*

As Angus explains, these systems "are good for overcoming forgetfulness, or the doctor just having a bad day or being distracted."

More advanced warning systems represent the holy grail of sepsis, and researchers today are exploring more predictive biometrics, such as heart rate variability, while using machine learning to integrate large datasets into advanced algorithms that can more quickly identify sepsis patients.[27]

We programmed our sepsis alert to activate for two scenarios:

1. Two or more SIRS criteria *and* suspected infection*

2. Two or more SIRS criteria *and* elevated blood lactate or low blood pressure

Having studied the pitfalls of previous sepsis alert systems, we aimed for an alert that was sensitive enough to assist physicians without annoying or overwhelming them with false alarms. Excess alerts can often lead to a flood of pop-up windows on the computer, making routine patient care sometimes feel like flying an airplane with malfunctioning instruments.

As Angus describes it, "I would use the support tool that is least irritating . . . for example, I love Google Maps, but I hate Google Maps if I'm near my house."[28]

Our system depended on a combination of human and computer input, as neither was perfect in isolation. Similar to the system at CHOP discussed in chapter thirteen, we encouraged nurses and doctors to think outside the

---

* Suspected infections were identified by an active blood culture or antibiotic order already placed by a clinician. This is often called an *implicit* infection code, meaning that the suspicion of infection is inferred from the electronic health record data rather than explicitly documented.

box—to be vigilant against sneaky sepsis patients the alert might miss. We employed multiple strategies to strengthen our sepsis culture and awareness—many of which couldn't be quantified by data or tracked by an algorithm.

Crucially, once triggered, the alert provided a physician the option to press one of three buttons: "sepsis confirmed," "not sepsis," or "not sure."* Once an ER doctor had confirmed sepsis, the alert would provide an electronic link to a set of easy-to-use sepsis quick orders in the computer, allowing them to request everything they needed, including blood cultures, blood lactate levels, fluids, and antibiotics. This captured the foundation of quality improvement implementation: making it easy to do the right thing. By pairing the alert process with a straightforward pathway to complete the bundle, we maximized the chances that our ER doctors would use it.†

Once activated, the system released checklist alerts—small electronic programs that search for digital tags called smart data elements (SDEs) assigned to active orders, such as blood cultures. If a checklist alert didn't see the SDE for its assigned sepsis bundle element order, such as a blood lactate, it would trigger a pop-up alert reminding the physician to place the order.‡

On the nursing side, the activated sepsis alert displayed large banners in the chart, including SEPSIS CONFIRMED, a timestamp, and a pop-up alert prompting the nurse to print a paper checklist to help complete the bundles. Years later, we would convert this into an electronic nursing checklist in the computer system. The overall effect was to create an electronic sepsis notification process that brought a sepsis patient to everyone's attention and facilitated the rapid completion of critical sepsis bundle elements. This alert process served as a giant safety net, keeping the patient visible to everyone, like a collective electronic lifeguarding system.

When we weren't working on the computer alert, we canvassed our hospitals to connect people with the cause. I attended physician department meetings, nursing and other healthcare staff gatherings, and educational conferences. Meanwhile, under the tireless and indispensable leadership of our sepsis nursing

---

* The "not sepsis" button retires the alert, while the "not sure" button dismisses the alert for thirty minutes.

† Alert fatigue is a common problem with healthcare computer systems. Providers often dismiss alerts without looking at them. It's crucial to measure user acceptance of alerts to ensure that they are being used properly.

‡ We built a checklist alert for each of the SEP-1 bundle elements.

leaders, our committee organized a series of public service announcements and educational activities, including a carnival of events every September for Sepsis Awareness Month: informational booths, sepsis trivia, and patient simulators.

Sepsis touches every corner of the hospital: the emergency room, the laboratory, and the medical wards. It also involves *everyone* in the hospital: nurses, medical assistants, pharmacists, administrators, data analysts, physicians, laboratory technicians, and environmental services workers, to name just a few. It takes a village to run a sepsis program, so we had to connect everyone to this story.

I always enjoyed visiting the ancillary services departments—they were often the most interested in sepsis. Laboratory staff would pepper me with questions, ranging from the microbiology of specific bacteria to whether tourniquets during blood draws could skew lactate levels. (They don't, if done correctly.) One of my favorite visits was to the hospital's environmental services (EVS) team. When I asked, "Who fights sepsis in this hospital?" an EVS worker confidently raised his hand and replied, "We do—by keeping this place clean!"

He was right—prevention is one of the pillars of sepsis care. It often relies on the unglamorous daily infrastructural work such as sanitation, infection control, and antibiotic stewardship.

———

Watts remembers Mickey as "one of those sneaky sepsis cases." At first glance, he appeared deceptively alert, conversant, and even charming. It was hard to appreciate how seriously ill he was until his blood pressure took a plunge.[29]

He was also the kind of patient who, in Watts's words, "used up every ounce of reserve holding out at home." Mickey was stoic and did not want to go to the hospital. As a result, his sepsis had festered for too long, dragging his system to the brink of shutdown. Once he'd finally arrived at the emergency room, it was only a matter of minutes before the floor dropped out from under him.[30]

Sepsis patients often experience significant delays before arriving at the emergency room. In a 2007 study involving over two thousand pneumonia patients, Angus and colleagues found that the average patient had been unwell for several days before coming to the hospital.[*][31] Additionally, a 2018 study led

---

*   When Angus and colleagues measured the patients' blood cytokine levels, they found that the levels had already peaked when they were finally seen in the emergency room.

by Dr. Vincent Liu from Kaiser Permanente Northern California examined forty-six thousand sepsis hospitalizations and found that nearly half of all sepsis patients visited a clinician during the week before their hospital admission.[32]

Thus, while urgent treatment in the emergency room is crucial, Angus believes we may be missing a huge opportunity to intervene even sooner.

He suggests, "The better area to focus on is three days earlier when that patient wasn't feeling well." Angus goes on, "This notion that sepsis arises as a sudden emergency is just not true. For me, one of the big untapped frontiers, which might become available because of iPhones and wearables, is this whole lead time before you get to the hospital."[33]

Mickey was also an *undifferentiated* patient—he didn't have an exact diagnosis, and there was no definitive evidence of infection yet. Patients might show classic signs of inflammation or be in shock, but it's not always clear if they have an infection. In other cases, sepsis patients might have no obvious evidence of inflammation *or* infection. They may be weak, appear confused, or show other vague signs and symptoms.

There is no "sepsis test," and confirming an infection takes time. As a result, clinicians must often act on suspicion alone.[34] Rapid assessment is critical—not just to initiate timely treatment if it is sepsis, but also to rule out other life-threatening conditions. This demands considerable clinical sleuthing and, at times, decisive action—administering antibiotics even when the picture is incomplete. In this fog of war, the line between treatment and overtreatment can easily blur.

The undifferentiated nature of sepsis patients has raised concerns among experts about the effectiveness of sepsis bundles and quality measures. The Infectious Diseases Society of America (IDSA) has only intermittently endorsed the Surviving Sepsis Campaign (SSC) guidelines and has consistently opposed SEP-1.* This is partly due to concerns that the time-sensitive nature of the bundles, combined with the diagnostic uncertainty surrounding sepsis patients, makes it too easy to overprescribe antibiotics. The IDSA argues:

"SEP-1's requirement to immediately administer antibiotic therapy to all patients with possible sepsis risks excessive and unnecessary antibiotic prescribing, as doctors may feel pressured to comply with the measure in patients who might not truly have sepsis."[35]

IDSA experts believe that hastily treating a suspected sepsis diagnosis could

---

* The IDSA endorsed the 2012 and 2021 SSC Guidelines.

lead to unnecessary harm to patients and delays in accurately diagnosing other conditions. This concern is compounded by the growing threat of antimicrobial-resistant organisms and *C. difficile* infections spreading through hospitals.

Some of this can be traced back to history. In 2003, CMS adopted a pneumonia quality measure, time to first antibiotic dose (TFAD), which required physicians to administer antibiotics within four hours to pneumonia patients. The decision was driven by two large retrospective observational studies, which suggested that faster antibiotic administration improved survival rates. By 2006, CMS had reinforced the measure by incorporating it into quality reporting programs that laid the groundwork for future pay-for-performance initiatives.[36]

The results were unsettling. The measure inadvertently drove antibiotic overuse, with some physicians prescribing antibiotics to patients with little or no evidence of pneumonia and, in some cases, for viral illnesses—simply to avoid failing the measure.[37] Within a few years, prospective or forward-looking clinical trials would show that the measure failed to improve patient survival while also increasing *C. difficile* infections—a dreaded consequence of antibiotic overexposure.[38]

As it turned out, the original pneumonia studies had significant flaws. Both studies were retrospective, meaning they analyzed past cases where bacterial pneumonia had already been confirmed. This created a hindsight bias, making it easy to link early antibiotic use with survival—after the diagnosis was already known. However, these studies overlooked the challenge of distinguishing bacterial pneumonia from other respiratory illnesses in real time.[39] When researchers later conducted *prospective* studies, the observed benefit of early antibiotics vanished amid the intricacies of diagnosing pneumonia in everyday practice.

Sepsis patients can be even trickier to sort out, often presenting with a combination of abnormal signs and symptoms without an obvious source of infection.[40] This makes them difficult to separate from patients with noninfectious diagnoses, such as cardiogenic shock or pulmonary embolism, which complicates matters for the average ER physician. As a result, focusing too much on sepsis can lead to inappropriate antibiotic prescribing and may also cause physicians to overlook other serious conditions that mimic sepsis—a cognitive error known as premature closure that you learned about in chapter thirteen.

Sepsis overdiagnosis might be more common than we would like. In a 2013 Dutch study, investigators retrospectively analyzed hospital charts of patients admitted with sepsis. They found an alarming 13 percent had almost no chance of infection, while 30 percent had only a possible chance.[41] Other observational studies have shown similar findings.[42]

At the same time, when a patient arrives at the hospital with sepsis, it's crucial to treat it as a true medical emergency. By 2017, consistent data showed that with each hour of delay in antibiotic administration, mortality increased. In cases of septic shock, this risk could rise to as much as 1.8 percent per hour.[43] Put differently, every hour without antibiotics could result in one additional death for every fifty-five patients, adding up to tens of thousands of preventable deaths each year in the US alone. In this context, when it comes to antibiotic timing for sepsis, if we're going to err, it may be safer to err on the side of overtreatment rather than undertreatment.

We should also remember that the emergency room is a hectic environment, filled with complex issues that pull doctors and nurses in multiple directions at once.

According to Watts, "There's always so much other stuff going on. Maybe you don't find out about the change in vital signs or their mental status until thirty or forty minutes later because the nurse is tied up with three other patients, and you're tied up with five other patients yourself."[44]

It is now routine for the healthcare system to shower medical professionals with constant interruptions and distractions across various electronic platforms, including patient monitors, alerts, chat messages, and hands-free voice communicators.

As Watts describes, "There's always something flashing, dinging, or beeping at you."[45]

Even more disturbingly, any one of these loud alarms or interruptions could signal a developing catastrophe, such as a falling oxygen level or dangerous arrhythmia. It's a concerning trend in modern medicine that undoubtedly disrupts doctors' and nurses' ability to care for patients.

Most sepsis patients first present to emergency departments, which have some of the highest rates of interruptions. In one study, emergency doctors were interrupted an astonishing twelve times per hour while trying to complete vital patient care tasks, such as reviewing patient data and writing medication prescriptions.[46] Another study showed the chilling effect of such distractions: in almost one in five cases of being interrupted, the emergency doctor failed to complete the original task.[47] Interruptions can also reduce a doctor's ability to detect meaningful clinical findings. For instance, a study examining chest

X-ray interpretation showed that when interrupted, radiologists were less accurate at detecting subtle findings on the X-ray.[48]

Watts recalls how, on one harrowing night, she was caring for a patient while receiving repeated calls on her hands-free communicator about another sick patient, text messages on her work phone about a potential transfer from an outside hospital, and an electrocardiogram handed to her for immediate review to rule out a potentially life-threatening myocardial infarction on an ambulance patient.

After all that, it's not uncommon to wonder, *what was I just doing?*[49]

Nurses face similar challenges. One study showed that nurses were distracted and interrupted every two minutes while administering medications to patients.[50] In a related study, interruptions resulted in a 12 percent increased risk of a medication error per interruption.[51]

Due to the recent surge in computerized alerts, patient monitors, hand-held communication devices, and alarm systems, noise and distraction have become ingrained in the healthcare system. A 2014 study revealed that patient care monitors in one academic hospital's intensive care units produced an astounding 2.5 million alerts in a single month, averaging 187 warnings *per* patient per day. Even more disturbing was that most of these warnings were false alarms.[52] Despite growing recognition of this issue and increased calls for change from patient safety advocates, little has been done to address this daily cacophony faced by healthcare workers.*

In the era of modern healthcare, the space for practicing medicine has been slowly shrinking.

In a recent interview, one of my emergency medicine colleagues and one of our sepsis champions, Dr. Melissa Denny, said, "I find value in the protocols and processes, but I also feel there has to be made space just for you to be a clinician, trust your gut, and take care of the patient."[53]

One of my most cherished memories from residency was training with the late Larry Osborn, an interventional cardiologist of rare composure. Osborn seemed to move through the hospital in his own time continuum, unaffected by the frantic pace around him. As an interventionalist, his call schedule could have easily led to a tightly wound existence, yet he always emanated a calm and meditative presence. His office was filled with towering stacks of medical

---

*   Ironically, many distracting alerts and alarms result from well-intentioned systems that aim to detect problems like sepsis.

journals and well-worn books on Shotokan Karate and Zen Buddhism. And his eyes had a soft glint, as if he had unlocked the secret to the universe.

Whenever we reached a diagnostic impasse during table rounds, Osborn had a simple solution: *go see the patient.* At the bedside, his ability to connect was uncanny. Within minutes, he made his patients feel understood while effortlessly diagnosing that quiet heart murmur we had all missed.

But what stood out the most was his ritual before performing a physical exam. He would close the door, take time to position the patient carefully, and then, for a moment, simply sit—eyes closed, breathing. One day, he turned to us and said, "Always be in the moment when you perform your physical exam. Otherwise, you'll miss the subtle findings."

Sepsis occurs when the body's response to infection makes an elusive switch from normal to abnormal, attacking its organ systems. It can be challenging to detect the precise moment this happens by looking at routine vital signs and laboratory tests. This means that doctors and nurses must maintain a high suspicion of it and, like the lifeguards at Huntington Beach, be on constant watch for any signs of distress. Like Dr. Osborn, they must also practice *in the moment* with awareness and intentionality.

Yet the modern healthcare system has created an environment filled with distractions and false alarms, which steal their attention, decrease diagnostic accuracy, and increase the risk of medical errors.

———

Mickey's blood cultures came back positive for *E. coli* the next day. After an exhaustive workup, the ICU team found no apparent source for the microbe. An infectious disease specialist was consulted on the case and believed the bacterium was likely introduced through microscopic entry points in Mickey's gut lining, a phenomenon called gut translocation. With a severely compromised immune system and no remaining neutrophils, Mickey was at high risk of any number of opportunistic microbes invading through various portals in his body. After establishing a foothold, the gram-negative bacteria had gone unchecked for days, multiplying as they'd invaded his bloodstream and triggering endotoxic shock syndrome reminiscent of that seen in mid-twentieth-century hospitals. Yet Mickey had been aided by a swift response from Dr. Watts and the Westside emergency room team. Despite having almost no reserves to work with, the ER had shifted the odds in his favor, thwarting what could have ended up being a total system collapse.

All that said, nothing came easy. It took days to wean Mickey off vasopressor life support. In the process, he developed secondary pneumonia. His respiratory system almost failed, requiring a brief period on a BiPAP ventilator mask. Initially, the ICU doctors didn't know if he would make it; even if he did, they weren't sure he would be the same person. He suffered from terrible delirium—what we now recognize as sepsis-associated encephalopathy—brain dysfunction caused not by the infection itself, but by the body's intense inflammatory and metabolic response.*[54] At one point, he even remembered being transported into the *Ray Donovan* television series. The early days were the hardest, but he had a lot of people in his corner, including Watts, who would often stop by after her shifts to see how he was doing.

In the end, Mickey pulled through. But survival came at a cost. He was left battered and frail, a shadow of his former self. He had lost twenty-seven pounds, his appetite had faded, and his muscles had withered. Even the simple act of getting out of bed had become a feat. At first, he wondered if this was how it would always be. Claudette was worried sick. Neither of them knew what would happen next.

As discharge neared, the thought of leaving felt distant and abstract, almost implausible. Home had become a vague memory, a place he could no longer picture. His focus now shifted from the question of survival to the uncertainty of what survival would look like. *What's left of me?* he wondered anxiously.

In time—and with tough love and kindness from nurses like Ron and Khristina, the devoted care of their nurse assistant, Alex, and the steady guidance of a physical therapist named Damien—Mickey gathered enough strength to leave the hospital. On November 27, seventeen days after his admission, he was wheeled outside into a crisp, sunny Portland morning on his way to a skilled nursing facility for rehabilitation. Within days, he was walking on his own. A few days after that, he was back home. After eight more weeks of dedicated physical therapy, he finally began to feel normal again.

---

* Sepsis-associated encephalopathy (SAE) results from widespread brain dysfunction that accompanies sepsis in the absence of direct infection of the brain itself. Poorly understood, it is thought to result from microscopic injury to brain tissue, disruptions in the brain's microcirculation, altered brain metabolism, and impaired neurotransmission. Patients who experience SAE may suffer lasting cognitive and functional defects.

Mickey soon found a new calling as a patient advocate for Kaiser Permanente. His experience had, among other things, underscored the importance of communication and compassion in healthcare. He began regularly visiting Westside Medical Center, meeting with staff and expressing gratitude to those who had helped him. He was always met with warmth and described feeling "nothing but love" every time he returned to the hospital.

———

I first met Mickey in 2018 when he spoke at our Fall Sepsis Summit. Listening to his story was a powerful reminder of why our sepsis work mattered. As I sat there, I couldn't help but reflect on my own experience years earlier, being pulled from the rip current by Emily and the California lifeguards at Huntington Beach. Just as I had been rescued by dedicated professionals working within a coordinated system that day, our work was about pulling our patients back from the brink.

When asked today what sepsis is from his perspective, Mickey reflects, "It was a failure of my immune system. Something happened, which threw that whole system into complete disrepair. That's all I understand in reality. That's it."

As the conversation turns to his experience now as a survivor, he continues, "I can't isolate sepsis as a specific place on the map the way a cancer survivor has a certain relationship to cancer. I only think of it as an array of things that happened. The word 'cascade' makes sense; so many things led to other things. Sepsis is almost more like a scenario than a disease. You can't locate it."[55]

CHAPTER SIXTEEN

The Pandemic

Even after the pandemic, many of the effects the pandemic has had on the healthcare workforce will likely persist. Addressing these impacts as well as the underlying challenges that pre-dated the pandemic can help build a stronger and more resilient health care system for the future.

—DEPARTMENT OF HEALTH AND HUMAN SERVICES, Office of the Assistant Secretary for Planning and Evaluation, issue brief, May 3, 2022[1]

ON SUNDAY, FEBRUARY 23, 2020, forty-six-year-old Hector Calderon arrived at the emergency room at Kaiser Westside Medical Center in Hillsboro, Oregon, with flu-like symptoms and respiratory distress. His condition deteriorated rapidly, and within days, he was on a ventilator, battling for his life.[2]

Calderon was the first person in Oregon to test positive for SARS-CoV-2, the virus responsible for COVID-19. As he had had no contact with travelers in the weeks preceding his illness, he was also the second person in the United States to contract the virus through community spread. This meant SARS-CoV-2 was now rampantly multiplying throughout Oregon.

A flood of text messages, emails, and alerts soon followed as state public health officials, infectious disease specialists, and hospital administrators braced for a tidal wave of infected patients.

Calderon's ICU nurse, Eric Cathey, recalls thinking, "Wow, this is really happening. It's here. We can't contain it."[3]

On January 7, 2020, Chinese health officials identified a novel strain of coronavirus responsible for a severe pneumonia outbreak in Wuhan, China. Genetically similar to SARS CoV-1—the virus that had caused the 2002 SARS epidemic—it was named SARS-CoV-2, and the disease it caused was named COVID-19.* By March 11, 2020, there were close to 120,000 documented infections across 114 countries, causing just over four thousand deaths, prompting the World Health Organization (WHO) to declare a global pandemic.[4] Within just a few weeks, there were upwards of eighty thousand new infections *daily*, resulting in around five thousand deaths per day worldwide.[5]

By its official end on May 5, 2023, the pandemic had led to just over 765 million documented infections, killing nearly seven million people and leaving tens of millions of survivors debilitated with long COVID syndrome.[6] It also led to widespread economic instability, increasing unemployment rates, income loss, worsening societal inequality, disrupted global supply chains, and rising inflation.[7]

COVID-19 is a case study for sepsis, highlighting many of the themes discussed throughout the book, such as prevention, early intervention, and the nuances of frontline sepsis care. It also painfully underscores the tension between large-scale public health initiatives and individual autonomy regarding vaccination programs, shutdowns, social isolation, and mask mandates. Additionally, the pandemic eviscerated an already ailing healthcare front line, leaving it severely compromised, with consequences that will reverberate for years to come.

SARS-CoV-2 has a remarkable proclivity for causing sepsis by dysregulating the body's immune response—the cytokine release syndrome referred to in chapter six. The ensuing barrage of inflammatory mediators can rain on the body's systems like a firestorm, resulting in widespread organ injury, most often involving the lungs.

A 2023 study published in the open-access journal *JAMA Network Open* estimated that, in the pandemic's first thirty-three months, nearly 30 percent of hospitalized COVID-19 patients developed sepsis, and almost a third of

---

* SARS stands for severe acute respiratory syndrome, owing to the virus's ability to rapidly cause a severe inflammatory reaction in the lungs.

them died.* In that five-hospital system, the virus accounted for about one in six sepsis cases.[8]

At the same time, the risk of severe illness, hospitalization, and death from COVID-19 varied significantly across the population, with low-risk individuals having an average risk of hospitalization as low as 0.5 percent and higher-risk individuals having an average risk over ten times greater at around 6 percent.[9] Individual characteristics, such as age, underlying chronic diseases, and socioeconomic status, were among the most crucial host factors contributing to a person's risk of severe illness.† In the end, for most individuals, COVID-19 led to mild to moderate disease without hospitalization, sepsis, or death, but for many others, it led to devastating illness.

Due to their novelty, early SARS-CoV-2 strains were particularly treacherous.‡[10] This meant that most of the global population lacked immunity to the virus during the first wave, making it highly transmissible and more harmful or virulent to those infected.

SARS-CoV-2 has an estimated introductory reproductive rate or R0 (pronounced "R naught") between 2 and 4, meaning that, on average, an infected person will infect between two and four *additional* people.[11] Even on the low end of that range, the number of infections will double each round, leading to an exponential rise in cases and quickly resulting in millions of infections.

As a result, even if the virus's *average* mortality rate is relatively modest, when multiplied by the entire infected population, it translates into countless deaths—and that's exactly what we saw during the pandemic. By the spring of 2023, the estimated average case fatality rate was about 1 percent. Yet by that point, there had been over one hundred million infections in the US and, by extension, well over a million deaths.§[12]

---

* Over time, mortality improved as the result of enhanced treatment strategies and greater immunity from vaccination, reaching a baseline of around 14 percent, close to the current observed overall sepsis mortality rate in the US.

† Recall from chapter five that a patient's baseline characteristics, or host factors, are one of the most important predictors of whether someone will get sepsis and how severe that sepsis response will be.

‡ One study from Wuhan, China, showed that only 4 percent of the population had antibodies to the virus during the first pandemic wave.

§ The case fatality rate (CFR) represents the mortality rate in confirmed cases, while the infection fatality rate (IFR) estimates the proportion of deaths among all infected individuals. Early in the pandemic, limited testing capacity meant that those tested often represented the sickest patients presenting to hospitals, thereby likely overestimating the CFR.

Another consequence of its high infectivity is that SARS-CoV-2 was able to swiftly overload our healthcare system with sick patients in only a matter of weeks. Hospitals have a finite number of staffed beds available to care for patients. In the United States, this number hovers around nine hundred thousand.[13] Additionally, many hospitals aren't equipped or staffed to handle a large surge of patients. Consequently, even the 1 to 2 percent average hospitalization rate we saw during the pandemic could quickly overwhelm our hospital bed capacity. In the most extreme case, a pandemic can grind the healthcare system to a halt, which means that every other emergency disease will be impacted as well: heart attacks, strokes, trauma, and bacterial sepsis, among others.* One study showed that between March 7, 2020, and April 30, 2021, about two-thirds of US hospitals reported significant emergency room and ICU overcrowding.[14] In another study, one in five American households reported experiencing delays in medical care or an inability to receive crucial medical services during the pandemic.†[15]

In the world of patient safety and quality improvement, the pandemic revealed just how fragile our prevention systems can be during a crisis. At the hospital level, this translated into declining SEP-1 performance—driven by emergency room overcrowding, resource constraints, and staffing shortages, all of which contributed to a decline in care standards. More troubling was a concurrent rise in overall sepsis mortality rates observed during this period, particularly in late 2020 and early 2021.

On the national level, COVID-19 exacerbated other sepsis-related problems, such as increased rates of antimicrobial resistance and healthcare-associated infections related to a breakdown in infection control standards and widespread overuse of antibiotics in COVID-19 patients. In fact, the US CDC reported a 15 percent increase in resistant hospital-acquired infections in the first year of the pandemic.[16]

----

* Recall from chapter ten how overcrowding in hospitals and emergency rooms had severe downstream effects on sepsis outcomes during the late 1990s and early 2000s.

† Some of these delays resulted from hospitals postponing so-called elective or non-emergency surgeries to shore up staffing and bed capacity for infected patients. The net result was a backlog of surgical cases, some for essential treatments, such as cancer resection.

Prevention is our most crucial strategy against sepsis, particularly during COVID-19 and other viral pandemics. Evidence shows that COVID-19 vaccines were (and still are) effective at preventing severe infection, hospitalization, and death. One 2022 study published in *The New England Journal of Medicine* showed that Pfizer's BNT162b2 mRNA COVID-19 vaccine demonstrated 96 percent efficacy in preventing hospitalization. Moreover, immunization maintained a similar efficacy against severe infection throughout the study, dropping to only 89 percent at seven months.*[17] Vaccinated individuals also have a lower risk of acquiring long COVID.[18]

The cumulative effect of worldwide vaccination campaigns was nothing short of impressive. A study published in *The Lancet* estimated that vaccines prevented close to twenty million excess deaths due to COVID-19 in the first year of the pandemic alone.[19]

Individual risk assessment becomes essential when discussing the effects of vaccines and other treatments on reducing the severity of COVID-19 and other viral illnesses. Persons at higher risk of severe disease are more likely to benefit from the vaccine or specific medical therapies. As a result, older adults, individuals with chronic health conditions, or those at high risk for severe disease should be prioritized for vaccines as early as possible and continue to receive regular boosters.

COVID-19 mRNA vaccines have become some of the most rigorously monitored and evaluated therapies in history and have an excellent safety profile.† However, as with any vaccine or medication, rare complications, such as severe allergic or inflammatory reactions, can occur, and there are specific contraindications for a small subset of people.‡[20] Importantly, events such as myocarditis are rare after vaccination and, in most populations, occur

---

* Efficacy is often reported as a *relative* risk reduction (RRR), which tells us how much the risk of severe infection or hospitalization decreased relative to what it was at its baseline. For example, if the baseline or absolute risk of hospitalization is 10 percent, the mRNA vaccine reduces that risk by about 95 percent, down to half a percent—an impressive *absolute* risk reduction of 9.5 percent, which translates to one prevented hospitalization for every ten people vaccinated. However, if the baseline risk is only 1 percent, the absolute risk reduction would only be 0.95 percent, translating to one prevented hospitalization for every 105 vaccinated people.

† The Johnson & Johnson adenovirus vaccine was based on a different mechanism (not mRNA), and its use was paused by the US FDA in 2021 due to reports of a rare complication, cerebral venous sinus thrombosis, and low platelet counts. It is no longer available in the US.

‡ People who should not receive the COVID-19 vaccines include those with a history of severe allergic reactions to previous mRNA vaccines or one of the vaccines' components, such as polyethylene glycol.

far more often after COVID-19 *itself* than after mRNA vaccination.[21]

While these vaccines are largely safe, SARS-CoV-2 is an unpredictable virus with the potential to cause severe illness, sepsis, and even death. In survivors, it can also cause a debilitating and mysterious post-infectious syndrome: long COVID.[*][22] As a physician who regularly cares for patients infected with SARS-CoV-2, I recommend regular vaccination as a strong preventive measure against COVID-19-related sepsis, particularly for those at higher risk of severe infection.

When it comes to the broader question of vaccine mandates, lockdowns, and other sweeping public health measures, COVID-19 has taught us that we need a more nuanced discussion. Public health policy must weigh both scientific evidence and human values without conflating the two.[†][23] To public health officials, the data were compelling: vaccines save lives, and mandates boost vaccination rates. Thus, mandates were framed as the only scientifically correct path to prevent mass death and preserve the healthcare system, while opponents of mandates were often labeled "anti-science." But this framing was oversimplistic, as in reality, their objections often stemmed from value-based concerns. After all, the decision to impose a mandate isn't purely scientific—it also reflects a value judgment: *in order to save lives, we have to sacrifice autonomy and, in some cases, our financial or social well-being.*[24]

For many people, mandates were seen as an unacceptable violation of their personal freedom. They also had concerns about the new vaccines, particularly due to the rapid pace at which they were developed. The blurry line between the pharmaceutical industry and the government didn't help matters. This was represented notably by individuals such as Dr. Scott Gottlieb, former US FDA commissioner and Pfizer board member, who frequently appeared on television news during the pandemic.[‡][25] These concerns caused many to question, and at times reject, the science behind the vaccines, with some even believing and spreading harmful vaccine misinformation.[26]

---

[*] Long COVID is itself a heterogeneous syndrome likely encompassing many causes and factors.

[†] Physician-writer Kristen Panthagani summarizes this nicely in a recent online article, "Science, Policy, and Values."

[‡] While Dr. Gottlieb is widely regarded as a highly competent and principled healthcare professional, his simultaneous roles—as Pfizer board member and a frequent media commentator on vaccine policy—underscore the ongoing challenge of perceived conflicts of interest between government regulators and the pharmaceutical industry.

In public health discussions, it is crucial to maintain a sharp distinction between scientific data and human values. As physician-writer Kristen Panthagani explains, "It is critical that we are very clear about what we're doing: when we are communicating objective facts and when we are layering our values on top of those facts."[27]

Additionally, while protecting life is the most important core value, it must still be balanced against other values, such as preserving autonomy. Public health officials should be open and honest about the challenges and uncertainties and respect differing value systems.

———

COVID-19 also aggravated a silent epidemic of burnout among medical professionals, taking a measurable toll on the morale of doctors and nurses nationwide. For example, by the end of 2021, 63 percent of physicians surveyed exhibited signs of burnout, compared to only 38 percent in 2020.[28] Notwithstanding its impact on providers themselves, burnout can considerably affect how patients are treated, as higher rates of burnout are associated with lower quality of care and increased medical errors.[29] And while it has improved somewhat since the pandemic, burnout still affects over *half* of all doctors in certain specialties, such as emergency medicine.[30]

In the wake of the pandemic, there was a significant increase in staff turnover. In a study published in *JAMA Health Forum*, when comparing 2018 to 2020, the exit rate for healthcare workers increased from 6 percent to 8 percent per year (a 2 percent absolute increase and a 33 percent relative increase).[31] This increase also persisted through 2021. Given the nearly nineteen million healthcare workers in the United States, the absolute difference translates to around 380,000 people dropping out of the workforce each year.*

Hospitals have been able to offset some of these losses by hiring new staff, but the damaging effects persist. Turnover can disrupt the continuity of patient care, and it requires significant time and resources to onboard new hires.

---

* This may explain the decrease in burnout cited in a 2023 survey by the American Medical Association, as more burned-out physicians likely dropped out of the workforce, thus lowering the overall average.

On a positive note, the pandemic served as an accelerated test lab for human innovation. With the rapid coalescing of research collaboratives worldwide, real-time sharing of best practices, and millions of cases to examine new medical treatments, we saw our knowledge and capabilities evolve at a speed nearly matching that of the pathogen we were fighting.

Platform trials, which test multiple drugs simultaneously, proved highly useful in testing COVID-19 therapies. For example, the REMAP-CAP trial—originally established in 2014 to study treatments for pneumonia and sepsis—was uniquely positioned to pivot when the pandemic struck and quickly demonstrated the benefits of the interleukin-blocking drugs tocilizumab and sarilumab in treating the COVID-19 cytokine release syndrome. These trials are designed to study diseases, not specific therapies, making them extremely versatile and perfectly structured to quickly accelerate knowledge during pandemics.[32] They will also prove to be game changers for future sepsis research.[33]

I was privileged to be part of a unique collaboration between multiple specialties within our organization. Together, we rapidly developed treatment guidance to support our frontline doctors and nurses. One key product of that effort was a COVID-19-specific sepsis pathway, emphasizing rapid diagnosis, early blood pressure support, and, most importantly, the avoidance of *over-resuscitation* with fluids. COVID-19 patients are particularly susceptible to complications from fluid overload—a powerful reminder that context matters when it comes to sepsis treatment.

Over time, as a global community, we expanded vaccination programs, implemented masking and social isolation practices to control the spread of the virus, and developed rapid and effective treatment protocols, including corticosteroids to tame the inflammatory response in the lungs, while also developing innovative approaches to intravenous fluid resuscitation and ventilator techniques to resist the virus's assault. Between early 2020 and mid-2022, global in-hospital mortality from COVID-19 dropped by roughly 50 percent, saving millions of lives worldwide.[*][34]

---

[*] At least some of this decrease in mortality is also related to a natural shift in the severity of subsequent SARS-CoV-2 variants, such as Omicron, and an increase in natural immunity across the population.

About two months into his grueling hospitalization, Hector Calderon began showing signs of improvement. Shortly afterward, his team was able to wean him off life support. He was eventually discharged from the hospital on May 5, 2020.[35] After weeks of rehabilitation in a skilled nursing facility, he returned home. When asked later about his ordeal, Calderon describes going into a coma shortly upon arriving at the hospital and not waking up for three months.[36]

Today, we're still putting the pieces back together. We have seen many hospitals struggle to staff their beds while the healthcare system is still recovering from a massive backlog of medical procedures and conditions that went untreated during the pandemic. Public trust in medical science has waned, making it more challenging to convince people to participate in vaccination and other preventive health efforts.[37] We have also seen a rise in antimicrobial-resistant organisms and hospital-acquired infections, showing us that when our prevention systems break down, we lose ground in the fight against infections and sepsis. Moreover, our frontline healthcare professionals are burned out yet still responsible for caring for patients in an increasingly complex and fragile healthcare system.

There is a misconception that COVID-19 unleashed a cascade of new problems in the healthcare system. In reality, many of these problems—overcrowded emergency rooms, rising health inequality, lack of emergency preparedness within healthcare organizations, inadequate personal protective equipment, inconsistency in quality improvement and patient safety, and provider burnout—had existed for decades, first surfacing in the 1970s and 1980s.[38] This underscores the vital role of unglamorous infrastructure in maintaining a smoothly run healthcare system. It also suggests that we should double down on the twenty-first-century patient safety and quality improvement renaissance.

Although the pandemic is officially over, we must remain vigilant. With emerging variants and periodic surges worldwide, SARS-CoV-2 may continue to impact us for the foreseeable future. We should continue vital public health measures, including virus tracking, genomic surveillance, and vaccine development.[39]

Meanwhile, urbanization, deforestation, and poorly regulated live animal and wet markets continue to pose a significant risk of zoonotic spillover, increasing the likelihood of emerging pandemic coronaviruses and other infectious threats.*[40]

Finally, the specter of another catastrophic influenza pandemic looms menacingly. US public health officials and infectious disease experts have recently become concerned over the spread of H5N1 avian influenza in livestock and agricultural workers in the United States. Already, there are worrisome signs that we haven't learned from our experience with COVID-19, as the initial response to this threat has left much to be desired. Lack of coordination between federal health agencies and uncertainty around jurisdictional boundaries have hindered a unified response to this threat. At the same time, a hesitation among farmers to cooperate with government agencies has impeded viral testing efforts, with many refusing health officials access to their livestock and personnel.[41] As a result, the actual number of cases involving dairy and agricultural workers remains unknown, and agencies like the US CDC have had to resort to testing samples of water runoff from farms and milk in supermarkets to track viral spread.[42] Making matters worse, the complex legal and sociopolitical environment around vaccines, much of which erupted during the COVID-19 pandemic, may significantly hamper future efforts to fast-track vaccine development, like Operation Warp Speed, in the event of another pandemic.[43]

As I write this in late winter 2025, H5N1 is still considered a low risk for the public. However, according to Dr. Nirav D. Shah, the CDC's former principal deputy director, "100 percent, that could change. This is a dangerous virus."†[44]

Historically, around half of all confirmed H5N1 infections in humans have been fatal, according to the World Health Organization, though most of those deaths occurred during earlier outbreaks.[45] The mortality figures in the United States have so far been far lower, but we still have much to learn about this evolving pathogen.

In North America, the currently circulating H5N1 group or *clade* 2.3.4.4b recently acquired mammalian-adaptive mutations and was linked to fatal infections in a thirteen-year-old girl in British Columbia and a sixty-five-year-old individual in Louisiana. In both cases, genomic analyses revealed additional mutations that enhanced the virus's ability to infect humans and cause severe illness. Meanwhile, from June 2024 to January 2025, the number of reported

---

*   See chapter six for more discussion on zoonotic spillover.

†   This is Nirav D. Shah, former acting principal deputy director of the US CDC, not former NY State Health Commissioner Nirav R. Shah from chapter fourteen.

human H5N1 cases increased twentyfold, from three to sixty-seven, emphasizing how quickly the situation could change.[46]

Such developments could represent a prelude to another pandemic. Yet according to James Lawler from the University of Nebraska's Global Center for Health Security, "where those were really supposed to trigger accelerated and amplified actions at the federal, state, and local levels, we've just kind of shrugged when each milestone has passed."[47] This confluence of events and a glaring lack of preparedness could usher in a pandemic disaster scenario that could make COVID-19 look like a walk in the park.

In addition to the infrastructural work being done by agencies like the CDC, another crucial pandemic preparedness strategy is public education. We need an army of trusted messengers and a massive media campaign to connect people with the science and history of vaccines, the germ theory of disease, and public health.[48] We should use these platforms to demystify what happens within the walls of hospitals so that the public can appreciate the ravages of viral sepsis from respiratory infections like COVID-19 and influenza. And we need better partnerships between government agencies and the public they serve—a fusion of science with values and idealism with pragmatism—to craft nuanced pandemic response systems for the future. This can't wait. We must do these things now because, when it comes to the threat of deadly pandemics, the past is prologue.

CHAPTER SEVENTEEN

What Really Matters

*Humans, by their nature, seek purpose—to make a contribution
and to be part of a cause greater and more enduring than themselves.*

—DANIEL PINK[1]

TODAY'S MEDICAL PROFESSION FACES IMMENSE challenges: healthcare inequality, the rising burden of chronic diseases, antimicrobial resistance, viral pandemics, and increasing burnout among frontline staff. Providing quality care has become more difficult, and finding fulfillment in this demanding environment can feel like an uphill battle.

Whenever I feel discouraged by the state of healthcare, I remind myself of the profound impact we have on our patients and their families. As Dave Schmidt noted years ago, healthcare professionals hold the unique privilege of improving lives—not only through direct patient care but also by building better systems through initiatives like the Surviving Sepsis Campaign. Thinking of this connects me to a greater purpose.

Like many of her colleagues, Amy Watts hit a wall toward the end of 2020. The COVID-19 pandemic showed no signs of letting up, and each shift brought an unending stream of sick and dying patients into the emergency room. Many of her teammates were burned out; some had already quit.[2]

Then, one evening in December, she unexpectedly received a three-page handwritten thank-you letter from Mickey. In it, he recounted an incredible journey through the hospital three years earlier, personally thanking Watts for her exceptional and compassionate care. With each line she read, his words warmed her. She later described it as "the most incredible thank you [she had] ever received from a patient." She immediately emailed Mickey to express her gratitude for the letter, then tucked it away in her bag, occasionally pulling it out to lift her spirits after tough shifts.[3]

As many of us clawed through that first pandemic winter, I felt even greater pressure to stay on track with our sepsis efforts. At times, I was of a single mind about reducing sepsis mortality. By then, our new sepsis alert system was in full force across our two metropolitan hospitals. The only question that remained was whether our efforts were truly making a difference.

In the spring of 2021, I teamed up with colleagues from Kaiser Permanente's Center for Health Research to examine whether the alert system had a measurable effect on our SEP-1 bundle performance and patient survival. We conducted a before-and-after analysis comparing risk-adjusted outcomes from patients seen two years before we launched the alert (2017 to 2018) with those seen two years after (2019 to 2020).[*]

I anxiously waited as our data analysts processed the numbers, finally unveiling a spreadsheet filled with tables and graphs, quantifying years of effort into numbers and percentages. As I scanned the results, I felt a surge of pride seeing that our SEP-1 rate had improved from 72 to 81 percent between the two time periods.[†][4] Yet, to my disappointment, our overall sepsis mortality remained unchanged at 7 percent.[‡][5]

---

[*] Sepsis patients were identified as those for whom the computer alert was activated or, in the case of the *before* patients, using the objective sepsis trigger criteria of our computer alert system. (See chapter fifteen.) Risk adjustment was performed using the Comorbidity Points Score (COPS), which assigns a score to patients based on the number of high-risk diagnoses they have. COVID-19 and influenza patients were excluded from this analysis.

[†] By comparison, the Medicare average SEP-1 performance at that time was 58 percent, while the Oregon state average was 54 percent.

[‡] The average *overall* in-hospital sepsis mortality in the US currently falls somewhere between 15 and 20 percent depending on the study, with a recent study estimating it at around 15 percent.

However, when we examined subgroups of patients, an important signal emerged. Looking at septic shock patients alone, their average mortality had dropped from 27 to 23 percent between the two periods, translating to one additional life saved for every twenty-five patients treated.* As one might expect, a subgroup analysis of non-shock sepsis patients showed that their mortality remained unchanged at 4 percent.†[6]

So, while the average result across our entire sepsis population showed no mortality improvement, embedded within the data was a subgroup of septic shock patients who appeared to benefit. This is consistent with other studies showing that the treatment effect of the bundles is most pronounced in the septic shock population.‡

What can we conclude from the lack of benefit in non-shock patients? For one, this group of patients already had very low baseline mortality. Thus, it's possible that our performance had plateaued in this population, making it difficult to decrease its mortality to less than 4 percent. Since this group made up most of our sepsis patients, the *overall* average mortality of our cohort remained unchanged.

The results also raise the issue of sepsis heterogeneity. Our sepsis population represented a diverse group of patients with an assortment of medical comorbidities and underlying infections—many subgroups of patients, each no doubt with different physiology and varying responses to common sepsis treatments. In the end, our results may reflect the problem of averages first discussed in chapter seven, with our treatment strategy benefitting some groups of patients but not others.

It also brings up another possibility—one I often dread. What if improving our SEP-1 performance in *non*-shock sepsis patients benefited the same number of patients it harmed? The net average result would be no benefit, but hidden within that result could be a harmful effect on some patients. Such effects could be hard to detect. Patients can sometimes die months after their

---

* There was also no difference in the average COPS score between the two groups.

† Some experts suggest caution when interpreting studies that cite such low overall sepsis mortality rates, as they may not be generalizable to the broader population. Our mortality rates are benchmarked closely against Kaiser Permanente Northern California.

‡ The system had a 27 percent positive predictive value or hit rate, meaning that just over one in four computer alerts was real. It also had a 99.5 percent negative predictive value, meaning patients had less than a 1 percent chance of developing sepsis if the alert didn't fire. By industry standards, that's about as good a result as possible.

first hospitalization. In these cases, how could we be sure it wasn't something we had or *hadn't* done that contributed to their death? How could we know if the treatment had been enough, too much, or the wrong formula? Questions like this would often keep me up at night.

There was another interesting finding worth noting. In cases where the ER doctor's final response to the alert was either "not sepsis" or "not sure," patients almost never developed sepsis. So, while our ER doctors were outstanding at spotting sepsis patients, they were also exceptional at recognizing when patients *didn't* have it. Thus, it was precisely the right move to give our frontline staff the ultimate say in who had sepsis. In other words, experience mattered, and we had now successfully combined clinical gestalt with a computer alert system.

Ultimately, I concluded that our electronic sepsis alert had led to a measurable improvement in SEP-1 bundle performance and was associated with decreased septic shock mortality. Our analysis suggests that the mortality benefit in septic shock patients was likely related to more timely sepsis care, as reflected through improved bundle performance, rather than differences between the patients themselves. I could also say that improving bundle performance was not associated with lower mortality in non-shock patients, and this may have been related to the heterogeneity of this population as well as its already low baseline mortality. Finally, the success we *did* have resulted from a blend of computer algorithms *and* human judgment, showing us that the best strategy was to combine the two.*

Our results align with decades of evidence showing that earlier, systematic treatment leads to better outcomes in sepsis patients. Historically, this benefit has been most visible in patients with septic shock—those who are the most severely ill and require the most urgent treatment. Larger databases also show that non-shock sepsis patients benefit from early treatment, though the signal here is weaker, with a smaller treatment effect.

SEP-1 allowed us to codify self-evident principles of sepsis care into routine medical practice, finally creating a standard operating procedure for these patients. This helped us more reliably deliver these basic principles of sepsis care.

The real question is, did SEP-1 have anything to do with our septic shock results? A purist would say this is unknown. *Causation versus correlation.* This

---

* Our data also showed that while the number of sepsis diagnoses (aka the denominator) increased over the first two years, it decreased over years three and four.

is often the issue in medical research. While our data are encouraging, they are purely observational. Without randomization, it's impossible to account for all the variables that could have influenced the results. All we can say is that improved SEP-1 performance correlated positively with better outcomes.

And while our before-and-after study was valuable in evaluating the computer alert's effect on SEP-1 performance, it could not fully account for the broader impact of our sepsis program. The computer alert was just one piece of a much wider effort, which included months of quality improvement committee work, countless meetings, emails, and presentations, and a massive sepsis awareness campaign.

In this sense, SEP-1 was more than just a performance measure or treatment paradigm; it became a catalyst, attracting attention and rallying support, driving meaningful change in sepsis care. Thus, the SEP-1 success rate may have served as an excellent proxy marker for our hospitals' *overall* structure and performance, positively tracking with other variables, such as faster screening and antibiotic and fluid administration rates.

But it takes more than just a system. The sepsis we currently refer to is a highly complex syndrome. Patients are often undifferentiated and can sometimes have vague signs and symptoms. Questions often remain: Do they have a bacterial infection? Is it viral? Is it something noninfectious, like congestive heart failure?

While a standard operating procedure like SEP-1 can help enable a systematic approach to sepsis patients, it cannot account for every detail, patient-specific factor, or clinical decision made by frontline providers, and it may sometimes be too blunt to apply in the same way to every patient. Much of the critical care must still happen at the bedside.

I'm reminded of a patient I cared for a few winters ago while working a late hospital shift. That night, a rapid response nurse called me to evaluate a seventy-year-old man named Joseph, who had developed a fever and severe respiratory distress two days after hip fracture surgery. Joseph's medical chart indicated that he had chronic congestive heart failure, meaning he had a severely weakened heart pump, making him especially vulnerable to fluid overload (the buildup of excess fluid in the lungs and cardiovascular system). After reviewing his chest X-ray, it was clear that Joseph was suffering from hospital-acquired pneumonia complicated by sepsis. Meanwhile, his blood pressure had plummeted, and his heart was racing. His blood lactate level, which the rapid response nurse had already ordered, was also elevated at 3.4 mmol/Liter.

I quickly ordered blood and sputum cultures and broad-spectrum antibiotics, including coverage for the type of resistant bacteria often seen in hospitals. Based on Joseph's cardiac history and my assessment that he needed intravenous fluid, I asked his nurse to administer a fluid bolus immediately. However, instead of the prescribed 30 milliliter/kilogram fluid bolus, which would have amounted to three liters of fluid, I asked her to give only *one* liter, hoping this would reduce the risk of fluid overload.

Joseph had also developed a terrible delirium and kept pulling off his oxygen mask. This exacerbated his labored breathing, and I feared his respiratory system would soon fail. On top of everything, he had a do-not-resuscitate or -intubate order, so he didn't want to be on life support or a mechanical ventilator, even if his life depended on it. This meant that we had a very narrow margin of error. Even the slightest misstep could lead to his death.

After confirming Joseph's wishes with his family over the telephone, I realized that my only hope was to sedate him just enough to help him tolerate his oxygen mask so he could weather the initial storm of his pneumonia. I knew this would be risky, so I called one of my ICU colleagues, Marty, for help.

Marty and I devised a plan to admit Joseph to the ICU for closer monitoring. We also provided a light dose of anxiety medication to help him tolerate the oxygen mask. Additionally, Marty developed a tailored pulmonary hygiene plan with the respiratory therapist to help clear Joseph's airways of mucus and other secretions.

Within an hour, Joseph was calmer and breathing comfortably with his mask. His blood pressure, heart rate, and lactate levels had all improved after the one-liter bolus, and a careful examination of his body's fluid status revealed that we had managed to thread the needle perfectly with that amount of fluid. By morning, he was breathing well without additional support and was less confused. Later that day, his blood cultures came back positive for a resistant strain of the gram-negative bacterium *Pseudomonas aeruginosa*—a common hospital-acquired pathogen. Fortunately, we had anticipated this possibility when prescribing the initial antibiotics. A few days later, he was discharged to a rehab facility and was home in another week, where he celebrated the arrival of a new grandson.

In medicine, no single recipe works for every patient. There can be dozens of moment-to-moment decisions rarely captured by clinical trials or observational data. In Joseph's case, there were at least a handful of clinical judgments that, had they been different, could have spelled disaster. While a framework is essential, we must also preserve space to practice medicine at the bedside, and the only way to do that is to infuse clinical autonomy and judgment into every corner of our healthcare system. Let both coexist. Surviving sepsis involves using systems to support experienced clinicians.

———

Hospitals have significantly improved their upfront sepsis care over the past decade, but certain patients still consistently fall through the cracks. As the broader sepsis movement has gained momentum in recent decades, experts have shifted their focus toward vulnerable groups and social determinants of health.

In 2020, a group led by epidemiologist Mohsen Naghavi from the University of Washington published a landmark study on the global burden of sepsis. In it, investigators carefully examined the World Health Organization's extensive Global Burden of Disease patient database in search of likely sepsis cases both inside and outside hospital settings.* The results were startling, with new figures surpassing previous estimates by over 100 percent, reaching a staggering forty-nine million annual sepsis cases and eleven million deaths worldwide. Additionally, this burden was disproportionately affecting low- to middle-income countries, which were often those most challenged in preventing, detecting, and treating sepsis.[7]

Geographic health disparities exist not only between nations but also in high-income countries like the United States. A 2008 study revealed that the risk of sepsis increased for Americans living in ZIP codes linked to higher poverty rates.[8] Sepsis and sepsis-related deaths are also more prevalent among US patients with publicly funded health insurance, such as Medicaid or Medicare, compared to those with private plans.[9]

Racial disparities continue to impact sepsis patient outcomes. Some of the discrepancies are linked to higher rates of chronic illness and poor access to primary and preventive care, while others stem from racial biases embedded within medical practice and technology.[10] For example, a large 2022 study

---

* This is the same Global Burden of Sepsis study discussed in chapter five.

published in *Critical Care Medicine* found that pulse oximetry—one of the primary tools for measuring blood oxygen levels—systematically overestimated blood oxygen levels in Asian, Black, and Hispanic patients compared to White patients.[11]

Health disparities have profound implications for both sepsis treatment and research. In this light, sepsis is not just a medical syndrome—it is also a social issue. It calls to mind the immortal words of French surgeon Jacques Tenon: "Hospitals are a measure of civilization."[12]

To truly combat sepsis, experts and policymakers must recognize the crucial role of social determinants of health in sepsis prevention. This means shaping societal infrastructure and allocating resources to close gaps in essential health services, such as access to clean drinking water, essential vaccinations, and primary care, while addressing racial disparities in sepsis detection and treatment.

As we saw in chapter ten, rich or poor, healthy or unhealthy, we all suffer the consequences of societal inequality.

———

Recent work into health disparities has also highlighted another vulnerable population: maternal patients. While numerous anatomical, physiological, and psychosocial factors make pregnancy a risky proposition, infections acquired during or shortly after pregnancy top the list in terms of these dangers.

For more than a decade, researchers have sounded the alarm over maternal sepsis. It is now recognized as the third leading cause of maternal death worldwide, responsible for about one in five deaths.[13] The numbers are similar in the United States. Even more troubling, nearly two-thirds of maternal sepsis deaths are preventable.[14]

Maternal sepsis underscores the challenge of detection in its purest form. The unique physiology of pregnancy means that the "normal" parameters that health professionals are used to seeing—a total white blood cell count, heart rate, or even blood pressure—are shifted drastically outside their normal ranges. For example, it isn't unusual for a healthy maternal patient to have a white blood cell count of 12,000 or a heart rate in the 90s, which would be considered positive SIRS criteria in a non-maternal patient. This reality makes traditional sepsis screening tests ineffective at detecting maternal sepsis—much like a lifeguard struggling to spot a distressed swimmer in turbulent waters.

Furthermore, pregnant and postpartum patients have often exhausted much of their body's reserves to sustain the pregnancy, leaving them particularly vulnerable during a medical emergency. As a result, once sepsis develops, it can rapidly escalate to septic shock, with devastating consequences. This stark reality is underscored by the alarming mortality rate of maternal septic shock, which exceeds 50 percent in some cases.[15]

Maternal patients also face significant health disparities, such as a lack of access to prenatal care and emergency reproductive medicine—gaps that are more likely to impact younger women and women of color.[16]

Too often, these individuals also become casualties of a society caught between competing values in reproductive health policy. On June 24, 2022, the US Supreme Court's decision in *Dobbs v. Jackson Women's Health Organization* overturned *Roe v. Wade*, effectively ending the Constitutional right to abortion. Experts immediately warned that this decision would raise maternal sepsis and mortality rates due to restricted access to critical healthcare during pregnancy-related emergencies.[17]

A recent investigation by ProPublica reported that, in the two years since Texas's abortion ban took effect, maternal sepsis rates have surged by a staggering 50 percent.[18] This alarming statistic underscores the urgent need to consider the real-world consequences of limiting reproductive healthcare access.

In 2016, responding to growing calls for urgency, the World Health Organization convened an expert panel to propose a global definition for maternal sepsis and provide guidance and support for sepsis programs worldwide.[19]

Meanwhile, the California Maternal Quality Care Collaborative (CMQCC), a multi-stakeholder organization formed in 2006 to prevent death, disability, and racial disparities in California maternal patients, began convening experts to develop toolkits for use in hospitals and clinics across the state to identify and treat maternal sepsis patients more quickly.

Unfortunately, the pandemic quelled early attempts to spark a meaningful transformation in maternal sepsis care.

So, when I received a call from our hospital's regional maternal nursing director in the spring of 2021 asking if I was interested in spearheading a Northwest regional maternal sepsis initiative, I was ecstatic. We got to work quickly, analyzing the problem, assembling a team of stakeholders, and developing screening criteria and treatment guidance tailored to the unique physiology of maternal patients.

A few years later, our program joined an expanding global movement, launching one of the first maternal sepsis initiatives in history—around two centuries after pioneers such as Alexander Gordon, Oliver Wendell Holmes, and Ignaz Semmelweis began sounding the alarm on puerperal sepsis.

———

By the summer of 2021, all eyes once again turned to the National Quality Forum (NQF) for SEP-1's scheduled maintenance review—a process that promised either continuance of the measure or its early retirement. The stakes were high. By then, sepsis had become recognized as a matter of public welfare, intersecting with the interests of government agencies, patients and families, physicians, hospitals, and the commercial industry. It was no longer an obscure syndrome compartmentalized to hospital wards.

As expected, there was vigorous debate between the measure's supporters and opponents.

Many academic experts, such as those in the Infectious Diseases Society of America (IDSA) and the American College of Emergency Physicians (ACEP), remained hesitant about the evidence backing the measure.* They felt that the wider sepsis population was far too heterogeneous to benefit from SEP-1's one-size-fits-all nature, which they felt overlooked the nuances of sepsis care. They also worried that it could result in antibiotic overuse and dangerous overtreatment with intravenous fluids.†[20] Their proposal? Modify the measure to focus only on septic shock patients—those who, based on the data, were the least undifferentiated on initial presentation and stood to benefit the most from the measure.‡[21]

At the same time, there were concerns that as the measure's arbiters, many

---

* They were joined by the American Hospital Association, Pediatric Infectious Disease Society, Society for Healthcare Epidemiology of America (SHEA), Society of Hospital Medicine, and Society of Infectious Disease Pharmacists.

† By 2021, Rivers and Townsend had already revised the measure to allow for an exception to the prescribed 30 mL/kg fluid bolus, which they announced during the review process on June 24, 2021.

‡ This is simplified but captures the general position. I encourage readers to delve deeper into the ACEP and IDSA position on SEP-1, which will be discussed in the next chapter. This coalition also proposed simplifying the time zero definition and removing serial lactate measurement from SEP-1.

of the NQF committee members lacked the expertise to fully appreciate the intricacies of sepsis and the measure's impact. Fueling these worries, several prominent sepsis experts on the panel had recused themselves from the deliberations due to conflicts of interest, leaving the remaining group deficient in content expertise on the measure's impact.[22]

Simultaneously, the measure's supporters, including a large coalition of patient safety and advocacy groups, such as the Sepsis Alliance and prominent patient safety organization the Leapfrog Group, stood strong with SEP-1's reported ability in large observational studies to reduce sepsis mortality, by extension saving potentially thousands of lives each year nationwide.[23] They called for its full re-endorsement.

Then came the meetings themselves—a real-life drama unfolding as the committee deliberated the merits of a measure that stood to either save or do little to nothing to help thousands of patients. Rivers and Townsend remained a strong presence throughout the review process. Their role was to be content experts, answering questions on the technical nature of the measure and the data. However, they quickly shifted their tenor, and as if battling for the very lives of the patients they hoped to save, waged an impassioned and at times heavy-handed defense of SEP-1.*[24]

Ultimately, the measure survived. The NQF voted to re-endorse it for another cycle. The decision was quickly appealed and then upheld in a subsequent vote the following spring.[25] At least for the time being, SEP-1 was here to stay.

Yet, with its complexity, ferocity, and devastation, sepsis had again managed to shock and dismantle even our most structured procedures for understanding and addressing it. In the end, the NQF's process broke down, leaving the medical community and many other stakeholders divided and disillusioned.†[26]

Stories about medical progress are also stories of the human condition. In *The Laws of Medicine,* Siddhartha Mukherjee writes, "Even as we train massive machines to collect, store, and manipulate data for us, humans are the final

---

*   According to NQF procedure, the measure's developers are present as content experts to respond to questions from the committee. They are not to argue for or against the measure. However, this did not happen, as the developers advocated heavily in favor of keeping the measure. During a committee meeting, one NQF member even asked if the measure's developers could be muted.

†   The CMS representative attending an October 13, 2021, meeting, Reena Duseja, stated, "You know, I think you need to take this back to NQF in terms of process. Because I'm observing this whole meeting, and we're not following the process here." A series of resignations followed the proceedings. By 2023, CMS had severed its relationship with the NQF.

observers, interpreters, and arbiters of that data."[27] Medicine's history is filled with conflicts, strong personalities, and sometimes questionable conduct.

Looking back, I think the more important story was that we were now debating in the public square over how to best care for sepsis patients rather than wondering why so many of them were dying. Years of sepsis awareness campaigns had finally shifted our attention upstream to a point earlier in the course of infection, either before patients developed sepsis or very early in their body's response to infection—so much so that in some cases, it was unclear whether they had sepsis at all.

And gradually, the collective impact of our efforts was becoming clearer. Sepsis registries worldwide demonstrated that frontline providers were saving thousands of additional lives each year. Awareness was growing. Success stories were spreading throughout the global community of sepsis programs, showing us that we were making a difference.

———

In the late summer of 2021, I was preparing a sepsis presentation for frontline physicians when I encountered a remarkable milestone: in the four years since 2017, the total number of sepsis survivors between our two Portland metropolitan hospitals had reached ten thousand. By then, our incremental efforts had slowly cut our overall mortality rate to approximately 10 percent below the average for Medicare patients nationwide. This translated to roughly a thousand additional lives saved over four years compared to the national average.*

I stopped what I was doing and just sat there for a moment. I thought about how a hundred years earlier—before antibiotics, vaccines, and infection control programs—sepsis had been almost invariably a death sentence. During my training two decades earlier, by the time we'd *seen* sepsis patients, their odds of survival had been no better than 50 percent. Now, in 2021, most of our patients lived to tell the tale. We had fundamentally changed how we approached this syndrome. Just like California lifeguards, we were forging a renaissance.

I found myself thinking more about our survivors—people like Mickey. Their stories brought me back to my own experience being rescued years earlier at Huntington Beach. At the same time, I thought about our frontline

---

* This estimate assumes an absolute mortality reduction of 10 percent.

providers, many of whom, like me, were exhausted and demoralized eighteen months into the pandemic. The relentless challenges had begun to erode our sense of purpose.

I realized it was time to share this extraordinary story. It wasn't just about the sepsis measure, the science, or the medicine—it was about the patients. Just as much as we were helping them, they were helping us, connecting us to something bigger than ourselves.

I scrapped my presentation and started over. After pulling together a few new slides, I called our Westside sepsis nursing leader, Jill, and asked: "Hey, this might be short notice, but do you think you could ask Mickey to come back and speak to our doctors this September?"

———

On Wednesday, September 1, 2021, I powered up my laptop to lead a virtual September Sepsis Awareness Month presentation. Our frontline hospital and emergency doctors were there, along with Mickey, who had accepted our invitation to speak. After a brief introduction, I quickly reviewed my files and began sharing my slide deck, presenting data on the cumulative impact of years of collective effort: *thousands* of lives saved.

Afterward, I shared my lifeguard rescue story, holding back tears as I recounted the ordeal—how it felt to be pulled back from the brink of death. I concluded:

"For those lifeguards, it was just another day at the office, but for me, it was the most significant day of my life."

Then I introduced Mickey. From the moment he began speaking, he captivated us with his powerful story. His passionate words cut through the numbness that had settled over so many of us during the past year and a half. He spoke about Amy Watts and the profound impact her care had had on him.

Moments later, Amy turned on her webcam, watching intently, her eyes misty with emotion. We all followed her lead one by one, switching on our cameras as if breaking through the cold distance of our virtual space. In that instant, we were connected to each other, bound by a shared truth: What we do every day matters. It matters to Mickey and thousands of others.

I continue to share this story with our frontline staff. Whether it's running a blood lactate result in the lab, sterilizing a hospital bed, attending an infection control meeting, crunching performance data, making moment-to-moment clinical decisions on the front line, or even washing our hands, we each contribute to a system that watches over and protects us. When we take a step back to see this larger structure, we're connected to something bigger than our individual existence.

Former New York Health Commissioner Nirav Shah once said, "There is a great power of interdependence . . . the sum can be greater than its parts, and when we share responsibility, real progress can be made."[28]

And when we get it right, it shines—just like that first glimpse of Emily swimming toward me at Huntington Beach, or when New York hospitals saved thousands of lives within two years of launching their state sepsis initiative. Something is out there keeping us safe, and we're building it together.

CHAPTER EIGHTEEN

Getting It Right

I am not here to be right. I am here to get it right.

—BRENÉ BROWN[1]

TO UNDERSTAND THE STATE of sepsis care today, you have to talk to critical care physicians—those who witness the syndrome at its most advanced stages. And lately, ICU doctors have been asking a surprising question: "Where's all the sepsis we used to see?"[2]

As recently as the early 2000s, sepsis often went unrecognized until it was too late. Patients would arrive at the ICU critically ill—or die in the hospital without ever receiving a diagnosis. But as our understanding deepened, we came to see sepsis not merely as an infection, but as the body's overwhelming and dysregulated response to one. That shift in perspective paved the way for systems designed to detect the syndrome in its earliest, most treatable stages.

Earlier recognition, better diagnostics like lactate testing, and more objective definitions helped shift the paradigm. We began catching cases sooner, treating them faster, and seeing improved outcomes. Sepsis emerged not just as a catastrophic ICU condition, but as a broad continuum ranging from organ dysfunction to life-threatening shock.

As Laura Evans reflects, "In 1999, sepsis patients came to the ICU on death's door. Today, they arrive looking very different—thanks to earlier treatment in the ED."[3]

In that sense, our understanding and perception of sepsis has evolved.

It is now the third decade since the Surviving Sepsis Campaign's (SSC) Barcelona Declaration. We have established a standard of care centered on early recognition and treatment and are seeing more sepsis patients surviving each year. In the United States, we have adopted a national sepsis measure, more states like New York are passing sepsis regulations, and most hospitals have dedicated sepsis programs. Patient advocacy groups are also bringing the syndrome to the forefront of public discourse. These days, more patients, families, and healthcare professionals are routinely asking the question, "Could it be sepsis?" In short, we're making progress.[4]

But we're far from the finish line. On average, nearly one in five sepsis patients dies worldwide. While the Centers for Medicare and Medicaid Services (CMS) has made sepsis management a part of US federal policy with SEP-1, adherence to sepsis treatment bundles has been suboptimal at around 60 percent, with huge variation in performance between hospitals.[5] The disparity in sepsis outcomes is also startling, with the average mortality rate ranging from as low as 4 percent to as high as 25 percent across healthcare systems.[6] What's more, of the 1.3 million sepsis survivors each year in the United States, many are left with lifelong disability, 25 percent are readmitted to the hospital within three months, and nearly half die within five years—outcomes that rival those of many common cancers.[7]

Doctors still disagree on how to define and measure sepsis. Though many experts attribute improved patient outcomes to timelier sepsis bundles, others worry that it's a statistical mirage. This, combined with the potential for unintended consequences, such as misdiagnosis and antibiotic overuse, has led multiple medical societies to continue opposing the rigorous adoption of these bundles, as well as quality measures like SEP-1.

Meanwhile, we're faced with an increasingly complex modern healthcare system, an aging population with soaring medical comorbidities, shortages in healthcare staffing and resources, persistent health inequity, an ever-growing list of dangerous drug-resistant pathogens, and a continuing threat of deadly viral pandemics. Each of these stands to contribute to a rising sepsis burden in one way or another, making sepsis a true case study for our entire healthcare system and society.

So, where do we go from here?

The evidence tells us we *can* make a difference. Decades of research have shown that most sepsis patients die simply because we're late to the game when treating them. By looking for objective signs of the body's abnormal response to infection, we've begun to identify the proverbial sepsis tipping point sooner, leading to faster treatment, which, for the most part, has led to improved survival. In just twenty-five years, we've seen the enormous impact that sepsis quality improvement programs have had on the lives of our patients.

But we still need to do this more reliably and identify patients earlier in the course of their illness. Today, our best definition of sepsis still requires the presence of organ injury, and isn't that already a little too late?[8]

We've also realized that sepsis is a complex and heterogeneous syndrome arising from a multitude of infections, each with its own way of triggering the body's defense systems while affecting a diverse range of patients. Thus, it is crucial that we not only improve the speed of recognition but also enhance our ability to identify precisely what it is we're treating.

This will require a high level of coordination among academic medical societies, government agencies, the medical industry, patients, and families. It means innovation married with good science, ethics, and regulation—and learning lessons from history. It will demand greater collaboration between health systems and healthcare professionals across diverse regions, significant increases in research funding, and sepsis advocacy. It's what the former head of the Institute for Healthcare Improvement, Dr. Kedar Mate, calls a socio-technical problem—one that requires a combination of technology, science, and people-centered solutions.[9]

Now more than ever, we must unite in our efforts to improve healthcare delivery while sustaining this commitment into the foreseeable future. All the pieces are in place; we just need to bring them together. We have to do this because it matters to our patients, families, and future.

In the words of Dr. Ronald Kline, Chief Medical Officer of the CMS Quality Measurement and Value-based Incentives Group, "This is a fight worth having."[10]

———

Measuring what we do in medicine is crucial, but the measurements must be calibrated constantly. Even minor measurement errors can lead us astray. As much as we want to believe that our intuition with sepsis will always match reality—that our quality improvement efforts are categorically working—I think it's important to be honest about the data's limitations. This doesn't necessarily mean we should abandon quality measures like SEP-1, but it does suggest that we should strive to improve our measurement standard so we can capture better data to help draw the right conclusions.

While large initiatives like the SSC have linked falling sepsis mortality rates to the timely delivery of sepsis bundles, this might not be the whole story. These programs have also raised sepsis awareness, identifying more cases involving less severely ill patients. This could skew the data toward lower mortality, leading us to overattribute the outcome results to our interventions while also concealing any potential harm signals buried in the data.[*][11]

We have a wealth of data showing that early sepsis treatment leads to better survival, but it's not black and white.[†][12] For example, what kind of infection was it? Did the physician select the correct antibiotic? Was it appropriately dosed? Was the fluid resuscitation adequate? Was it too much? When it comes to *urgency* in sepsis treatment, there's a one-size-fits-all strategy: *do it now*. But as we've seen, dozens of uncaptured details exist within that urgent response. We need a general framework to help us approach this condition quickly, but we also need to create the space for clinical judgment on a case-by-case basis.

Measuring our sepsis efforts comes with inherent challenges. Patients and hospitals are different, and as observers, we are biased. We need a way to measure sepsis we can agree on, so at the end of the day, we're all talking about the same thing.

When measuring the quality of our sepsis care, we should consider not only process but also outcomes. We should also look at the structures or systems in place to deliver care—so-called structural measures—while considering potential unintended consequences or balancing measures.

Sepsis bundles exemplify process-based care—a standard operating procedure for sepsis that promotes the rapid delivery of lifesaving therapies like

---

[*]   Patients with higher medical complexity have higher baseline mortality. Thus, when the data show us an association between low bundle compliance and high mortality, we must ask ourselves: is low bundle compliance itself causing death, is it a correlation, or is it both? While researchers have attempted to rigorously adjust for such factors using sophisticated statistical tools such as propensity matching, many of these confounders can still lurk in the data, potentially skewing the results.

[†]   Sepsis bundles are more difficult to complete in sicker patients with higher medical complexity. Such patients tend to have vaguer symptoms and lack classic signs of infection, such as fever, leading to delays in diagnosis and treatment. Physicians may also withhold certain therapies, such as fluids, in sicker patients to avoid precipitating complications, such as fluid overload.

antibiotics and intravenous fluids. In the words of one of the SEP-1 developers, Sean Townsend, "[They are] a structured way of thinking about the disease to help people maneuver and start treating it."[13] I hope the stories in this book have shown how crucial it is to have a systematic approach to sepsis. Process measures like SEP-1 have held hospitals and staff accountable for having these practices in place.

Yet for all their merits, sepsis bundles, and by extension, SEP-1, have produced mixed results. As we saw in chapter seventeen, improved SEP-1 compliance at Kaiser Permanente Northwest was linked to lower mortality in patients with septic shock, but *overall* sepsis mortality remained unchanged. The national experience has mirrored this pattern: while compliance rates have risen, consistent improvements in patient outcomes across the broader sepsis population have largely failed to materialize.

Is it that bundles are fundamentally problematic? Not likely. A better explanation is that sepsis treatment is highly nuanced. Each patient brings unique pathogens, host factors, and potential complications. If bundles aren't paired with sound clinical judgment, they may not work for every patient and can result in unintended consequences, such as fluid overload. Physicians should be granted leeway to craft a tailored approach to individual patients. This suggests that we may need to reimagine rigid, *all-or-nothing* bundles, like SEP-1, to allow for greater flexibility in how they are delivered.

For instance, there's little doubt that sepsis patients need urgent resuscitation with intravenous fluids, but data on the exact *formula* are unclear. Studies show that up to half of sepsis patients may not respond favorably to fluid boluses at all.[14] Large fluid boluses may also lead to fluid overload in some sepsis patients, such as those with congestive heart failure.*[15] When it comes to administering intravenous fluids in sepsis, context matters. This syndrome may be too

---

* Small randomized clinical trials have shown that protocolizing prescribed fluid boluses may harm certain patient populations, particularly those in low-resource settings or with underlying conditions such as malnutrition. Caution is warranted, however, when generalizing these findings to the broader sepsis population. For example, sepsis expert Dr. Hallie Prescott has noted that in one African trial (SSSP-2), many patients were likely underweight—inferred from mid-upper arm circumference measurement, since scales were not available. As a result, the prescribed fluid boluses may have amounted to 50 to 80 milliliters per kilogram, disproportionately large for their body size, and far greater than the 30 milliliter per kilogram bolus recommended by the SSC. In the context of severe malnutrition, with fragile vasculature and reduced oncotic pressure, such large fluid boluses could predispose patients to capillary leak and fluid overload.

heterogeneous for a prescribed fluid approach.*[16] Today, most sepsis experts agree that while a larger, weight-based fluid bolus is a reasonable approach in many cases, it's not the right therapy for *all* patients.

Ambiguity around fluid resuscitation has led to significant recent changes in the sepsis landscape. The SSC recently downgraded the prescribed 30 milliliter per kilogram fluid bolus from a strong to a *weak* recommendation based on the low quality of evidence supporting the practice.[17] Commensurately, in 2021, the SEP-1 developers relaxed the fluid bolus requirement in the national sepsis measure, permitting physicians to withhold or modify the therapy based on their discretion as long as they also document an exception in the medical chart. Such exceptions to the rules give physicians credit for using their clinical judgment.

As for antibiotics, physicians must balance the need for urgent antimicrobial therapy with the potential harms of overexposure. In addition, many suspected sepsis patients are undifferentiated in the early stages, without a clear diagnosis. This makes it difficult for physicians to avoid overtreating some of them. In fact, studies now show that as many as a third of patients treated for "possible sepsis" end up having viral infections, which don't require antibiotics, or *non-infectious* conditions that were never sepsis in the first place.[18]

In its most recent position paper, the Infectious Diseases Society of America (IDSA) cited several observational studies showing increased use of broad-spectrum antibiotics in hospitals after SEP-1 was implemented.[19] This suggests that doctors are more willing to prescribe so-called "big-gun" antibiotics in response to the added time pressure of the national measure and a desire to cover for all possible pathogens (as recommended by the SSC).

The largest of these studies, led by researcher Amy Pakyz from Virginia Commonwealth University, looked at 111 academic hospitals and showed that there was a short-term increase in the use of antibiotics by 1.4 percent immediately after SEP-1 was released, driven mainly by a 2.3 percent increase in broad-spectrum antibiotics targeting multi-drug-resistant bacteria. This was

---

*   There are also many hidden variables confounding the data on fluid resuscitation. For instance, sepflation could disguise a harmful signal in the data by averaging out healthier patients with sicker patients, making it seem that a prescribed approach works when it harms a small subgroup within the group. This could skew the data in favor of a more aggressive fluid approach. On the other hand, septic shock patients are more likely to receive fluids earlier because they're more obviously sick. Since shock patients are also more likely to die, this could tilt the data against early fluid administration.

followed by a smaller long-term increase in multi-drug-resistant antibiotic use of 0.4 percent per month.[20]

Other data suggest that sepsis bundles don't always lead to antibiotic overuse. A recent 2022 study examining over 270,000 sepsis patients across 152 hospitals showed that between 2013 and 2018, the time to first antibiotic dose decreased by an average of thirty-seven minutes, while overall antibiotic use *also* decreased in the same period.* The authors concluded that increasing antibiotic urgency didn't necessarily lead to indiscriminate antibiotic use.[21]

Antibiotic overprescription is a legitimate concern, but it must be understood within the context of a complex clinical reality. For one, studies examining antibiotic prescribing are vulnerable to any number of confounders. As a case in point, antimicrobial resistance has been a problem for decades. Thus, increased use of broad-spectrum antibiotics could reflect greater awareness of antimicrobial resistance irrespective of sepsis. One of the studies the IDSA cited in their recent sepsis position paper showed a preexisting trend toward increased broad-spectrum antibiotic use, independent of SEP-1.[22]

It should also be noted that, while there's a tendency to blame only antibiotic overuse for antimicrobial resistance, the situation may be more complicated. Many forms of antibiotic misuse can contribute to resistance.[23] For example, physicians can make errors in antibiotic dosing, administration route, treatment duration, or class of antibiotic used.

Finally, and perhaps most importantly, until we have more sophisticated tests to rapidly diagnose suspected sepsis patients, overtreatment may be a necessary price to pay so that we save that one *additional* patient like Rory Staunton. Considering this, we should all ask ourselves: even if the evidence is low quality, would we rather risk overtreating or undertreating patients?

Ultimately, the preponderance of evidence suggests that bundles, like those embodied in SEP-1, can be effective instruments for encouraging rapid antibiotic administration for sepsis patients. However, they work best when hospitals combine them with antibiotic stewardship programs and decision-support tools to assist physicians in selecting and dosing antibiotics.

In this light, US government agencies have recently assumed a more active role in guiding antibiotic therapy. In 2014, the CDC published *Core Elements of Hospital Antibiotic Stewardship Programs*, which provides resources and direction

---

* Specifically, antibiotic use within forty-eight hours, total days of antimicrobial therapy, and receipt of broad-spectrum antibiotics all decreased.

to hospitals as they develop antibiotic stewardship programs (ASPs).[24] One year later, the federal government released its *National Action Plan for Combating Antibiotic-Resistant Bacteria*, which included expanding evidence-based practices for reducing antibiotic resistance, such as requiring ASPs for all federally funded hospitals.[25] Through partnerships with other organizations, like the National Quality Forum and the Joint Commission, the CDC has fostered a surge in antibiotic stewardship nationwide, with 85 percent of hospitals boasting high-quality ASPs by 2018.*[26] Meanwhile, the Agency for Healthcare Research and Quality (AHRQ) has also developed antibiotic stewardship toolkits, including "Four Moments of Antibiotic Decision Making," to help embed high-quality antibiotic prescribing practices into the daily routine of frontline medicine.[27]

We now see evidence that antimicrobial resistance rates can decrease when sepsis programs are tied to good antibiotic stewardship. The Pakyz study also showed that *C. difficile* rates decreased by just over 7 percent during the same period. This suggests that any negative effects from the observed increase in antibiotic prescribing may have been offset by hospital infection control and antimicrobial stewardship programs.[28] In addition, when the CDC recently analyzed antimicrobial resistance trends across a large cohort of 890 US hospitals, it found that the incidence of hospital-acquired infections involving multiple resistant bacterial species declined between 2012 and 2017.† Although its authors didn't specifically examine the reasons for this reduction, they speculated that it was most likely due to enhanced hospital infection-control procedures.[29]

While we're at it, we might want to focus on lower-hanging fruit when addressing the general problem of antibiotic overuse. For instance, 85 to 95 percent of human antibiotic use in the United States occurs *outside* the hospital.[30] The numbers are similar in Europe.[31] According to the CDC, out of the roughly 256 million antibiotic prescriptions dispensed each year from US community pharmacies, about a third are unnecessary.[32] If you consider the risk-benefit analysis of withholding antibiotics in a clinic patient with a common cold, it's much more palatable than that of a sepsis patient in the hospital or emergency room who might, on average, have a 20 percent chance of dying.

---

* In 2019, CMS also issued a federal regulatory requirement for hospitals to have antimicrobial stewardship programs.

† Another large study looking at 138 US Veterans Affairs Medical Centers from 2007 to 2022 showed a significant drop in antibiotic resistance across multiple bacterial species, correlating with the expansion of infection control and antimicrobial stewardship programs. (See endnote 29.)

Furthermore, as mentioned in chapter five, the lion's share of antibiotic use worldwide is in industrial farming. In the US, there has been some progress toward regulating antibiotics in this context, with the FDA banning certain antibiotics in poultry and providing nonbinding guidance to farmers to refrain from using antibiotics as growth promoters. European regulators have taken further steps by banning antibiotics for livestock growth promotion.*[33]

———

On February 1, 2023, CMS announced the decision to move SEP-1 into its Value-Based Purchasing program, which ties hospital payments directly to sepsis bundle performance—a move that signaled a strong commitment to improving sepsis quality nationwide.

Dr. Kline, who leads CMS's sepsis work, says, "When you attach money to things in hospitals, people start paying attention."[34]

Supporters of SEP-1 have applauded the decision, as they believe it will further boost efforts to improve sepsis recognition and treatment and, by extension, save more lives. Yet multiple medical societies have opposed the move, primarily citing concerns over the low quality of evidence backing the measure, the risk that it could lead to financially-motivated overtreatment, and because it could encourage hospitals to further divert resources away from more comprehensive approaches to sepsis care as they strive to improve compliance.[35]

Tension between the measure's potential and the realities of the data has long fueled the SEP-1 debate, with clinical studies failing to definitively show that improving compliance leads to better outcomes. Controversy continues to this day, with newer studies raising more questions than answers. For instance, a large systematic review of seventeen studies published in February 2025 in the *Annals of Internal Medicine* failed to show any moderate- or high-quality evidence linking SEP-1 compliance to sepsis mortality.[36] It's also important to note that, as we've seen throughout this saga, for a multitude of reasons—the vast heterogeneity of sepsis patients being the most prominent—it has often

---

*   Such restrictions may constrain farmers and increase food prices. However, the return on investment may justify this action, as experts estimate that even a 1 percent reduction in antibiotic efficacy could levy costs of $600 billion to $3 trillion in lost human health. These savings could be shared with farmers as subsidies for better antimicrobial stewardship.

been very challenging to consistently link timely bundled care to improved outcomes. Nevertheless, medical societies like the IDSA believe that the evidence supporting SEP-1 is simply not there.

As for the issue of financially-driven overcompliance, as we painfully learned from past measures like the TFAD pneumonia measure, pay-for-performance programs can come with unintended consequences. At the same time, frontline physicians want to do what's best for patients, and as we learned in chapter seventeen, experienced doctors have the clinical gumption to know when and when *not* to initiate specific therapies. Recent data also suggest that physicians have since learned from their experience with programs like TFAD and are less likely to overtreat patients just to meet the metrics.* So it's not a foregone conclusion that it will happen.

There is little doubt that building and maintaining the systems necessary to deliver timely sepsis bundles, combined with the resources necessary for data reporting, have placed a significant burden on hospitals, particularly those in low-resource settings. Introducing financial penalties for undercompliance could exacerbate this problem. It may also risk further diverting resources from other crucial hospital programs, such as ASPs, as well as shifting the focus of hospitals away from a more comprehensive approach to caring for sepsis patients.

There are also many nonclinical issues that impact SEP-1 compliance. The healthcare front line is a complicated environment with many moving parts, and sepsis is a complex syndrome. SEP-1 is also one of history's most intricate quality measures—recall that the measure's original specifications manual for hospital data abstraction was a mind-boggling 51 pages long, with a 393-page supplemental guidebook. If you ask any sepsis leader like myself, we can cite any number of nonmedical and sometimes flat-out inane reasons why hospitals fail the bundle, including documentation errors and computer glitches. While a hardship for many healthcare systems, this reality may present an existential challenge to smaller hospitals with fewer resources, leaving them vulnerable to significant revenue loss related to value-based purchasing programs.[37]

Additionally, in a small but significant subset of patients, it is simply unsafe

---

* One argument in favor of this is that, while adherence to SEP-1 has improved in recent years, overall average compliance rates have remained low at around 60 percent, suggesting that doctors are unwilling to comply with the measure just to pass. But some experts believe this could change once there are financial incentives in place.

to complete the bundles because it could harm the patient. Early on, this was a much larger issue when the measure lacked appropriate exceptions for safety concerns such as fluid overload. Yet, even today, because of the measure's all-or-nothing nature, it is a common explanation for lower compliance rates.

Almost a decade after its release, SEP-1's developers have significantly modified the measure to better accommodate the realities of frontline medicine. Hospitals are also adapting and developing new systems, like our computer sepsis alert at Kaiser Permanente Northwest, to meet the measure's requirements. Meanwhile, innovative companies are emerging to help hospital systems meet the measure and track performance.

All that said, SEP-1 has only been the first iteration of a national sepsis measure—a prominent example of the SSC bundles put into a regulatory framework. It may be a bit clunky and convoluted. But that's partly due to the nature of regulations, which often function like rigid fragments of law.[38] This is not to mention the fact that the measure has aimed to define and tackle one of the most elusive syndromes of all time—no easy task.

Meanwhile, SEP-1 has undeniably led to greater attention to sepsis and catalyzed the growth of sepsis programs across the country. And while the data are mixed, there are many studies linking bundle compliance to improved mortality, particularly in septic shock patients. In our experience in the Northwest, bundles helped us improve the reliability of our sepsis care, and this was also associated with reduced septic shock mortality.

SEP-1 is not the end, but the beginning. While it's clear that hospitals should be held accountable for their sepsis care, moving forward, the real questions are: What should that accountability look like? How should it be enforced? And how can we fine-tune our measures to better reflect the realities of the front line?

For example, instead of focusing on tedious processes like a highly specific 30 milliliter per kilogram intravenous fluid bolus, as well as all the documentation required to stay in compliance, perhaps we could implement a broader "time to recognition and treatment" metric that measures how fast hospitals identify and treat a sepsis patient, without requiring a prescribed approach. Maybe it's also time to start looking at other ways of gauging success besides process measures.

This brings us to outcomes. In July 2022, CMS announced its plans to develop a sepsis mortality measure, which now falls under its electronic Clinical Quality Measures (eCQM) program. The measure is still in the development phase and, once approved, will require participating hospitals to electronically report risk-adjusted sepsis mortality as a performance measure.* In principle, the adjustment should allow for an apples-to-apples comparison of sepsis survival across different hospitals in the United States. Its electronic nature would also make it a more objective and less burdensome method of reporting performance than manual hospital data abstraction.[39]

Many experts and organizations have praised this move, as they feel that an outcome measure may better indicate a hospital's *overall* sepsis performance.[40] If you're demonstrably saving lives, then you're likely acing sepsis. Instead of focusing only on a specific set of proficiencies in complying with process measures like SEP-1, hospitals would have to harness their *entire* system, from emergency room triage to hospital discharge, to ensure that patients are recognized early, treated promptly, and adequately cared for throughout their stay, thus enabling the best possible outcomes.

Nevertheless, there are important considerations with such an outcome measure, none more important than the issue of how we define sepsis for reporting purposes. As we've seen throughout this book, harmonizing sepsis definitions, the so-called apples-to-oranges comparison problem, has repeatedly stifled sepsis clinical research and quality improvement efforts. The current CMS sepsis definition requires a patient to have two out of four SIRS criteria, an ICD-10 infection diagnosis code, and objective evidence of organ dysfunction. However, the issue with this definition is that SIRS, while a fairly good screening test for severe infection and *possible* sepsis, does not provide enough specificity to confidently identify sepsis patients and may result in too many false positives. Additionally, as we saw in chapter fifteen, relying on diagnosis codes to identify sepsis patients could be problematic due to sepflation.

This also ties into the risk adjustment component of an outcome measure, which works by assigning risk scores to patients based on medical comorbidities

---

* Many outcome measures use thirty-day mortality as the outcome, which is feasible when focusing on Medicare beneficiaries, but it may lead to long lag times for results involving non-Medicare patients. The proposed sepsis outcome measure, which was developed by the CDC in partnership with Harvard Pilgrim Health Care Institute, uses *in-hospital death or discharge to hospice* as the outcome, which allows for faster turnaround and feedback to hospitals while including a broader patient population. Studies show that this proposed outcome measure has a strong correlation with thirty-day sepsis mortality.

and diagnosis codes, similar to the COPS score from chapter seventeen.[*] Risk adjustment scores are used to adjust the raw mortality, depending on how sick patients look on paper.[†] One unintended consequence of this is that hospitals with more efficient clinical documentation programs can game the system through better bookkeeping. This means that, on average, the individual risk scores assigned to their patients would be higher, making their patients appear sicker and resulting in lower *adjusted* mortality scores.[41]

To address some of these challenges and facilitate better identification of sepsis cases in hospitals, the CDC recently developed a sepsis surveillance definition called the Adult Sepsis Event (ASE).[‡][42] The ASE was designed as an epidemiologic sepsis definition using only objective criteria—not diagnosis codes—thus filtering out subjectivity and gaming, which can skew data toward softer sepsis diagnoses (aka sepflation).[§][43] It also excludes SIRS criteria from the definition, as the CDC feels that SIRS is far too common and nonspecific to accurately identify sepsis patients. CMS is now working closely with the CDC to align its definition of sepsis with the ASE.[¶][44]

Electronic outcome measures are also limited by the data quality in the analyzed databases and the compatibility or "interoperability" of the different computer systems used. For instance, when Harvard researchers applied risk adjustment models to two large deidentified patient databases—Cerner

---

[*]   See chapter eight for a discussion on the mortality ratio.

[†]   Risk-adjustment scores can also consider objective disease-severity markers, like those captured by the APACHE score from chapter eight.

[‡]   An astute observer might point out that there seem to be many *types* of sepsis definitions. According to US CDC sepsis expert Dr. Raymund Dantes, it may be "appropriate to have multiple definitions of sepsis for different purposes." In fact, when a group of high-level sepsis experts met in 2016 to discuss a framework for defining sepsis, they concluded that there were several different areas within the broader sepsis campaign—for example, clinical care, basic research, surveillance, and quality improvement—each of which required slightly different definitions of the syndrome.

[§]   ASE criteria: (1) Presumed serious infection (blood culture and administration of antibiotics (including at least one parenteral/intravenous antibiotic) within +/- two days of blood culture day and continued for ≥ four days or until ≤ one day before death, discharge to another hospital or hospice, or transition to comfort care), and (2) Organ dysfunction (≥ one of the following within +/- two days of blood culture day): (a) Initiation of vasopressors, (b) Initiation of mechanical ventilation, (c) Doubling in serum creatinine or a decrease of ≥ 50% of estimated glomerular filtration rate relative to baseline, (d) Total bilirubin ≥2 mg/dL and doubling from baseline, (e) Platelet count <100,000 and a ≥50% decline from baseline (baseline must be ≥100,000), (f) Serum lactate ≥2.0 mmol/L.

[¶]   Even the ASE has limitations—for example, its requirement for a blood culture order in the chart may result in missed cases where no blood cultures were obtained.

HealthFacts and HCA Healthcare network—they found data elements often missing, such as vital signs and blood lactate results.[45] Recall that one of the more critical technical barriers to the widespread adoption of the 1980s APACHE II risk prediction tool from chapter eight was that it was incompatible with many existing hospital electronic health record systems.[46]

Fortunately, according to US CDC sepsis expert Dr. Raymund Dantes, significant recent advances in data interoperability have occurred. The agency is tapping into these improved data interoperability standards, such as Fast Healthcare Interoperability Resources (FHIR), which allows patients, clinicians, and quality improvement leaders to rapidly and securely access health record data. In fact, the CDC's National Healthcare Safety Network (NHSN) is currently leveraging FHIR to develop digital quality measures such as the proposed sepsis outcome measure, allowing electronic data to flow automatically from hospital electronic health record systems into the CDC's national surveillance platform. Experts are also imagining ways FHIR could be optimized for research purposes. The future thus holds great promise in granting quality improvement leaders and researchers better access to patient data—enabling them to draw better conclusions about sepsis treatment effects and keep patients better informed about their healthcare.[47]

Another drawback to a mortality outcome measure is that mortality is not necessarily the only way to measure success or failure in sepsis treatment.[48] Sepsis is deadly, but it's also associated with organ and limb injury and physical, cognitive, and emotional disability. Focusing only on survival may underemphasize these other outcomes. This has led some experts, like Laura Evans, to suggest that we should continue to measure and improve our performance when it comes to sepsis processes like bundles while fine-tuning our approach as the data evolve.[49]

Eventually, we must move beyond the goal of merely *surviving* sepsis and begin to measure what comes after. *Functional* outcomes, such as physical recovery, cognitive function, and quality of life, should become central to how we evaluate success. Expanding the time horizon to include longer-term mortality, hospital readmissions, and post-discharge impairments will give us a fuller picture of sepsis's lasting impact and help us design systems that support patients not just in the hospital, but throughout their recovery.*[50]

---

*   There is emerging evidence that multidisciplinary rehabilitation programs may benefit sepsis patients after discharge from the hospital. One recent program based in North Carolina,

Sepsis researcher Colonel Ian Stewart said it best during the 2023 End Sepsis National Sepsis Forum: "One of the issues with sepsis is that we view it as this one thing when it's clearly a continuum . . . the chronic morbidity associated with it is still a phase of sepsis."[51]

Even if you do everything right, you are still dealing with significant injury to patients, often leaving those who survive the initial phase of treatment with lasting impairment. Many sepsis patients also have other comorbidities, like diabetes, heart failure, and chronic kidney disease. This means there may be a ceiling in terms of the benefits of sepsis treatment. Thus, the next phase of sepsis innovation might involve *post-acute* sepsis care—after the initial hospitalization.

In the words of Derek Angus, "Now we need a get-up and get-out-of-bed juice for these patients."[52]

Regulators are beginning to recognize this need. CMS recently contracted with Yale New Haven Health Services Corporation's Center for Outcomes Research and Evaluation (CORE) to develop a sepsis readmission measure. In theory, such a measure would expand hospital accountability beyond discharge, reflecting a more integrated view of sepsis patients as they move through the healthcare system.[53]

I would be remiss if I didn't also acknowledge one of the hardest lessons I've learned in practicing medicine: for some patients, a diagnosis of sepsis marks the beginning of an end-of-life scenario. In such cases, our interventions may do little more than delay the inevitable, and it becomes essential to have an honest, compassionate conversation about death and dying.

Meanwhile, it's time for a national *pediatric* sepsis measure. Until now, SEP-1 has excluded children, as there has historically been limited evidence supporting best practices in pediatric sepsis. But times have changed. In 2020, the Surviving Sepsis Campaign (SSC) released its first international sepsis guidelines for children. Four years later, an international task force of pediatric sepsis experts developed the most comprehensive definition of pediatric sepsis in history, the Phoenix Sepsis Criteria.[54]

The Children's Hospital Association—an integrated network of pediatric hospitals across the United States—recently published results of a large-scale quality improvement initiative called the Improving Pediatric Sepsis Outcomes Collaborative, looking at the association between sepsis bundle compliance

---

called Sepsis Transition and Recovery (STAR), is showing promising preliminary results such as improved sepsis mortality after discharge.

and survival in pediatric sepsis. It showed that, as bundle compliance improved, the mortality rate in suspected sepsis patients dropped by a third, while it was cut in *half* in patients with septic shock.[55] Armed with this guidance, we're well-positioned for a national pediatric sepsis measure.

At the same time, a small but significant subset of children dies from sepsis despite our best treatment strategies. This special group of patients who develop sepsis with multiple-organ dysfunction syndrome (MODS) represents around 20 percent of all cases and keeps pediatric intensive care researchers like Scott Weiss awake at night. According to Weiss, most children with sepsis improve with rapid, early basic therapies, such as antibiotics and fluids. However, despite those therapies, children with MODS often fail to improve.

As Weiss, whose research focuses on mitochondrial dysfunction as a contributor to MODS in sepsis, explains, "Many of these kids just don't get better, and that's the group for whom there is a pathophysiology that we don't entirely yet understand, and that we're not targeting with our current therapeutic armamentarium."*

Weiss believes additional research will identify "new therapeutic targets that could save some children." He says, "I wish there were more attention from granting agencies and philanthropies paid to that subset of children."[56]

We still need to do more. Quality improvement is about making it easy to do the right thing. Government payers should incentivize healthcare systems to develop decision support systems that streamline quality improvement initiatives and help frontline healthcare workers meet requirements for important measures like SEP-1. This includes sepsis screening systems, computerized order entry systems, and documentation tools to help physicians and nurses quickly navigate the tricky process of ordering and completing bundle measures like antibiotics and fluids while making it easy to meet documentation requirements.

These systems should be intuitive and user-friendly, like smartphone apps—not bulky and archaic, like most current electronic health record systems. Organizations like the Institute for Healthcare Improvement have long advocated for such human-centered digital systems, which may one day function as seamlessly as familiar computer operating systems like Microsoft Windows or Apple's iOS.[57]

---

* Recall from chapter nine that mitochondria are the energy factories of cells and can fall into dysfunction during sepsis.

With this, we arrive at measuring structure and systems. As the "savior of mothers," Ignaz Semmelweis, learned so painfully in the nineteenth century, *implementation* makes or breaks any quality improvement initiative. The hidden reality behind sepsis process and outcome measures is all the tedious work that goes into running a sepsis program. Public health initiatives like the SSC have catalyzed the organization and expansion of an unprecedented global and local sepsis apparatus while focusing the eyes of hospitals and emergency rooms on sepsis patients. But as we've seen throughout the book, the magic comes from the tireless and unglamorous behind-the-scenes quality improvement work.

The US CDC has also caught on to this idea and, in 2023, published its *Hospital Sepsis Program Core Elements,* which summarizes essential components of high-quality sepsis programs, including the provision of dedicated administrative time to local sepsis leaders, multi-stakeholder engagement, and the implementation of structures and processes for systematically identifying and treating sepsis patients, to name a few.[58] In a 2022 CDC survey of over five thousand hospitals, 73 percent had sepsis committees, while just over half provided dedicated administrative time to sepsis program leaders.[59] Using a framework similar to that found in its *Core Elements of Hospital Antibiotic Stewardship Programs,* it hopes to improve these numbers while working with other quality improvement agencies to provide hospitals with more guidance and oversight in building sepsis programs.[60] This effort received funding through the 2023 Omnibus Appropriations bill, largely the result of the Stauntons' advocacy work. We've come a long way compared to when Orlaith and Ciaran first confronted the CDC back in 2014.*

Lastly, we should closely monitor so-called balancing measures such as antimicrobial resistance rates, *C. difficile* infections, and blood culture contamination rates. Most hospitals already track these metrics, but this work should be integrated with programs to assess the potential unintended consequences of bundle compliance. For instance, if a hospital improves bundle compliance by 5 percent but also observes a 10 percent increase in *C. difficile* infections, this could indicate a potential downstream harm linked to increased antibiotic use, prompting leaders to reinforce sensible antibiotic prescribing practices.

---

*   CMS is currently evaluating a proposed structural sepsis measure that would assess hospital adherence to the CDC's Hospital Sepsis Program Core Elements. The Joint Commission also provides a sepsis-focused certification, which incorporates evidence-based standards for sepsis recognition and treatment, as well as sepsis program oversight.

As of this book's publication, significant changes may be on the horizon in the sepsis regulatory world. CMS's electronic sepsis outcome measure has been moved to the Measures Under Consideration (MUC) list, meaning it has formally entered the process for potential inclusion in an upcoming measurement cycle. While no final rulemaking or implementation timeline has yet been confirmed, the measure has the potential to replace—or at least diminish reliance on—SEP-1.[61]

While I fully support introducing a sepsis outcome measure, I worry that by retiring SEP-1, we could lose something by shifting our focus exclusively toward mortality outcomes and away from process. For all the reasons already discussed, we should have a multifaceted approach to measuring performance when it comes to a condition as complex and deadly as sepsis. Each individual measurement strategy has its strengths and drawbacks.

Some experts would say that SEP-1's primary contribution has been to draw greater attention to sepsis while leveraging healthcare systems to enhance their own structures and processes around sepsis recognition and treatment. As Laura Evans puts it, "When you pay attention to a condition, it changes how you manage it, and it's very clear that sepsis quality improvement efforts have changed how we approach sepsis care."*[62] Perhaps, in that sense, SEP-1 has accomplished its purpose and now it's time to fine-tune our national approach to measuring sepsis care.

It's also possible that the data have been telling us that you simply can't find a reliable sepsis process that works for every hospital or patient, so it might be best left to those individual systems, and the providers working within those systems, to determine an approach that fits each situation.

Even if SEP-1 goes away, I would still encourage individual hospitals, healthcare systems, and even states to continue tracking sepsis process measures while investing heavily in systems to deliver timely sepsis care reliably. I hope this book has shown that systems have enormous potential to improve survival, and process measures like SEP-1 encourage us to build and improve upon those systems.

When thoughtfully crafted and based on the latest evidence, measures can

---

* This phenomenon is sometimes associated with the Hawthorne effect.

drive meaningful outcomes—becoming, in a way, almost transcendent in their ability to protect patients. We can bicker about the data, but on balance, if sepsis bundles are associated with even a slight benefit, they are going to save lives. Thus, I fully support using them until we have a better process in place. There are simply too many lives at stake.

We also need to sustain this progress. Quality improvement initiatives are like gardens—if you don't tend to them constantly, they wither and die. If we dial down our efforts or retire SEP-1, we risk backsliding to an era when urgency was an afterthought. Right now, we should double down while continuously fine-tuning our processes to keep them feasible and in line with the realities of everyday medicine.

—————

I want to end this chapter by returning to New York State, which recently released updated figures indicating that between 2015 and 2019, its state sepsis initiative saved another sixteen thousand lives, bringing the total to nearly twenty thousand since its inception.[63] What began with Rory Staunton's death has now rapidly expanded into a movement that has reportedly saved tens of thousands of people.

This tells us something profound. If the results seen in New York can be generalized to broader populations, the potential for these systems to save lives around the world is extraordinary. The mere possibility of such an impact should inspire our entire community to come together and amplify these efforts. As leading sepsis expert Kevin Tracey noted during the 2023 End Sepsis National Sepsis Forum, "You're hearing about thousands of lives saved in New York State. Imagine multiplying that [to] all fifty states, which we have to do, and then imagine multiplying that to every country in the world. The multiplier effect on lives saved will be uncountable."[64]

We should fiercely emulate successful tactics, shamelessly borrow proven methods, and pull on every lever to push down our mortality rates. And if we find ourselves off course, we must do everything in our power to improve our process and measurement standards. The goal is not to be right but to *get it* right, even if that means rethinking our approach entirely. We owe this to our patients and to our entire community.

Even small incremental improvements—when multiplied across hospitals, states, and nations—can lead to astonishing results. Just think where we could be in another twenty years . . .

Hereafter

Tomorrow belongs to those who can hear it coming.

—DAVID BOWIE[1]

IT'S WEDNESDAY, MARCH 1, 2046, and an eight-year-old girl named Serena arrives via ambulance at an undisclosed emergency department with fevers and lethargy. The ER staff rapidly assembles an advanced life support and monitoring apparatus—gathering crucial biometric data, such as temperature, heart rate, blood pressure, heart rate variability, and an extensive panel of biomarker tests.

Minutes later, an AI system calculates a 97 percent probability of bacterial sepsis with the delta response phenotype, while metagenomic sequencing identifies a resistant strain of *Streptococcus pyogenes* as the causative microbe.[2]

A "code sepsis" is called.

Within seconds, a dedicated response team is deployed, led by a physician specialized in sepsis care: a *sepologist*.

Meanwhile, the ER physician orders an antibiotic specifically targeting the identified *Streptococcus* strain. After that, she uses an advanced handheld imaging system to assess Serena's blood volume and orders a precise amount of fluid based on the system's readings.

The sepsis team arrives minutes later and transports Serena to a sepsis treatment unit (STU), where additional advanced diagnostic testing determines that she's a steroid-responsive patient with a low level of activated protein C.

The team administers a customized formula of advanced supplemental drug therapies, including the steroid hydrocortisone and recombinant activated protein C (aka Xigris).

Within two hours, Serena's vital signs stabilize, and a repeat battery of tests, analyzed by the AI system, shows a significant decrease in her sepsis response. She's transferred to the pediatric step-down unit, where a pediatric hospitalist takes over. The physician updates Serena's family, informing them that their daughter will likely walk out of the hospital in a few days.

———

Fiction aside, Serena's story isn't too far off from where we might one day find ourselves when caring for sepsis patients. The next few decades hold immense promise—technological advancements and an understanding of medical science on a level never seen before.

Yet, to ensure the future we all want, we must first better understand the biological mechanisms underpinning sepsis as a syndrome and identify the crucial sepsis tipping point sooner. We should also improve our reliability in rapidly treating the sepsis patients we identify while enhancing our ability to diagnose the specific infections causing it. Furthermore, we must embrace sepsis heterogeneity and begin to catalog the syndrome's many different faces so that, like cancer, one day, doctors will be able to tailor therapy to a specific sepsis phenotype.

Many unanswered questions remain. For example, we know treatment must be urgent—particularly in septic shock—yet the optimal thresholds are still being refined. Large observational trials suggest we should treat sepsis as quickly as possible, and as we'll see shortly, a massive clinical trial is underway to answer this question.

One of the other quandaries with sepsis is that we don't always know *what* we're treating—is it bacterial pneumonia, viral pneumonia, or something noninfectious? While advanced diagnostic tests could be game changers here, thus far they have fallen short.

We still don't have a good way to identify the precise moment a patient becomes septic. Right now, our definitions are all over the place, with some, like SIRS, identifying a much too general response to infection (or any injury, for that matter), while others, like the latest Sepsis 3 definition, wait until the patient is already faced with life-threatening organ dysfunction. Better bio-marker tests and AI systems could help identify the sepsis tipping point before the presence of life-threatening organ injury or shock, but our understanding of sepsis is evolving, and there is still much work to be done.

We've also seen how the heterogeneous nature of sepsis has thwarted our ability to develop advanced sepsis therapies, leading to the sepsis clinical trials conundrum. We're just beginning to understand all the different sepsis finger-prints. Sophisticated machine learning systems are starting to pattern-match many of these phenotypes, which may soon help us identify more precise strategies for treating them via so-called enhanced therapies—using drugs like Xigris in cases where we *know* patients will respond favorably.

I hope this book has also made the case that, no matter what the future holds, our greatest untapped resource for reducing the sepsis death toll is still *preventing* infections in the first place.

———

Sepsis continues to suffer from a brand recognition problem. These days, if an average person thinks of a heart attack, she knows exactly what that means, what the signs are, and who treats it. With sepsis, we're still not connecting all the dots. While two-thirds of US adults are aware of the syndrome, only 15 percent can identify its most common symptoms.[3] Groups like End Sepsis, the Sepsis Alliance, and the Global Sepsis Alliance aim to change this through advocacy. End Sepsis has even partnered with the American Federation of Teachers to develop a comprehensive K–12 sepsis curriculum for children.[4] It also recently secured a grant from the US government agency known as the Biomedical Advanced Research and Development Authority (BARDA) to develop educational materials for maternal sepsis.[5] Public health agencies also play a crucial role, with the US Centers for Disease Control and Prevention (CDC) recently launching its Get Ahead of Sepsis campaign to educate healthcare professionals and patients. But we need to do more to expand this awareness.[6]

Then there's ownership. Because sepsis afflicts a wide variety of patients while damaging many different organ systems, it's often treated by physicians across multiple specialties. This makes it what pioneering researcher Emanuel Rivers called the "orphan disease" because it isn't "owned by the major players out there like heart attacks, cancer, and stroke."[7]

Given its sheer complexity and death toll, I'm still puzzled why sepsis doesn't yet have its own dedicated medical specialty—"sepology," perhaps—or specialized "code sepsis" teams ready to respond in every hospital the moment a sepsis patient arrives at the emergency room, as we do for heart attacks and strokes.

This brings us to another major challenge in sepsis research: financial resources. Sepsis expert Laura Evans states, "The funding landscape hasn't been there for sepsis."[8]

As the orphan disease, until recently, sepsis hadn't enjoyed a snug place at the National Institutes of Health in the same way as, say, cardiovascular disease or neurodegenerative disorders like Alzheimer's disease. It only recently found a home within the agency at the National Institute of General Medical Sciences. Yet it only makes up a small part of that research portfolio.

As Evans says, "Proportionally, the amount of funding going to sepsis has been pretty darn low."[9]

In recent years, groups like End Sepsis have intensely advocated to lawmakers to increase sepsis funding, and this is starting to pay off. For the first time in history, sepsis funding was included in the $1.7 trillion Omnibus spending bill passed by Congress and signed by President Joe Biden in January 2023. This included allocating funds to the AHRQ to conduct sepsis epidemiologic studies and requiring CMS to work hand in hand with the CDC to continue developing strong sepsis quality measures.[10] The US House of Representatives reintroduced "Lulu's Law" on April 18, 2024, named after four-year-old Lulu Haynes, who died unexpectedly from sepsis in 2014 following appendix surgery. The bill calls for the development of a national sepsis strategy—standardizing its definition, designating it a nationally notifiable condition, and creating a network of sepsis information repositories across the country.[11] On September 11, 2024, US Senators Chuck Schumer, Susan Collins, and Bob Casey introduced the SEPSIS Act. If passed, it would enhance CDC efforts to educate the medical community on sepsis, improve pediatric sepsis data collection, and develop and implement a sepsis outcome measure.[12]

———

For over a decade, observational data have shown that the most critical variable in sepsis survival is *time*, with earlier treatment resulting in better outcomes. In 2018, in response to accumulating data, the Surviving Sepsis Campaign (SSC) updated its guidelines with a new "hour-1" bundle to reflect an even greater need for urgency.[13] However, this move was immediately met with resistance from the medical community, whose members felt that the evidence supporting such a change needed to be of higher quality and that increased time pressure on frontline physicians would result in misdiagnosis and overtreatment.[14] While some hospitals have adopted the hour-1 bundle, most haven't. The national SEP-1 measure has also kept with the three- and six-hour time windows in the original SSC bundles.

Now underway is one of the most ambitious sepsis clinical trials in history: the Assessment of Implementation Methods in Sepsis and Respiratory Failure (AIMS). Led by SSC cofounder Mitchell Levy, AIMS was initiated in 2022 and is set to run through mid-2027. It's a massive trial, which plans to enroll about ten thousand patients across eighteen carefully selected hospital settings, ensuring a highly diverse and representative sample of patients generalizable to the broader sepsis population.* As a large randomized clinical trial, it hopes to answer today's most essential sepsis questions: Is a one-hour sepsis bundle more effective than a three-hour bundle at reducing sepsis mortality?† What implementation tactics can frontline sepsis programs use to improve bundle compliance? Lastly, can specific sepsis fingerprints or phenotypes influence the treatment effect of either sepsis bundle?[15]

Urgency aside, doctors still face the challenge of the *undifferentiated* patient—when it is not immediately clear what we are treating. As infectious disease expert David Gilbert, coauthor of the IDSA sepsis position papers, explains, "We need to know what's wrong with you, and we need to know it quicker."[16]

As discussed in chapter five, advanced metagenomic and molecular assays have the potential to quickly identify pathogens, facilitating earlier, more tailored therapy. Just as importantly, they can reveal when a patient's illness stems from more benign causes, reducing the risk of unnecessary antibiotic use.

Gilbert continues, "We have the diagnostic tools, and they're being increasingly refined. We can quickly get back information within hours, if not minutes, telling us if we're dealing with a viral process, bacterial process, or

---

*   Study planners consulted with ED leadership to ensure hospital emergency rooms in the study were representative.

†   AIMS is actually a cluster-randomized trial (CRT). CRTs randomize groups or "clusters" of patients and are useful for studying different methods or approaches to patient care, such as bundles.

[one that isn't] bacterial or viral."[17]

When asked if now is the right time to pivot toward advanced diagnostic testing, Gilbert says, "Absolutely. That's going to be our salvation, but we have to get the people who are funding the research, [and] the application of the research to clinical use, to reimburse."

He goes on, "The hard thing to convince the regulators is that you're saving money and drugs. You're using less empiric antibiotics."*[18]

Others, like Laura Evans, caution that we're not there yet.[19] These tests still face important clinical limitations. One such challenge is coinfection—when a sepsis patient harbors both a bacterial *and* viral pathogens. In community-acquired pneumonia, for instance, it is not unusual to isolate a bacterial organism such as *Streptococcus* alongside a common cold virus like rhinovirus.[20] Sometimes the viral infection precedes the bacterial one; at other times, the reverse is true. Even if a sepsis patient tests positive for a virus, clinicians cannot safely rule out a concurrent bacterial coinfection, especially in the first few hours in the emergency room. For this reason, the SSC continues to recommend prompt administration of antibiotics to cover *all* possible pathogens when sepsis is strongly suspected or when patients are critically ill with shock—with de-escalation once further diagnostic information becomes available.[21]

The ultimate clinical value and cost-effectiveness of advanced diagnostic tests remain to be proven, and at least for now, isolation and direct testing of viable pathogens are still the gold standard for confirming resistance. Still, Evans and others predict that one of the significant evolutions in sepsis practice over the next decade will be more reliable pathogen diagnostics, offering physicians greater certainty about what they are treating.[22]

Meanwhile, advanced sepsis-response biomarkers hold the promise of detecting the molecular signature of sepsis far earlier than current methods, ideally before life-threatening or disabling organ injury occurs. Early efforts focused on single inflammatory proteins, such as C-reactive protein or interleukin-6. More recently, researchers have turned to panels of biomarkers and host gene-expression patterns to better distinguish a normal response to

---

* Currently, third-party carriers charge for this kind of testing by the individual pathogen test. However, during a typical undifferentiated respiratory infection, there may be dozens of potential candidates for which to test. Biotech companies such as bioMérieux have developed multiple-pathogen test panels. Gilbert explains, "If you could get insurers to pay for the thirty-target panel, the percentage of emergency room patients [receiving] unnecessary antibiotics would plummet."

infection from the dysregulated response that defines sepsis.[23]

Single biomarker tests have so far struggled to demonstrate real-world benefit. A key reason is limited sensitivity—the ability of a test to correctly identify patients with the disease. Procalcitonin, a precursor of the hormone calcitonin, illustrates the challenge. Normally, it is nearly undetectable in the bloodstream. During bacterial sepsis, however, inflammatory cytokines trigger its overproduction by multiple tissues throughout the body, raising procalcitonin levels.[24]* This led some to propose its use in diagnosing or excluding bacterial sepsis. Yet its sensitivity is only about 77 percent, meaning nearly one in four patients with bacterial sepsis could test negative.[25] Faced with such significant risk, clinicians are understandably reluctant to withhold antibiotics based on a single biomarker. Unsurprisingly, randomized trials of procalcitonin-guided sepsis protocols have failed to demonstrate any survival benefit over standard care.[26]

On April 3, 2024, the FDA granted De Novo authorization for Prenosis's Sepsis ImmunoScore, the first AI-driven sepsis prediction tool cleared to aid clinicians in assessing a patient's sepsis risk. The system uses twenty-two clinical and molecular biomarkers to generate a stratified risk score for patients already undergoing evaluation for sepsis. Prenosis claims it has built a proprietary biobank of over one hundred thousand blood samples and is using machine learning to analyze the data for patterns that can be used to refine its algorithm.[27]

Prenosis isn't alone in this space. For example, Cytovale's IntelliSep is an advanced machine learning algorithm that can analyze a sample of blood and within minutes identify structural changes in white blood cells seen during an early sepsis response.[28]

As for published data, systems like the Sepsis ImmunoScore are beginning to show promise, with some demonstrating better predictive abilities than existing tools such as SIRS or SOFA. Others have been associated with reductions in hospital mortality and length of stay, but to date, no conclusive randomized trials have shown mortality benefit.[29]

AI systems have the potential to improve overall sepsis care in hospitals by facilitating earlier diagnosis and serving as a buddy system for frontline

---

* Procalcitonin is normally produced in the thyroid and rapidly converted to calcitonin. During bacterial infection, however, it is released by other tissues such as the lung and intestines. When produced outside the thyroid, it isn't cleaved into its usual end products. As a result, calcitonin levels remain unchanged while *procalcitonin* levels rise sharply.

providers, reminding them to complete important processes like antibiotic administration and fluid resuscitation. But given the myriad factors that go into treating patients at the bedside, it's unlikely they'll replace frontline clinical judgment anytime soon.

These systems are also still in their early stages, and like humans, they're susceptible to blind spots and biases. For instance, an early AI model designed to predict the risk of death in pneumonia incorrectly and dangerously concluded that asthma patients with pneumonia were less likely to die.[30] Analysis later showed that the hospital in which the model was tested had a preexisting policy to admit all asthma patients with pneumonia directly to the intensive care unit, leading to timelier care and better mortality outcomes for patients treated at that center. When the AI system studied the data, it erroneously concluded that "asthma" was a protective factor in pneumonia when it was actually a correlation.[31]

As discussed in chapter fifteen, early warning systems might only move the needle a little when it comes to sepsis recognition in the emergency room, as most of these departments are already heavily focused on upfront sepsis identification.

As Derek Angus explains, "All they're going to do is get upstream of when the ball dropped, or the lightbulb went off for the clinician . . . and there's not much upstream to be had."[32]

However, as a *supplement* to existing clinical processes, these tools could potentially identify sepsis cases that might otherwise go unnoticed by the clinician or, in the case of other computerized tools like our Kaiser Permanente Northwest sepsis alert, support clinicians in remembering to order all the appropriate therapies.

One area where AI-based early warning systems may be beneficial is so-called hospital-onset sepsis—when sepsis develops or finally manifests itself *after* the patient has been admitted. Recall from chapter three that hospitals are noisy places, filled with distractions and blaring alarms, and a ripe environment for sepsis to emerge. Caregivers are also anchored to patients' existing diagnoses and not always expecting something *else* to go wrong. As one might expect, hospital-onset sepsis is associated with significantly higher delays in recognition and treatment compared to sepsis in the emergency room. Systems like Sepsis ImmunoScore could thus help physicians detect danger signals in hospitalized patients, where the difference in recognition time could be as much as several hours or days.[33]

Another exciting area in AI sepsis research is pre-hospital sepsis recognition. Recall from chapter fifteen that many sepsis patients presenting in the emergency room have already been sick for several days. Many have also seen a provider in the outpatient clinic the week before their illness. AI-based tools can tap into existing databases, such as wearable devices and smartwatches, to identify sepsis warning signs days in advance. There could be widespread applications for such systems, including hospital-at-home programs, kidney dialysis centers, and chemotherapy clinics. One medical startup, Sepsis Scout, which Cytovale recently acquired, is inching us closer to this futuristic *Star Trek* universe. It's developing wearable devices—such as smartwatches—programmed with deep learning algorithms that continuously monitor patients' vital signs for early signs of sepsis.[34]

Lastly, advanced AI systems and molecular diagnostic tests might make a huge difference in which sepsis therapy protocol or recipe to use. As in the AIMS trial, researchers are starting to examine patterns in the sepsis biochemical mix, which might tell them, for example, "This is sepsis phenotype X, which is more likely to respond favorably to therapy Y." This so-called "enhanced" therapy may add a layer of precision to our sepsis bundles, allowing doctors to tailor treatments to individual patients' needs—for example, more restrictive fluid therapy in patients who are deemed fluid nonresponders; steroid therapy in steroid-responsive patients; the original Rivers EGDT protocol for a subset of patients with profound shock on initial presentation; and even Xigris for patients who have reduced protein C activity.

This could also mean future sepsis definitions will involve further subclassifying the syndrome according to its responsiveness to specific therapies.

According to Angus, a potential Sepsis 4 definition could be "the dawn of a new era where we start to have subsets of sepsis for whom you need a particular diagnosis because you would give a particular therapy . . . Sepsis 4 is when you would move into the world of 'theranostics.'"[35]

———

I want to conclude this discussion with prevention. Since the beginning of the twentieth century, prevention has been our greatest ally in combating sepsis; however, many of us, including those in the medical field, often take this for granted. Even today, according to the World Health Organization, most sepsis cases are avoidable. Experts like Angus argue that prevention is still "our most important untapped resource."[36]

There are many ways to reduce the risk of sepsis on an individual level. Forgive the laundry list, but as a physician, I simply couldn't end this book without highlighting some of the most impactful lifestyle measures that anyone can implement today to improve their resistance to infections and sepsis.

It starts with adopting a balanced diet—eating sensibly, minimizing processed foods, washing produce, and ensuring meats and seafood are properly handled and cooked. Reducing sugar intake, avoiding or at least moderating alcohol consumption, and quitting tobacco and nicotine products, including vaping, are also crucial. Avoiding intravenous drug use is vital, but for those struggling with substance use disorders, seeking treatment while always using clean needles can help mitigate risks.

Regular exercise helps maintain a strong immune system, as do meaningful social connections and a supportive community. Practices such as mindfulness, meditation, faith, or spirituality can further strengthen overall well-being. Staying proactive with medical care, receiving recommended vaccinations, seeking trustworthy information about vaccine safety, and properly cleaning wounds are all essential in reducing the risk of sepsis.

And, of course, we should all seek *immediate* attention for suspected infections.

Improving sepsis prevention in the broader healthcare setting requires strengthening infection control procedures, surgical infection prevention protocols, hand hygiene practices, and hospital environmental services while supporting robust antimicrobial stewardship programs. These established safety systems have reduced rates of hospital-acquired infections and antimicrobial resistance. In contrast, the opposite trend emerged during the COVID-19 pandemic, when these systems broke down—underscoring the importance of infection prevention and the often-overlooked work of quality improvement and patient safety.

Meanwhile, we must continue to enhance the environment in which healthcare professionals work and protect the space for practicing medicine. This means improving decision support systems, hiring sufficient frontline staff, addressing factors that contribute to burnout, and investing more in quality improvement initiatives. Above all, it means building a healthcare system that makes it consistently easy to do the right thing.

We should embrace the reality that healthcare is, at its core, a team sport.

With the rapid democratization of medical knowledge, the rise of personal AI assistants, the proliferation of wearable health devices, and the expansion of home-based, virtual, and telemedicine services, we are living through another paradigm shift in the practice of medicine. In this new landscape, communication and partnership among patients, families, and providers are as essential to good care as the clinical guidelines themselves.

Crucially, patients and families must be empowered with the knowledge to recognize the signs and symptoms of sepsis and prepared to seek medical attention the moment these warning signs appear.

It is imperative to continue advocating for greater government investment in antimicrobial stewardship programs and the development of new antibiotics and advanced non-antibiotic antimicrobial therapies. One promising example is phage therapy—a novel approach that reengineers bacterial viruses (phages) to selectively target harmful bacteria while minimizing collateral damage to the host's microbiome. Technologies like this could one day replace broad-spectrum antibiotics and dramatically reduce the burden of antimicrobial resistance.

Bacterial vaccination also holds great promise in reducing the burden of antimicrobial-resistant bacterial diseases. Viruses are not the only "pandemic" threat. The Golden Staph Era taught us that resistant bacteria can also sweep across the world, silently decimating populations—and they remain an ever-growing danger. Today, vaccines are in development for several major pathogens, including *C. difficile*, *Mycobacterium tuberculosis*, *Salmonella*, and *E. coli*, among others.[37]

As a key component of the US Administration for Strategic Preparedness and Response (ASPR), BARDA currently oversees several public–private partnerships dedicated to addressing emerging infectious diseases, enhancing diagnostic testing, and developing new antimicrobial therapies.[38] On April 27, 2023, the US Senate introduced the bipartisan PASTEUR Act, which aims to strengthen antimicrobial research and innovation, provide grants to hospitals to bolster antimicrobial stewardship practices, and establish a multi-stakeholder Committee on Critical Need Antimicrobials to improve national antimicrobial stewardship guidelines. Both the US CDC and BARDA are designated to play key roles in the bill's implementation and oversight.[39]

Current projections estimate that by 2050, antimicrobial-resistant infections could claim 40 million lives and indirectly contribute to an additional 170 million deaths.[40] In addition to reinforcing antimicrobial stewardship and infection control programs, we could avert many of these tragedies by ensuring timely access to antimicrobial therapy for those who need it most.

We should also remember that, in the event of another cataclysmic viral pandemic, especially one involving influenza, secondary bacterial pneumonia—particularly from drug-resistant *Streptococcus* strains—could end up being the leading cause of death. We should shore up our existing antibiotics in preparation for this threat while improving our immunity to the bacterium through comprehensive *Streptococcus pneumoniae* vaccination programs.

This brings us to the general issue of viral pandemics, which still loom as an existential threat to our civilization. With COVID-19, we saw how a virus like SARS-CoV-2 could quickly surge out of control and threaten to shut down our healthcare system due to its high infectivity (R0). We also experienced how the pandemic divided our society over its conflicting values while forcing us to take drastic infection control measures, which themselves caused significant injury and trauma to our personal well-being and economic system.

We've since learned from this experience and will likely modernize our pandemic response strategies. This doesn't mean abandoning core principles of infection prevention—handwashing, masking, and social distancing. However, it does suggest that a more nuanced approach will better serve the needs of a complex and interconnected society—one in which many people, especially children and seniors—are vulnerable not only to infection but also to the social effects of isolation.

This is not a time to weaken our core public health institutions. The US CDC, like any organization, has had its shortcomings and blind spots. Yet, as this book has shown, it has consistently adapted in response to emerging evidence. Since its inception in 1946, it has pursued an unwavering mission to protect and improve lives, serving as a guiding star for public health around the world. The path forward lies in reform—strengthening what works, correcting what doesn't—while preserving the agency's essential role. Safeguarding the CDC and other public health agencies is central to protecting our collective future.[41]

Additionally, we must recognize that hospitals and emergency rooms are the tip of the spear during a viral pandemic. As highlighted in the Institute of Medicine's *Hospital-Based Emergency Care: At the Breaking Point*, shoring up our capacity to manage infected patients starts here—by improving emergency room throughput and expanding hospital bed capacity to withstand a pandemic wave.

That said, vaccination remains our best strategy for combating future pandemics.

Now more than ever, it is essential to connect the public with the history of medicine, our enduring battle against germs, and the technologies that can protect us now and in the years to come. Today, there are increasing efforts to reduce vaccine eligibility, undo longstanding childhood immunization requirements, and reduce funding for mRNA vaccine research.[42] Such actions risk exposing our population to a worst-case scenario should another deadly coronavirus or influenza virus emerge, or could reverse decades of progress by allowing previously controlled diseases, such as measles and polio, to resurge, needlessly taking the lives of countless children.

We must also expand viral and bacterial vaccination programs abroad and launch a massive global vaccine effectiveness and safety campaign. Vaccination remains the single most effective global public health strategy in history with a recent study published in *The Lancet* attributing 154 million saved lives to vaccination programs since 1974.[43] And even if we don't all agree that it's our moral responsibility to help others in need, the reality of our interconnected world means that devastating diseases like COVID-19 or Ebola will inevitably reach our doorstep. In that light, proactive action isn't just compassion—it's the most pragmatic approach.

Beyond that, we should continue to improve our food safety monitoring programs. Achieving this will necessitate strong partnerships between government agencies and the agricultural sector to promote safer and more sustainable livestock farming practices. This will ultimately help decrease the risk of antimicrobial resistance and outbreaks of foodborne illnesses.

We can also expect that, as long as health and social inequality exist, there will be a disproportionate population of underserved individuals suffering from sepsis, whether it's children with diarrheal sepsis in low- to middle-income countries or disadvantaged patients living in high-income countries like the United States or the United Kingdom.

As we learned in chapter ten, rich or poor, we're all in this together. We should address pockets of inequality throughout our society and worldwide, not only for those suffering within but also to preserve the health of our interconnected global community. The Global Burden of Disease Study showed us that, between 1990 and 2017, sepsis cases and mortality decreased around the world. This means we *can* make a difference.*[44]

Finally, we need participation. Whether on the front line, directly caring for patients as a provider; working in the clinical laboratory, hospital environmental services, pharmacy, or quality improvement committees; or outside the hospital, in the research laboratory, government organizations, or advocacy groups, we need more people to get involved and become a part of this story. Every contribution matters.

———

As I write this, the question "What is sepsis?" implies something far more profound and human than it once did. The book's title, *Blood Poison,* belongs to another era—one that saw only the surface of medicine's oldest and most enduring mystery. We've now peered into the depths to see it as the body's severe response to infection, a process that can harm, even destroy, the very life it's meant to protect.

Sepsis defies easy definition. It isn't a classical disease like a heart attack or stroke, with a clear cause-and-effect relationship. It's a syndrome—a shifting confluence of signs and symptoms, sometimes clear, sometimes elusive—an ongoing reminder of how complex the body's dialogue with infection can be.

The term "sepsis" encompasses many conditions: viremic sepsis, such as that seen with COVID-19; endotoxic sepsis, as in an *E. coli* bloodstream infection; pneumonia with sepsis and acute respiratory distress syndrome (ARDS); staphylococcal or streptococcal sepsis from a skin or wound infection; toxin-mediated sepsis or septic shock from a *C. difficile* infection; or even fungemic sepsis resulting from an invasive yeast infection. It also impacts a variety of hosts, leading to different phenotypes. We're just beginning to scratch the surface of this complexity, and there is still much to uncover. For now, our focus must remain on the fundamentals of prevention, early recognition, and timely treatment.[45]

We don't yet have a definitive "sepsis test," so we must operate with a high degree of suspicion whenever someone has a serious infection. It's crucial to use a system that helps us identify its early signs. The most well-known example of this is SIRS. However, while systems like SIRS can bring potential sepsis

---

* The study showed that the original projections were underestimates. However, the trend during that period still showed a decrease in cases and mortality.

patients to our attention, they don't provide a complete picture. We need to look for evidence of organ dysfunction before issuing an official sepsis alert, and we should continue to rely on our best clinical assessment when treating it. The optimal approach is to combine systems with good clinical judgment.

Reversing septic shock is like trying to disarm a bomb while it's exploding. Our best strategy is to act early or prevent it altogether. Because sepsis behaves like a cascade, doctors must often move swiftly with limited information. In the same way lifeguards treat the instinctive drowning response, they must intervene *before* the sepsis response amplifies beyond their ability to control it. Sepsis bundles are precisely designed for this purpose: to expedite treatment. And we've seen encouraging results—bundles save lives when faithfully applied, though their impact, like sepsis itself, resists simple measurement.

We're making progress—sepsis mortality rates are slowly declining—but we're still far from where we need to be, and outcomes remain uneven. New York State's program stands out for its remarkable results—a success story born of strong leadership, shared purpose, and all the devilish details of implementation. Other states have followed suit, and sepsis collaboratives are cropping up worldwide.

There are still many questions, and we still don't fully understand why patients die from sepsis or why it impacts survivors so severely. Is it because we didn't act quickly enough? Because the treatment was inadequate? Because it was too much? Was there a resistant organism we failed to detect? Was it simply the patient's time? Eventually, we will gain greater insight into these questions as we build more comprehensive databases, design better clinical trials, and form stronger collaborations.

Considering our increasingly overburdened healthcare system, the looming threat of another deadly pandemic, and the danger of multi-drug-resistant microbes, we have our work cut out for us. These are serious issues, and we must harness every part of our economy and information ecosystem to address them. We need more than just accountability; we need a sense of shared responsibility.[46] The future belongs to all of us.

During this journey, I reconnected with the history of medicine and rediscovered remarkable stories—like the germ theory of disease and how it helped humanity turn the tide against infection. It reminded me of the power of prevention and the countless, unglamorous actions that keep us safe every day. Looking back now at the sepsis saga, I see an extraordinary story of people coming together to improve our lives.

To the nonmedical reader, I hope this book inspires you to become more engaged in healthcare advocacy or even to consider a career in medicine. We could really use your help. To my fellow healthcare professionals, I hope these stories rekindle your sense of purpose and help you feel proud of your calling. I encourage more of you to join our quality improvement efforts—even a little bit goes a long way.

History teaches us that the arc of progress can be tortuous, yet it bends in our favor. In the words of David Gilbert, "Science will prevail."[47] We must see progress as a living structure that transcends the individual and any single period. It's a continuous thread of which we are each a small part.

Our security doesn't arrive quickly or easily. It doesn't come from superheroes or miracles. It arises from countless incremental improvements in medical care over the last two centuries, a pilot's checklist, a lifeguard's training, and millions of people devoted to public service worldwide. We won't notice this infrastructure until it begins to crumble. Only when something goes wrong will we realize that someone was supposed to be keeping watch.

I'm still counting our sepsis survivors. Most don't know who they are and perhaps never will. Maybe the true glory is no glory at all.

Save a Life, Save the World

IN MY FIRST YEAR AS a practicing physician, I cared for a sixty-year-old man with pneumonia. His condition was relatively mild, and he certainly didn't have sepsis—making his case fairly routine.

Each morning, after my assessment, I would pat him on the shoulder and say, "Things are moving in the right direction."

He would respond with a faint smile and a quiet "Thank you."

On the day of his discharge, I told him he was ready to go home. But this time, instead of his usual nod, he gripped my hand tightly and burst into tears.

"Thank you for saving my life," he said, his voice trembling.

I was so caught off guard that all I could manage was an uninspiring, almost reflexive, "It's my job."

As medical professionals, we often downplay the impact we have on our patients. For us, a typical hospital or emergency room shift involves spinning high-stakes, life-and-death situations into a routine set of well-rehearsed actions. Yet these moments serve as inconceivable inflection points in the lives of those we care for, not to mention their families.

Growing up, my mother taught me an old proverb, one echoed across many faith traditions. The Talmud puts it this way: "Whoever saves a single life is considered by scripture to have saved the world."[1] It's a reminder of the sanctity of every life—the truth that each person carries within them a universe of hopes, relationships, and aspirations. To save a life is to safeguard something immeasurable; to lose one is to lose an entire world.

Years ago, I found myself teetering at the edge of death at Huntington Beach. My story could have easily ended had things played out just a little differently. Had the lifeguards arrived a few minutes later, they might not have reached me in time. Had I been swimming in an unmonitored break, I could have just slipped away, unnoticed. I can't imagine the heartbreak my family would have endured.

For the lifeguards, it was just another routine rescue—another day at the office. But for me, it was the most pivotal moment of my life.

———

In the summer of 2022, as I was preparing to write this book, I reached out to the California State Lifeguards to learn more about my rescue experience. I had seen the striking parallels between aquatic safety and patient care, and I was convinced that, as healthcare professionals, we could learn a thing or two from lifeguarding.

A year earlier, I had witnessed the profound impact of Mickey and Amy Watts reuniting at our sepsis conference. That memory brought my thoughts back to Emily, the lifeguard who had saved me. The idea of reconnecting and expressing my gratitude to her and her team for saving my life felt like an essential piece of this story.

My first point of contact was a phone call with Superintendent Justin McHenry, an aquatic specialist based in Carlsbad, California. As I recounted my Huntington Beach rescue experience, he quickly warmed up to me and within minutes peeled away my glitzy conception of lifeguarding, revealing instead an intricate system of protocols and a rich tradition of public service.

I learned that while California lifeguards proudly report around ten thousand full-blown rescues per year, the real story lies in all the rescues that never have to happen. These events are classified as "preventive actions," and there are about a million of them per year.[2]

A few days later, to my surprise, a simple internet search led me to an old record from the United States Lifesaving Association Foster's National Lifeguard Championships. Listed among the competing lifeguards for August 2000 was a familiar name: Emily Hagan, Huntington Beach.[3]

A few keystrokes later, I stumbled upon a 2007 *Orange County Register* article about lifeguarding. There, among the featured lifeguards, was a photograph of Emily.[4]

"That's her!" I shouted, recognizing her instantly.

The following week, McHenry put me in touch with Sergeant Elisabeth Ward, a Huntington Beach lifeguard supervisor. Ward, a Huntington Beach native, comes from a long line of lifeguards dating back to her grandfather, Ray Bray, a local lifeguarding legend. Bray was one of the pioneers of the California lifeguarding renaissance of the 1950s and helped establish one of the world's first Junior Lifeguard Programs.[5]

Like many lifeguards, Ward began her training as a teenager, mastering the art of vigilant observation: learning to filter signal from noise, understanding the weather and tides, reading body language, and recognizing the subtle signs of a swimmer in distress. Over time, through experience and repetition, lifeguards acquire a refined intuition, which they combine with systematic surveillance methods.[6]

One such tactic, the perimeter defense system, entails overlapping zones of observation between lifeguard towers, creating redundancy, reducing the risk of missing a potential drowning victim. Simultaneously, lifeguards engage in continuous risk assessment, evaluating both the water conditions and individual swimmers' abilities.[7]

In fact, as a beachgoer, by the time you've even dipped your toes in the water, the lifeguard on duty has already assessed you, quietly estimating your odds of getting into trouble.[8]

At the end of our conversation, Ward invited me to attend the lifeguard training program the following spring. But the best part? She also personally knew Emily, who was still lifeguarding in Southern California. As we said our goodbyes, she promised to arrange for us to reunite.

———

On a gray and misty morning, June 12, 2023, I arrived at the Huntington State Beach Lifeguard Headquarters for a long-anticipated reunion with Emily and the California lifeguard team. At first, I was jittery, unsure what to expect.

But as I approached the entrance to the command center, my anxiety melted away. A uniformed officer stood at the doorway, waving with a bright smile. It was Sergeant Elisabeth Ward. She greeted me with a hug and immediately introduced me to her colleague Ennio Rocca, one of the training sergeants.

Half an hour later, I stood at the front of a classroom, facing two dozen lifeguard trainees, a handful of instructors, and Emily, who had walked in moments before my introduction. As I recounted my rescue experience, I realized that, even after all these years, I still hadn't fully processed what had happened that day. The weight of it all caught me off guard, making it hard not to choke up.

I closed by expressing my deepest gratitude to the lifeguards. Then Ward called Emily up to the front of the room. Her face lit up as she stepped forward, and when she reached me, I hugged her and handed her a plaque inscribed with the following words: *"Thank you for saving my life. In that moment, you were my whole world."*

It felt like such a small gesture compared to the immeasurable gift she had given me more than two decades ago.

When the presentation ended and the class went on break, I had a chance to meet the other instructors. Many simply wanted to thank me for sharing my story. One remarked, "These kids need to hear stories like this." Recruitment, he explained, had been declining recently, and new trainees needed to be reminded why their work mattered.

Afterward, we toured the training site, watching lifeguard trainees practice rescue drills. Huntington Beach is a mecca for lifeguard training, and its waters are among the most challenging and treacherous in the world.

During the tour, Emily and I talked.

"You know, I think I remember you," she said.

"That's interesting. Just meeting you again has jogged a lot of memories from that day for me as well," I replied.

"Now that I think about it, we're standing in front of Tower 8. This was my tower back then. I think this is where it all happened."

She was right. There it was—*Tower 8.*

It was hard to believe. After all this time, I had finally come full circle—back to the very spot where my life had almost ended.

I've often wondered what it really means to save a life. When I nearly drowned, my greatest fear wasn't death itself—it was the feeling of being left behind. But the lifeguards were there for me that day. They saw me. And in that moment, there was kindness. It felt as if they had pulled me back from the void. In doing so, they didn't just save my life—they opened my eyes to something bigger than myself.

When families of sepsis victims describe their grief, they express more than just sorrow over the tragic loss of their loved ones. They remember feeling unheard and abandoned.[9] The painful common thread in so many stories like Rory's is that the patients were left behind by the very system meant to protect them.

We are all searching for something to hold on to—a sense of security, a sign that we are part of a grand design. Saving a life isn't only about preventing death; it's also an assurance that we're watching over and protecting one another. It's more than a single act—it's about building and sustaining a system, a community, that leaves no one behind.

Before heading back to the lifeguard station, I took a short walk along the beach alone. The ocean roared in the background, steady, indifferent. I reflected on how incredibly lucky I was to have been saved from its grip years ago.

My thoughts drifted to Rory. He had wanted to change the world. Orlaith once told me that she and Ciaran still come home wanting to tell him about their advocacy work, as if he were still there, waiting to hear the latest updates.

We lost someone extraordinary the day Rory died. Yet, even in death, his legacy lives on. His spirit stretches far beyond his own life, carried forward by the boundless love of his parents—transforming grief and anger into something deeply meaningful.

I wish Rory could see how far we've come in understanding and treating sepsis, the New York Sepsis Initiative, and the thousands of lives it's saved. I think he would be pleased.

I turned back one last time to look at the ocean. It wasn't mesmerizing like it had been that fateful day over twenty years ago. Come to think of it, there was nothing remarkable about it at all—except, perhaps, for what didn't happen to me there.

Acknowledgments

I AM INDEBTED TO MANY INDIVIDUALS. First, my life partner, Anna Spangler, for her tireless support as a first reader, a bringer of common sense, emotional support, and at times, for pulling me out of the depths of a writer's darkness.

I could not have been in the position to embark on such a project without the unconditional love and support of my parents, Jamileh and Mohsen Shahinpoor, sister, Sheerin Shahinpoor Haubenreich, brother, David Shahinpoor, and their families. My father deserves special thanks for introducing me to science and teaching me reason and critical thinking. In addition, I would not have my sanity if not for the love and friendship of my closest friends, Joaquin Sanchez, David Sheski, Hannah Hillebrand, Peter Carty, Stephanie Kaplan, Scott Forman, Greg Brown, Jason Kist, and Nazy Sharifi.

I am sincerely grateful to those who reviewed and helped shape the book in its ideas, content, and writing. First, my best friend, Joaquin Sanchez, who was my closest advisor, voice of reason, and my earliest and most dedicated reader. My other first readers, Sheerin Shahinpoor Haubenreich, Laurel Berge, Foster Gesten, and Nirav Shah, left their indelible mark on this project through their selflessness, brilliance, and love.

Thanks to my production editor, Brandon Coward, whose sharp intellect and steady guidance shaped this project from manuscript to finished form, and whose belief in the book sustained it through its final stages; editors Ray Sylvester and Carolyn Allard for their tireless, meticulous work polishing every page; designer Caitlin Smith, who created a truly beautiful book both inside and out; and my book coach, Jessica Sindler, who helped me become a stronger narrative writer.

Deep thanks also are in order to the many expert reviewers who dedicated time out of their lives to review the book and/or individual chapters: James Ford, Foster Gesten, David Gilbert, Vinnie Liu, John Marshall, David Mosen, Hallie Prescott, Chanu Rhee, Elaine Rinicker, Eric Walter, Scott Weiss, Joost Wiersinga, and Elisabeth Ward—as well as the many experts around the world who granted me interviews, helping me develop my thinking around complex topics, while sharing their incredible perspectives: Derek Angus, Martin Blaser, Ray Dantes, Peter Eichacker, Laura Evans, Foster Gesten, David Gilbert, Niranjan "Tex" Kissoon, Ron Kline, William Knaus, Mitchell Levy, Vinnie Liu, John Marshall, Justin McHenry, Naomi O'Grady, Bruce Quinn, Chanu Rhee, Elaine Rinicker, Emanuel Rivers, Jonathan Sevransky, Nirav Shah, Sean Townsend, Eric Walter, Elisabeth Ward, Scott Weiss, Joost Wiersinga, and Donald Yealy.

I must thank my mentor, David Schmidt, for opening my eyes to sepsis leadership work and serving as a role model and consummate academic pragmatist, as well as my colleagues who shared their personal stories and perspectives: Briar Ertz Berger, Laurel Berge, Elizabeth Ehrlich, Melissa Denny, "Amy Watts," Anne Ramey, and Jonathan Rettmann.

I also want to thank Emily Hagan for saving my life, and the California lifeguards, particularly Justin McHenry, Elisabeth Ward, and Ennio Rocca, for welcoming me to their program and teaching me about their incredible profession.

I am also thankful for my organization's support for this project, and in particular for colleagues such as Joel Womack, Eric Poolman, Cylia Amendolara, David Parsons, Eric Roth, Farah Pakseresht, Marcus Cassar, Micah Thorp, Mary Giswold, Leong Koh, Maria Ansari, Sean Briggs, and Molly Herrmann. And of course, special thanks to Jennifer McBride and the Kaiser Permanente Northwest Librarians for their invaluable help in researching this topic, pulling archaic centuries-old medical journal articles, sometimes written in original French or German (and thank you to my good friend Bruce Filardi for helping translate German text). Beyond that, I owe deep gratitude to my sepsis quality improvement team and all the physicians, nurses, and healthcare professionals who work on the front lines daily to care for our patients.

Lastly and most importantly, I am profoundly indebted to the patients and their families, most notably the Staunton family, who offered tireless and passionate support for this project, helped me develop the stories and content, and opened my mind and my heart throughout the process. I must also thank "Mickey," who granted me permission to share his entire story, and Carl Flatley and the Sepsis Alliance, for bringing Erin Flatley's tragic story to the public consciousness and continuing to advocate year after year for sepsis awareness.

Notes

Epigraph

1   Donald Berwick, excerpted from plenary address at Institute for Healthcare Improvement 16th Annual National forum on Quality *Improvement in Health Care*, December 2004.

Prologue

1   Rory Staunton's story was written based on interviews with the Staunton family between 2022 and 2025, as well as the incredible reporting work by the late Jim Dwyer of *The New York Times*. The following are references for both factual content and quotes: Jim Dwyer, "An Infection, Unnoticed, Turns Unstoppable," *The New York Times*, July 11, 2012, https:// www.nytimes.com/2012/07/12/nyregion/in-rory-stauntons-fight-for-his-life-signs-that-went-unheeded.html; Jim Dwyer, "Death of a Boy Prompts New Medical Efforts Nation-wide," *The New York Times*, October 25, 2012, https://www.nytimes.com/2012/10/26/nyregion/tale-of-rory-stauntons-death-prompts-new-medical-efforts-nationwide.html; "Medical Documents in Sepsis Death," *The New York Times*, July 11, 2012, https://archive.nytimes.com/screenshots/www.nytimes.com/interactive/2012/07/11/nyregion/medi-cal-documents-in-depsis-death.jpg; "Ciaran and Orlaith Staunton," RTE Radio 1, *Sunday with Miriam*, November 6, 2022, https://www.rte.ie/radio/radio1/clips/22167937/.

Introduction: The Silent Killer

1   "European Societies Unite Against Severe Sepsis: The Barcelona Declaration," *Medscape Medical News*, October 2, 2002, https://www.medscape.com/viewarticle/442395.

2   R. P. Dellinger, A. Rhodes, L. Evans, et al., "Surviving Sepsis Campaign," *Critical Care Medicine* 51, no. 4 (2023): 431–444, https://doi.org/10.1097/CCM.0000000000005804.

3   L. Evans, A. Rhodes, W. Alhazzani, et al., "Surviving sepsis campaign: international guide-lines for management of sepsis and septic shock: 2021," *Intensive Care Medicine* 47, no. 11 (2021): 1181–1247, https://doi.org/10.1007/s00134-021-06506-y.

4 Brandon Coward, conversation with editor, March 14, 2025.

5 Mitchell Levy, interview, December 8, 2022.

6 C. Rhee, R. Dantes, L. Epstein, et al., "Incidence and Trends of Sepsis in US Hospitals Using Clinical vs Claims Data, 2009–2014," *JAMA* 318, no. 13 (2017): 1241–1249, https://doi.org/10.1001/jama.2017.13836; S. A. Sterling, et al., "The Impact of the Sepsis-3 Septic Shock Definition on Previously Defined Septic Shock Patients," *Critical Care Medicine* 45, no. 9 (2017): 1436-1442, doi: 10.1097/CCM.0000000000002512, PMID: 28542029, PMCID: PMC5693309.

7 Centers for Disease Control and Prevention, "Sepsis Program Activities in Acute Care Hospitals – National Healthcare Safety Network, United States, 2022," *Morbidity and Mortality Weekly Report* 72, no. 34 (August 25, 2023): 907–11, https://www.cdc.gov/mmwr/volumes/72/wr/mm7234a2.htm.

8 "Global Report on the Epidemiology and Burden of Sepsis," World Health Organization, September 9, 2020, https://www.who.int/publications/i/item/9789240010789; "WHO Calls for Global Action on Sepsis – Cause of 1 in 5 Deaths Worldwide," World Health Organization, September 8, 2020, https://www.who.int/news/item/08-09-2020-who-calls-for-global-action-on-sepsis---cause-of-1-in-5-deaths-worldwide.

9 "Global Report on the Epidemiology and Burden of Sepsis," World Health Organization.

10 Kevin Tracey, remarks during the 2023 End Sepsis National Sepsis Forum, September 13, 2023; D.W. Chang, et al., "Rehospitalizations Following Sepsis: Common and Costly," *Critical Care Medicine* 43, no. 10 (2015): 2085-93, doi: 10.1097/CCM.0000000000001159, PMID: 26131597, PMCID: PMC5044864.

11 "Global Report on the Epidemiology and Burden of Sepsis," World Health Organization.

12 T. G. Buchman, S. Q. Simpson, K. L. Sciaretta, et al., "Sepsis Among Medicare Beneficiaries: 3. The Methods, Models, and Forecasts of Sepsis, 2012–2018," *Critical Care Medicine* 48, no. 3 (2020):302–318, doi: 10.1097/CCM.0000000000004225, PMID: 32058368, PMCID: PMC7017950.

13 M. van den Berg, F. E. van Beuningen, J. C. Ter Maaten, and H. R. Bouma, "Hospital-related costs of sepsis around the world: A systematic review exploring the economic burden of sepsis," *Journal of Critical Care* 71 (2022): 154096, doi: 10.1016/j.jcrc.2022.154096.

14 David Schmidt, conversation with mentor, September 2011.

15 Atul Gawande, *The Checklist Manifesto* (Picador, 2009).

16 Ibid.

17 Stefanos Geroulanos, "Prehippocratic Epidemics and the Plague of Athens," lecture by Global Doctors' Hippocratic Institute, "Hippocrates Unites the Five Continents," YouTube, March 20, 2021, https://www.youtube.com/watch?v=XHnzfPsbIlM.

Chapter One: Bacterial Shock

1 Justice Potter Stewart, *Jacobellis v. Ohio*, 378 U.S. 184 (1964), https://constitution.congress.gov/browse/essay/amdt1-7-5-11/ALDE_00013812/; R. C. Bone, W. J. Sibbald, and C. L. Sprung, "The ACCP-SCCM consensus conference on sepsis and organ failure," *Chest* 101 no. 6 (1992): 1481–1483, https://doi.org/10.1378/chest.101.6.1481.

2 F. H. Millham, "A brief history of shock," *Surgery* 148, no. 5 (2010): 1026–1037, https://doi.org/10.1016/j.surg.2010.02.014.

3 Ibid.

4 Ibid.

5 N. Tripathi, M. Zubair, and A. Sapra, "Gram Staining" in *StatPearls* (StatPearls Publishing, 2025 Jan–) https://www.ncbi.nlm.nih.gov/books/NBK562156.

6 L. Weinstein, "Gram-Negative Bacterial Infections: A Look at the Past, a View of the Present, and a Glance at the Future," *Reviews of Infectious Diseases* 7, no. 4 (1985): S538–S544, https://doi.org/10.1093/clinids/7.Supplement_4.S538; Ed Yong, *I Contain Multitudes* (HarperCollins, 2016), 11.

7 Weinstein, "Gram-Negative Bacterial Infections: A Look at the Past, a View of the Present, and a Glance at the Future."

8 D. E. Rogers, "The changing pattern of life-threatening microbial disease," *The New England Journal of Medicine* 261 (1959): 677–683, https://doi.org/10.1056/NEJM195910012611401.

9 J. A. Barnett and J. P. Sanford, "Bacterial Shock," *JAMA* 209, no. 10 (1969): 1514–1517, doi:10.1001/jama.1969.03160230048012.

10 A. L. Flores-Mireles, J. N. Walker, M. Caparon, and S. J. Hultgren, "Urinary tract infections: epidemiology, mechanisms of infection and treatment options," *Nature Reviews Microbiology* 13, no. 5 (2015): 269–284, https://doi.org/10.1038/nrmicro3432; Minnesota Department of Health, Infectious Disease Epidemiology, Prevention and Control Division, *"Escherichia coli (E. coli),"* Minnesota Department of Health, accessed June 14, 2025. https://www.health.state.mn.us/diseases/ecoli/index.html.

11 Nicole Perkes, "But What Is Gestalt, Really?" *in-House*, February 28, 2017, https://in-housestaff.org/but-what-is-gestalt-really-626.

12 Mark Sheldon, discussion during cardiology rounds, 2003. This idiom is originally credited to English writer John Heywood.

13 W. J. Wiersinga and C. W. Seymour, eds., *Handbook of Sepsis* (Springer International, 2018), 3.

14 L. Chen, H. Deng, H. Cui, et al., "Inflammatory responses and inflammation-associated diseases in organs." *Oncotarget* 9, no. 6 (2017): 7204–7218, https://doi.org/10.18632/oncotarget.23208.

15 A. Scott, K. M. Khan, J. L. Cook, and V. Duronio, "What is 'inflammation'? Are we ready to move beyond Celsus?" *British Journal of Sports Medicine* 38, no. 3 (2004): 248–249, https://doi.org/10.1136/bjsm.2003.011221; J. M. Cavaillon, "Once upon a time, inflammation," *Journal of Venomous Animals and Toxins Including Tropical Diseases*, 27 (2021): e20200147, doi: 10.1590/1678-9199-JVATITD-2020-0147, PMID: 33889184, PMCID: PMC8040910; L. J. Rather, "Disturbance of Function (*Functio Laesa*): The Legendary Fifth Cardinal Sign of Inflammation, Added by Galen to the Four Cardinal Signs of Celsus," *Bulletin of the New York Academy of Medicine* 47, no. 3 (1971): 303–22.

16 Scott, Khan, Cook, and Duronio, "What is 'inflammation'? Are we ready to move beyond Celsus?"; L. J. Rather, "Disturbance of Function (*Functio Laesa*): The Legendary Fifth Cardinal Sign of Inflammation, Added by Galen to the Four Cardinal Signs of Celsus," *Bulletin of the New York Academy of Medicine* 47, no. 3 (1971): 303–22.

17 M. Protsiv, C. Ley, J. Lankester, T. Hastie, and J. Parsonnet, "Decreasing human body temperature in the United States since the industrial revolution," *eLife* 9 (2020): e49555, https://doi.org/10.7554/eLife.49555; P. A. Mackowiak, S. S. Wasserman, and M. M. Levine, "A critical appraisal of 98.6 degrees F, the upper limit of the normal body temperature, and other legacies of Carl Reinhold August Wunderlich," *JAMA* 268, no. 12(1992): 1578-1580.

18 S. Pellett, "Learning from the past: Historical aspects of bacterial toxins as pharmaceuticals," *Current Opinion in Microbiology* 15, no. 3 (2012): 292–299, https://doi.org/10.1016/j.mib.2012.05.005.

19 Ibid.

20 F. J. Erbguth, "Historical notes on botulism, Clostridium botulinum, botulinum toxin, and the idea of the therapeutic use of the toxin," *Movement Disorders: Official Journal of the Movement Disorder Society* 19, no. 8 (2004): S2–S6, https://doi.org/10.1002/mds.20003; Émile van Ermengem, "Ueber einen neuen anaeroben Bacillus und seine Beziehungen zum Botulismus," *Zeitschrift für Hygiene und Infektionskrankheiten* 26, no. 1 (1897): 1–56.

21 Catherine Offord, "Identifying a Killer, 1895," *The Scientist*, July 1, 2021, https://www.the-scientist.com/identifying-a-killer-1895-68861.

22 J. D. Williamson, K. G. Gould, and K. Brown, "Richard Pfeiffer's typhoid vaccine and Almroth Wright's claim to priority," *Vaccine* 39, no. 15 (2021): 2074–2079, https://doi.org/10.1016/j.vaccine.2021.03.017; Perri Klass, "How Science Conquered Diphtheria, the Plague Among Children," *Smithsonian Online*, October 2021, https://www.smithsonianmag.com/science-nature/science-diphtheria-plague-among-children-180978572/.

23 "Cholera," World Health Organization, December 5, 2024, https://www.who.int/news-room/fact-sheets/detail/cholera.

24 "Who First Discovered Vibrio Cholera," UCLA Department of Epidemiology, Fielding School of Public Health, July 21, 2024, https://www.ph.ucla.edu/epi/snow/firstdiscoveredcholera.html; Filippo Pacini, *Osservazioni microscopiche e deduzioni patologiche sul cholera asiatico* (Stamperia e Cartiere, 1854).

25 Williamson, Gould, and Brown, "Richard Pfeiffer's typhoid vaccine and Almroth Wright's claim to priority."

26 Ibid.

27 O. Westphal, "Bacterial endotoxins. The second Carl Prausnitz Memorial Lecture," *International Archives of Allergy and Applied Immunology* 49, nos. 1–2 (1975): 1–43; Eugenio Centanni, "Studio sulla febbre infettiva. Prima comunicazione. Il veleno della febbre nei batteri," *Riforma medica*, IX [1893], 4, 361–368; Giovanni Favilli, "Ricordo di Eugenio Centanni, patologo, ad un secolo dalla nascita," *Archivio "de Vecchi" per l'anatomia patologica e la medicina clinica* 46, no. 3 (December 1965): 819–836.

28 L. Mazgaeen and P. Gurung, "Recent Advances in Lipopolysaccharide Recognition Systems," *International Journal of Molecular Sciences* 21, no. 2 (2020): 379, https://doi.org/10.3390/ijms21020379.

29 S. Rezania, N. Amirmozaffari, B. Tabarraei, et al., "Extraction, Purification and Characterization of Lipopolysaccharide from *Escherichia coli* and *Salmonella typhi*," *Avicenna Journal of Medical Biotechnology* 3, no. 1 (2011): 3–9.

30 M. M. Parker and J. E. Parrillo, "Septic shock. Hemodynamics and pathogenesis," *JAMA* 250, no. 24 (1983): 3324–3327.

31 Ibid.

32 Dr. Elizabeth Ehrlich, conversation with colleague, March 20, 2023.

33 Siddhartha Mukherjee, *The Laws of Medicine* (Simon & Schuster, 2014), 45.

Chapter Two: Putrefaction

1 James Henry Breasted, *The Edwin Smith Surgical Papyrus: Published in Facsimile and Hieroglyphic Transliteration and Commentary in Two Volumes* (University of Chicago Press, 1930), 423.

2   Mukherjee, *The Emperor of All Maladies*, 40; Emma J. Edelstein and Ludwig Edelstein, *Asclepius: A Collection and Interpretation of the Testimonies*, Vol. 1 (Hopkins University Press, 1945); John F. Nunn, *Ancient Egyptian Medicine* (University of Oklahoma Press, 1996).

3   Seymour and Wiersinga, eds., *Handbook of Sepsis*, 4.

4   Mukherjee, *The Laws of Medicine*, 45.

5   Homer, *The Iliad of Homer*, trans. Andrew Lang, Walter Leaf, and Ernest Myers (The Modern Library, 1950), 453; S. Geroulanos and E. T. Douka, "Historical perspective of the word 'sepsis,'" *Intensive Care Medicine* 32, no. 12 (2006): 2077, https://doi.org/10.1007/s00134-006-0392-2.

6   Homer, *The Iliad of Homer*, 441.

7   R. Shedge, K. Krishan, V. Warrier, et al., "Postmortem Changes," *StatPearls*, StatPearls Publishing, 2024–, https://www.ncbi.nlm.nih.gov/books/NBK539741; Guido Majno, *The Healing Hand: Man and Wound in the Ancient World* (Harvard University Press, 1975), 131.

8   "EGYPTIAN AND CNIDIAN MEDICINE," *JAMA* 175, no. 10 (1961): 902–903, doi:10.1001/jama.1961.03040100066018.

9   Ibid.

10 Ibid.

11 Guido Majno, "The ancient riddle of sigma eta psi iota sigma (sepsis)," *The Journal of Infectious Diseases* 163, no. 5 (1991): 937–945, https://doi.org/10.1093/infdis/163.5.937; Professor John Baines, Oxford University, email correspondence, October 20, 2025.

12 "EGYPTIAN AND CNIDIAN MEDICINE," *JAMA*.

13 Majno, "The ancient riddle of sigma eta psi iota sigma (sepsis)."

14 Majno, *The Healing Hand*, 115; J. Yupanqui Mieles, C. Vyas, E. Aslan, G. Humphreys, C. Driver, and P. Bartolo, "Honey: An Advanced Antimicrobial and Wound Healing Biomaterial for Tissue Engineering Applications," *Pharmaceutics* 14, no. 8 (2022): 1663, https://doi.org/10.3390/pharmaceutics14081663.

15 Majno, "The ancient riddle of sigma eta psi iota sigma (sepsis)"; John E. Bennett, Raphael Dolin, and Martin J. Blaser, *Mandell, Douglas, and Bennett's Principles and Practice of Infectious Diseases*, 9th ed. (Elsevier, 2020), 22.

16 This exploration into ancient Egyptian papyri was inspired by Mukherjee's *The Emperor of All Maladies*.

17 Mukherjee, *The Emperor of All Maladies*, 40.

18 Ibid.

19 Majno, *The Healing Hand*, 101.

20 Ibid., 96–98.

21 Ibid., 96; James Henry Breasted, *The Edwin Smith Surgical Papyrus: Published in Facsimile and Hieroglyphic Transliteration and Commentary in Two Volumes* (University of Chicago Press, 1930), 424.

22 Majno, *The Healing Hand*, 99.

23 H. J. Thompson, "Fever: a concept analysis," *Journal of Advanced Nursing* 51, no. 5 (2005): 484–492, https://doi.org/10.1111/j.1365-2648.2005.03520.x.

24 Breasted, *The Edwin Smith Surgical Papyrus*, 4–5.

25 Majno, *The Healing Hand*, 104.

26 Francis Adams, *The Genuine Works of Hippocrates* (Sydenham Society, 1849), 313.

27 G. Henry and W. L. Garner, "Inflammatory mediators in wound healing," *The Surgical Clinics of North America* 83, no. 3 (2003): 483–507, https://doi.org/10.1016/S0039-6109(02)00200-1.

28 Majno, *The Healing Hand*, 102.

29 Ibid., 102.

30 J. A. Freiberg, "The mythos of laudable pus along with an explanation for its origin," *Journal of Community Hospital Internal Medicine Perspectives* 7, no. 3 (2017): 196–198, https://doi.org/10.1080/20009666.2017.1343077.

31 Ibid.

32 M. Turgut, "Ancient medical schools in Knidos and Kos," *Child's Nervous System* 27, no. 2 (2011): 197–200, https://doi.org/10.1007/s00381-010-1271-2.

33 G. Pappas, I. J. Kiriaze, and M. E. Falagas, "Insights into infectious disease in the era of Hippocrates," *International Journal of Infectious Diseases* 12, no. 4 (2008): 347–350, https://doi.org/10.1016/j.ijid.2007.11.003.

34 Stefanos Geroulanos, "Ancient Greek Medicine: Hippocratic Medicine," Hippocratic Lectures, International Hippocratic Foundation, https://hippocraticfoundation.org/images/hippocrat/pdf/lectueres/Hippocratic_Medicine_1_M_Goulandri_VVV_-_A.pdf; Hippocrates, *On the Sacred Disease*, in *Hippocratic Writings*, ed. G. E. R. Lloyd, trans. J. Chadwick and W. N. Mann (Penguin Books, 1983), 244–58.

35 M. Rossi, "Homer and Herodotus to Egyptian medicine," *Vesalius: Acta Internationales Historiae Medicinae*, (2010): 3–5; Homer, *Odyssey*, trans. Robert Fagles (Viking, 1996), 4.229–232; Herodotus, *Histories*, trans. Aubrey de Sélincourt, rev. John Marincola (Penguin Books, 2003), 2.84–86.

36 Majno, "The ancient riddle of sigma eta psi iota sigma (sepsis)."

37 Ibid.

38 Ibid.

39 Ibid.

40 Ibid.

41 Ibid.

42 John Redman Coxe, *The Writings of Hippocrates and Galen: Epitomised From the Original Latin Translations* (Lindsay and Blakiston, 1846), 88–89, 94, 96, 111–112, 114.

43 Thompson, "Fever: a concept analysis."

44 Coxe, *The Writings of Hippocrates and Galen*, 94.

45 P. A. Mackowiak, "Was This the Demise of the Food Critic?" *Clinical Infectious Diseases* 40, no. 5 (2005): 718, https://doi.org/10.1086/427702; John Chadwick and W. N. Mann, *The Medical Works of Hippocrates* (Charles C. Thomas, 1950), 50.

46 Mackowiak, "Was This the Demise of the Food Critic?"; Chadwick and Mann, *The Medical Works of Hippocrates*, 50.

47 Ibid.

48 Ibid.

49 Majno, *The Healing Hand*, 183.

50 Ibid.

51 Ibid.

52 Freiberg, "The mythos of laudable pus along with an explanation for its origin."

53 Ibid.

54 Ibid.

55 Majno, *The Healing Hand*, 184.

56 Freiberg, "The mythos of laudable pus along with an explanation for its origin."

57 Ibid.

58 Coxe, *The Writings of Hippocrates and Galen*, 463–464.

59 Freiberg, "The mythos of laudable pus along with an explanation for its origin."

60 D. E. Gyorki, "Laudable pus: historic concept revisited," *ANZ Journal of Surgery* 75, no. 4 (2005): 24, https://doi.org/10.1111/j.1445-2197.2005.03338.x.

61 Ibid.; Freiberg, "The mythos of laudable pus along with an explanation for its origin"; Theodoric Borgognoni, *The Surgery of Theodoric, ca. A.D. 1267*, trans. E. Campbell (Appleton, 1955); Henri de Mondeville, *Chirurgie: Traduction Contemporaine de l'Auteur*, French ed. (Forgotten Books, 2018); M. Donaldson, E. Alment, and A. J. Wright, "A Plea for Ignoring 'Laudable Pus' in the Treatment of Septic Wounds," *British Medical Journal* 2, no. 2904 (1916): 286–89, https://doi.org/10.1136/bmj.2.2904.286.

62 M. Siegler, "The progression of medicine. From physician paternalism to patient autonomy to bureaucratic parsimony," *Archives of Internal Medicine* 145, no. 4 (1985): 713–715, https://doi.org/10.1001/archinte.145.4.713.

Chapter Three: Germs

1 Timothy Ferris, *Coming of Age in the Milky Way* (Doubleday, 1988), 386.

2 D. J. Funk, J. E. Parrillo, and A. Kumar, "Sepsis and septic shock: a history. *Critical Care Clinics* 25, no. 1 (2009): 83–viii, https://doi.org/10.1016/j.ccc.2008.12.003; Siddhartha Mukherjee, *The Song of the Cell* (Scribner, 2022), 26–27; Douglas Anderson, "Galileo's Microscope," Lens on Leeuwenhoek, May 21, 2025, https://lensonleeuwenhoek.net/content/galileos-microscope.

3 Laura Poppick, "Let Us Now Praise the Invention of the Microscope," *Smithsonian Magazine*, March 30, 2017, https://www.smithsonianmag.com/science-nature/what-we-owe-to-the-invention-microscope-180962725/.

4 H. Gest, "The discovery of microorganisms by Robert Hooke and Antoni Van Leeuwenhoek, fellows of the Royal Society," *Notes and Records of the Royal Society of London* 58, no. 2 (2004): 187–201, https://doi.org/10.1098/rsnr.2004.0055.

5 Mukherjee, *The Song of the Cell*, 27.

6 N. Lane, "The unseen world: Reflections on Leeuwenhoek (1677) 'Concerning little animals,'" *Philosophical Transactions of the Royal Society of London: Series B, Biological Sciences* 370, no. 1666 (2015): 20140344, https://doi.org/10.1098/rstb.2014.0344.

7 Ibid.

8 Gest, "The discovery of microorganisms by Robert Hooke and Antoni Van Leeuwenhoek, fellows of the Royal Society."

9 Lane, "The unseen world: Reflections on Leeuwenhoek (1677) 'Concerning little animals'."

10 Ibid.

11 Ibid.

12 Gest, "The discovery of microorganisms by Robert Hooke and Antoni Van Leeuwenhoek, fellows of the Royal Society."

13 Jacques Tenon, *Memoirs on Paris Hospitals* (Science History Publications, 1996), 7; "Hôtel-Dieu, Paris," Wikipedia, last updated July 26, 2024, https://en.wikipedia.org/w/index.php?title=H%C3%B4tel-Dieu,_Paris&oldid=1235352183.

14 Guenter B. Risse, *Mending Bodies*, Saving Souls (Oxford University Press, 1999); Charles E. Rosenberg, *The Care of Strangers* (Johns Hopkins University Press, 1987); George Rosen, *A History of Public Health*, rev. ed. (Johns Hopkins University Press, 2015).

15 Tenon, *Memoirs on Paris Hospitals*, 7.

16 Ibid., 238.

17 Ibid., 167.

18 Ibid.,14, 17.

19 Phyllis Allen Richmond, "The Hôtel-Dieu of Paris on the Eve of the Revolution," *Journal of the History of Medicine and Allied Sciences* 16, no. 4, (1961): 335–353, https://doi.org/10.1093/jhmas/XVI.4.335.

20 Ibid.

21 Ibid.

22 Rosen, *A History of Public Health*, 77–80.

23 Majno, "The ancient riddle of sigma eta psi iota sigma (sepsis)."

24 Ibid.

25 J. S. Hernandez Botero and M. C. Florian Perez, "The History of Sepsis from Ancient Egypt to the XIX Century," *InTech* (2012): 14–15, doi: 10.5772/51484, https://www.intechopen.com/chapters/39638.

26 Mukherjee, *The Song of the Cell*, 56–57.

27 Rosenberg, *The Care of Strangers*, 20, 69, 75; Risse, *Mending Bodies, Saving Souls*, 300–305.

28 Mukherjee, *The Song of the Cell*, 56.

29 Emil Noeggerath and Abraham Jacobi, *Contributions to Midwifery and Diseases of Women and Children with a Report on the Progress of Obstetrics, Uterine and Infantile Pathology in 1858* (Baillièr Bros, 1859), 247.

30 Mukherjee, *The Song of the Cell*, 61; Irvine Loudon, *The Tragedy of Childbed Fever* (Oxford University Press, 2000).

31 Sarah Andrews, "Alexander Gordon, Puerperal Fever" in *Notes from the John Martin Rare Book Room*, Hardin Library for the Health Sciences, September 5, 2018, https://blog.lib.uiowa.edu/needtoknow/2018/09/05/alexander-gordon-puerperal-fever-september-2018-notes-from-the-john-martin-rare-book-room-hardin-library/.

32 Alexander Gordon, *A Treatise on the Epidemic Puerperal Fever of Aberdeen* (G.G. & J. Robinson, 1795).

33 Ibid.; I. M. Gould, "Alexander Gordon, puerperal sepsis, and modern theories of infection control--Semmelweis in perspective," *The Lancet Infectious Diseases* 10, no. 4 (2010): 275–278, https://doi.org/10.1016/S1473-3099(09)70304-4.

34 Ibid.

35 Ibid.

36 Ibid.; O. W. Holmes, "The Contagiousness of Puerperal Fever," *New England Quarterly Journal of Medicine and Surgery* 1 (1843): 503–530.

37 Danielle Ofri, *When We Do Harm: A Doctor Confronts Medical Error* (Beacon Press, 2020), 15.

38 Mukherjee, *The Song of the Cell*, 61.

39 Ofri, *When We Do Harm*, 16.

40 Ibid.

41 Ibid.

42 Ibid.; Mukherjee, *The Song of the Cell*, 61.

43 Mukherjee, *The Song of the Cell*, 62.

44 Ofri, *When We Do Harm*, 17.

45 Ibid., 16–17.

46 Ibid., 17.

47 V. Mouajou, K. Adams, G. DeLisle, and C. Quach, "Hand hygiene compliance in the prevention of hospital-acquired infections: a systematic review," *The Journal of Hospital Infection* 119 (2022): 33–48, https://doi.org/10.1016/j.jhin.2021.09.016; "Global Report on Infection Prevention and Control," World Health Organization, May 23, 2022, https://www.who.int/publications/i/item/9789240051164; V. Erasmus, T. J. Daha, H. Brug, et al., "Systematic Review of Studies on Compliance with Hand Hygiene Guidelines in Hospital Care," *Infection Control & Hospital Epidemiology* 31, no. 3 (2010): 283–294.

48 "Healthcare-Acquired Infections (HAIs)," PatientCareLink, August 28, 2023, https://www.patientcarelink.org/improving-patient-care/healthcare-acquired-infections-hais.

49 "Key Facts and Figures, World Hand Hygiene Day 2021," World Health Organization, July 26, 2024, https://www.who.int/campaigns/world-hand-hygiene-day/2021/key-facts-and-figures.

50 Mukherjee, *The Song of the Cell*, 57; Rosen, *A History of Public Health*, 40.

51 Mukherjee, *The Song of the Cell*, 66.

52 J. Lister, "On a New Method of Treating Compound Fracture, Abscess, etc., with Observations on the Conditions of Suppuration," *The Lancet* 89, no. 2299 (March 16, 1867): 326–329.

53 J. Lister, "Antiseptic Principle in the Practice of Surgery," *The British Medical Journal*, September 1867, https://www.ncbi.nlm.nih.gov/pmc/articles/PMC1841140/pdf/brmedj02129-0027.pdf.

54 W. W. Van Arsdale, "I. On the Present State of Knowledge in Bacterial Science in Its Surgical Relations (Continued): Sepsis," *Annals of Surgery* 3 no. 4 (1886): 321–333.

55 Ibid.

56 Seymour and Wiersinga, eds., *Handbook of Sepsis*, 5–6.

57 David A. Rennie, "1874–1882," *Sir Alexander Ogston, 1844–1929: A Life at Medical and Military Frontlines* (Edinburgh University Press, 2024), 21–34, https://doi.org/10.1515/9781399501330-005; Abigail Orenstein, "The Discovery and Naming of *Staphylococcus aureus*," 2006, https://www.researchgate.net/publication/237219827_The_Discovery_and_Naming_of_Staphylococcus_aureus; "Alexander Ogston (1884–1929)," *British Journal of Surgery* 52, no. 12 (1965): 917–92, https://doi.org/10.1002/bjs.1800521203.

58 Mukherjee, *The Song of the Cell*, 59.

59 Centers for Disease Control and Prevention, "Historical Perspectives Centennial: Koch's Discovery of the Tubercle Bacillus," *Morbidity and Mortality Weekly Report* 31, no. 10 (March 19, 1982): 121–23,

60 I. Barberis, N. L. Bragazzi, L. Galluzzo, and M. Martini, "The history of tuberculosis: from the first historical records to the isolation of Koch's bacillus," *Journal of Preventive Medicine and Hygiene* 58, no. 1 (2017): E9–E12.

61 Ibid.; "History of World TB Day," Centers for Disease Control and Prevention, December 5, 2024, https://www.cdc.gov/world-tb-day/history/?CDC_AAref_Val=https://www.cdc.gov/tb/worldtbday/history.htm.

62 Ibid.

63 S. M. Blevins and M. S. Bronze, "Robert Koch and the 'golden age' of bacteriology," *International Journal of Infectious Diseases* 14, no. 9 (2010): e744–e751, https://doi.org/10.1016/j.ijid.2009.12.003.

64 G. Budelmann, trans. Bruce Filardi, "Hugo Schottmüller, 1867–1936: The problem of sepsis," *Der Internist* 10, no. 3 (1969): 92–101.

65 Funk, Parrillo, and Kumar, "Sepsis and septic shock: a history."

Chapter Four: Magic Bullets and Murphy's Law

1 S. Y. Tan and Y. Tatsumura, "Alexander Fleming (1881–1955): Discoverer of penicillin," *Singapore Medical Journal* 56, no. 7 (2015), 366–367, https://doi.org/10.11622/smedj.2015105.

2 Wolfgang Saxon, "Anne Miller, 90, First Patient Who Was Saved by Penicillin," *The New York Times*, June 9, 1999, https://www.nytimes.com/1999/06/09/us/anne-miller-90-first-patient-who-was-saved-by-penicillin.html.

3 William Rosen, *Miracle Cure* (Penguin Books, 2017), 1.

4 I. Oransky, "Obituary: Orvan Hess," *The Lancet* 360, no. 9340 (2002): 1179, https://www.thelancet.com/journals/lancet/article/PIIS0140-6736(02)11230-X/fulltext.

5 "Medication Superstar Made Its U.S. Debut Right Here," Yale New Haven Health, September 7, 2017, archived at Internet Archive, capture date September 29, 2022, https://web.archive.org/web/20220929134206/https://www.ynhhs.org/publications/bulletin/archive/090717/medication-superstar-made-its-us-debut-right-here.

6 Ibid.

7 Carla Baranauckas, "Dr. Orvan W. Hess, 96, Dies; Developed Fetal Heart Monitor," *The New York Times*, September 16, 2002, https://www.nytimes.com/2002/09/16/us/dr-orvan-w-hess-96-dies-developed-fetal-heart-monitor.html; "Medication Superstar Made Its U.S. Debut Right Here," Yale New Haven Health; Rosen, *Miracle Cure*, 1.

8 Alexander Fleming, "On the Antibacterial Action of Cultures of a *Penicillium*, with Special Reference to Their Use in the Isolation of *B. influenzae*," *British Journal of Experimental Pathology* 10, no. 3 (1929): 226–36; H. W. Florey, E. Chain, N. G. Heatley, et al., "Further Observations on Penicillin," *The Lancet* 236, no. 6104 (1941): 177–89; Milton Wainwright, "The History of the Therapeutic Use of Penicillin," *History and Philosophy of the Life Sciences* 15, no. 3 (1993): 291–311; R. Quinn, "Rethinking antibiotic research and development: World War II and the penicillin collaborative," *American Journal of Public Health* 103, no. 3 (2013): 426–434, https://doi.org/10.2105/AJPH.2012.300693.

9 Rosen, *Miracle Cure*, 1.

10 Ibid., 2; Ivan Oransky, "Orvan Hess," *The Lancet* 360, no. 9343 (2002): 1124; John Parascandola, *The Development of American Antibiotics during World War II: What We Learned and What We Have Forgotten* (American Institute of the History of Pharmacy, 1980), 11–18.

11 Rosen, *Miracle Cure*, 2.

12 Ibid.

13 Ibid., 3.

14 Ofri, *When We Do Harm*, 2.

15 Centers for Disease Control and Prevention, "Achievements in Public Health, 1900–1999: Control of Infectious Diseases," *Morbidity and Mortality Weekly Report* 48, no. 29 (July 30, 1999): 621–29, https://www.cdc.gov/mmwr/preview/mmwrhtml/mm4829a1.htm.

16 "Life Expectancy in the USA, 1900–1998," Department of Demography, Berkeley University, accessed November 14, 2025, archived at Internet Archive, capture date July 2, 2016, https://web.archive.org/web/20160901114018/http://u.demog.berkeley.edu/~andrew/1918/figure2.html; Robert. H. Shmerling, "Why life expectancy in the US is falling," Harvard Health Publishing, October 20, 2022, https://www.health.harvard.edu/blog/why-life-expectancy-in-the-us-is-falling-202210202835.

17 D. Skinner and C. S. Keefer, "Significance of Bacteremia caused by *Staphylococcus aureus*: A study of one hundred and twenty-two cases and a review of the literature concerned with experimental infection in animals," *Archives of Internal Medicine* 68, no. 5 (1941): 851–875, doi: 10.1001/archinte.1941.00200110003001.

18 A. R. Felty and C. S. Keefer, "*Bacillus coli* sepsis: clinical study of twenty-eight cases of blood stream infection by the colon *bacillus*," *JAMA* 82, no. 18 (1924): 1430–1433, doi:10.1001/jama.1924.02650440024010.

19 Ibid.

20 T. J. Hommes, W. J. Wiersinga, and T. van der Poll, "The Host Response to Sepsis," in *Yearbook of Intensive Care and Emergency Medicine 2009*, ed. J.-L. Vincent (Springer, 2009), https://doi.org/10.1007/978-3-540-92276-6_4.

21 Felty and Keefer, "*Bacillus coli* sepsis: clinical study of twenty-eight cases of blood stream infection by the colon *bacillus*."

22 Mukherjee, *The Song of the Cell*, 56–57.

23 "History of Port Health," Centers for Disease Control and Prevention, May 15, 2024, https://www.cdc.gov/port-health/about/history-port-health.html.

24 Rosen, *A History of Public Health*, 72.

25 "1881–1896 cholera pandemic," Wikipedia, last edited October 27, 2025, https://en.wikipedia.org/w/index.php?title=1881%E2%80%931896_cholera_pandemic&oldid=1198515148; M. T. Phillips, K. A. Owers, B. T. Grenfell, and V. E. Pitzer, "Changes in historical typhoid transmission across 16 U.S. cities, 1889-1931: Quantifying the impact of investments in water and sewer infrastructures," *PLoS Neglected Tropical Diseases* 14, no. 3 (2020): e0008048, https://doi.org/10.1371/journal.pntd.0008048.

26 Centers for Disease Control and Prevention, "Achievements in Public Health, 1900–1999: Control of Infectious Disease," *Morbidity and Mortality Weekly Report* 48, no. 29 (July 30, 1999): 621–29, https://www.cdc.gov/mmwr/preview/mmwrhtml/mm4829a1.htm.

27 Ibid.

28 "A Century of U.S. Water Chlorination and Treatment: One of the Ten Greatest Public Health Achievements of the 20th Century," Centers for Disease Control and Prevention, November 26, 2012, https://stacks.cdc.gov/view/cdc/92155.

29 Ibid.

30 Centers for Disease Control and Prevention, "Achievements in Public Health, 1900–1999: Control of Infectious Disease."

31 Diane Whitmore Schanzenbach, Ryan Nunn, and Lauren Bauer, "The Changing Landscape of American Life Expectancy," The Hamilton Project, June 2016, https://www.hamilton-project.org/assets/files/changing_landscape_american_life_expectancy.pdf; Centers for Disease Control and Prevention, "Ten Great Public Health Achievements — United States, 1900–1999," *Morbidity and Mortality Weekly Report* 48, no. 12 (April 2, 1999): 241-256, https://www.cdc.gov/mmwr/pdf/wk/mm4812.pdf.

32 G. L. Armstrong, L. A. Conn, and R. W. Pinner, "Trends in infectious disease mortality in the United States during the 20th century," *JAMA* 281, no. 1 (1999): 61–66, https://doi.org/10.1001/jama.281.1.61.

33 Eileen M. Crimmins, Samuel H. Preston, and Barney Cohen, eds., "Explaining Divergent Levels of Longevity in High-Income Countries (Difference Between Life Expectancy in the United States and Other High-Income Countries)," National Academies Press, 2011, https://nap.nationalacademies.org/read/13089/chapter/3.

34 Bennett, Dolin, and Blaser, *Mandell, Douglas, and Bennett's Principles and Practice of Infectious Diseases*, 992.

35 Lewis Thomas, *The Youngest Science* (Viking, 1983), 40.

36 A. R. Reynolds, "Pneumonia: the new 'captain of the men of death.': its increasing prevalence and the necessity of methods for its restriction," *JAMA* XL, no. 9 (1903): 583–586, doi:10.1001/jama.1903.92490090031001k.

37 S. H. Podolsky, "The changing fate of pneumonia as a public health concern in 20th-century America and beyond," *American Journal of Public Health* 95, no. 12 (2005): 2144–2154, https://doi.org/10.2105/AJPH.2004.048397.

38 R. Austrian, "The Gram stain and the etiology of lobar pneumonia, an historical note," *Bacteriological Reviews* 24, no. 3 (1960): 261–265, https://doi.org/10.1128/br.24.3.261-265.1960; C. Friedlaender, "Ueber die Schizomyceten bei der acuten fibrösen Pneumonie," *Virchows Archiv* 87 (1882): 319–324, https://doi.org/10.1007/BF01880516.

39 Mukherjee, *The Song of the Cell*, 188.

40 Ibid., 188–190.

41 Ibid., 190.

42 A. Opinel and G. Gachelin, "French 19th century contributions to the development of treatments for diphtheria," *Journal of the Royal Society of Medicine* 104, no. 4 (2011): 173–178, https://doi.org/10.1258/jrsm.2010.10k069.

43 Klass, "How Science Conquered Diphtheria, the Plague Among Children."

44 A. R. Dochez and L. J. Gillespie, "A biologic classification of pneumococci by means of immunity reactions," *JAMA* 61, no. 10 (1913): 727–732, doi:10.1001/jama.1913.04350100005003.

45 M. Kalin, "Pneumococcal serotypes and their clinical relevance," *Thorax* 53, no. 3 (1998): 159–162, https://doi.org/10.1136/thx.53.3.159.

46 "Clinical Overview of Pneumococcal Disease," Centers for Disease Control and Prevention, February 6, 2024, https://www.cdc.gov/pneumococcal/hcp/clinical-overview/index.html.

47 Podolsky, "The Changing Fate of Pneumonia as a Public Health Concern in 20th-Century America and Beyond."

48 Ibid.; World Health Organization, *Laboratory Methods for the Diagnosis of Meningitis Caused by Neisseria meningitidis, Streptococcus pneumoniae, and Haemophilus influenzae* (World Health Organization, 2011), 63–66.

49 Podolsky, "The changing fate of pneumonia as a public health concern in 20th-century America and beyond"; Barbara Gutmann Rosenkrantz, *Public Health and the State: Changing Views in Massachusetts, 1842–1936* (Harvard University Press, 1972), 129–130.

50 This is an idea inspired by Siddhartha Mukherjee's 2020 article "What the Coronavirus Crisis Reveals About American Medicine," *New Yorker*, April 27, https://www.newyorker.com/magazine/2020/05/04/what-the-coronavirus-crisis-reveals-about-american-medicine.

51 Podolsky, "The changing fate of pneumonia as a public health concern in 20th-century America and beyond."

52 Ibid.

53 Ibid.

54 Ibid.

55 David M. Musher, Ronald Anderson, and Charles Feldman, "The Remarkable History of Pneumococcal Vaccination: An Ongoing Challenge," *Pneumonia (Nathan)* 14, no. 1 (September 25, 2022): 5, https://doi.org/10.1186/s41479-022-00097-y.

56 Podolsky, "The changing fate of pneumonia as a public health concern in 20th-century America and beyond."

57 Ibid.

58 Blake Stilwell, "The Real-Life Murphy and How 'Murphy's Law' Came to Be," Military.com, June 10, 2022, https://www.military.com/history/real-life-murphy-and-how-murphys-law-came-be.html.

59 Penn Nursing, "History of Hospitals," University of Pennsylvania, accessed November 10, 2025, https://www.nursing.upenn.edu/nhhc/nurses-institutions-caring/history-of-hospitals/.

60 Ibid.

61 "Total Number of Hospital Admissions in the U.S. from 1946 to 2019," Statista online, accessed November 10, 2025, https://www.statista.com/statistics/459718/total-hospital-admission-number-in-the-us/.

62 Gawande, *The Checklist Manifesto*, 19.

63 D. M. Musher and A. R. Thorner, "Community-acquired pneumonia," *The New England Journal of Medicine* 371, no. 17 (2014): 1619–1628, https://doi.org/10.1056/NEJMra1312885.

64 Ofri, *When We Do Harm*, 3.

Chapter Five: Changing Patterns of Infection

1   Rogers, "The changing pattern of life-threatening microbial disease."

2   Lori Wiviott Tischler, "Drug-Resistant Bacteria a Growing Health Problem," Harvard Health Blog, September 17, 2013, archived at Internet Archive, capture date September 24, 2013, https://web.archive.org/web/20131001215139/http://www.health.harvard.edu/blog/drug-resistant-bacteria-a-growing-health-problem-201309176677.

3   Rogers, "The changing pattern of life-threatening microbial disease."

4   Ibid.; W. R. McCabe and G. G. Jackson, "Gram-Negative Bacteremia: I. Etiology and Ecology," *Archives of Internal Medicine* 110, no. 6 (1962): 847–855, doi:10.1001/archinte.1962.03620240029006.

5   Rogers, "The changing pattern of life-threatening microbial disease."

6   Alexander Fleming, "Penicillin," Nobel Lecture, December 11, 1945, https://www.nobelprize.org/uploads/2018/06/fleming-lecture.pdf.

7   Steven Spielberg, *Jurassic Park* (Universal Pictures, 1993).

8   "2019 Antibiotic Resistance Threats Report," Centers for Disease Control and Prevention, July 16, 2024, https://www.cdc.gov/antimicrobial-resistance/data-research/threats/index.html.

9   M. I. Hutchings, A. W. Truman, and B. Wilkinson, "Antibiotics: past, present and future," *Current Opinion in Microbiology* 51 (2019): 72–80, https://doi.org/10.1016/j.mib.2019.10.008.

10 E. P. Abraham and E. Chain, "An enzyme from bacteria able to destroy penicillin," *Reviews of Infectious Diseases* 10, no. 4 (1988): 677–678.

11 C. H. Rammelkamp and T. Maxon, "Resistance of *Staphylococcus aureus* to the Action of Penicillin," *Proceedings of the Society for Experimental Biology and Medicine* 51, no. 3 (1942): 386–389, doi:10.3181/00379727-51-13986.

12 "2019 Antibiotic Resistance Threats Report," Centers for Disease Control and Prevention.

13 S. Gupta, A. Sakhuja, G. Kumar, et al., "Culture-Negative Severe Sepsis: Nationwide Trends and Outcomes," *Chest* 150, no. 6 (2016): 1251–1259, https://doi.org/10.1016/j.chest.2016.08.1460; N. J. Meyer and H. C. Prescott, "Sepsis and Septic Shock," *The New England Journal of Medicine* 391, no. 22 (2024): 2133–2146, https://doi.org/10.1056/NEJMra2403213.

14 Martin J. Blaser, Jeffrey I. Cohen, and Steven M. Holland, *Mandell, Douglas, and Bennett's Principles and Practice of Infectious Diseases*, 10th ed. (Elsevier, 2025), 942.

15 David Gilbert, telephone discussion, July 29, 2024.

16 "2019 Antibiotic Resistance Threats Report," Centers for Disease Control and Prevention.

17 Ibid.

18 "Antimicrobial resistance," World Health Organization Newsroom, November 21, 2023, https://www.who.int/news-room/fact-sheets/detail/antimicrobial-resistance.

19 "2019 Antibiotic Resistance Threats Report," Centers for Disease Control and Prevention.

20 Antimicrobial Resistance Collaborators, "Global burden of bacterial antimicrobial resistance in 2019: a systematic analysis," *The Lancet* 399, no. 10325 (2022): 629–655, https://doi.org/10.1016/S0140-6736(21)02724-0.

21 M. Naghavi, S. E. Vollset, K. S. Ikuta, et al., "Global burden of bacterial antimicrobial resistance 1990-2021: a systematic analysis with forecasts to 2050," *The Lancet* 404, no. 10459 (2024): 1199–1226.

22 Rosen, *Miracle Cure*, 301.

23 J. Morschhäuser, G. Köhler, W. Ziebuhr, et al., "Evolution of microbial pathogens," *Philosophical Transactions of the Royal Society of London: Series B, Biological Sciences* 355, no. 1397 (2000): 695–704, https://doi.org/10.1098/rstb.2000.0609.

24 D. R. Helinski, "A Brief History of Plasmids," *EcoSal Plus* 10, no. 1 (2022): eESP00282021, https://doi.org/10.1128/ecosalplus.esp-0028-2021.

25 S. Tao, H. Chen, N. Li, et al., "The Spread of Antibiotic Resistance Genes In Vivo Model," *The Canadian Journal of Infectious Diseases & Medical Microbiology (Journal Canadien des Maladies Infectieuses et de la Microbiologie Medicale)* 3348695 (2022), https://doi.org/10.1155/2022/3348695.

26 A. C. Shore and D. C. Coleman, "Staphylococcal cassette chromosome mec: recent advances and new insights," *International Journal of Medical Microbiology: IJMM* 303, nos. 6–7 (2013): 350–359, https://doi.org/10.1016/j.ijmm.2013.02.002.

27 Tao, Chen, Li, et al., "The Spread of Antibiotic Resistance Genes In Vivo Model."

28 Rosen, *Miracle Cure*, 301.

29 Madeline Barron, "The Gut Resistome and the Spread of Antimicrobial Resistance," American Society for Microbiology Online, June 13, 2022, https://asm.org/articles/2022/june/the-gut-resistome-and-the-spread-of-antimicrobial.

30 Hutchings, Truman, and Wilkinson, "Antibiotics: past, present and future," *Current Opinion in Microbiology* 51, (2019): 72–80, https://doi.org/10.1016/j.mib.2019.10.008.

31 Kai Kupferschmidt, "Resistance fighters," *Science* 352 (2016): 758–761, https://www.science.org/doi/10.1126/science.352.6287.758; R. I. Aminov, "A brief history of the antibiotic era: lessons learned and challenges for the future," *Frontiers in Microbiology* 1 (2010): 134, https://doi.org/10.3389/fmicb.2010.00134.

32 Rosen, *Miracle Cure*, 301–302.

33 K. E. Fleming-Dutra, A. L. Hersh, D. J. Shapiro, et al., "Prevalence of Inappropriate Antibiotic Prescriptions Among US Ambulatory Care Visits, 2010–2011," *JAMA* 315, no. 17 (2016): 1864–1873, https://doi.org/10.1001/jama.2016.4151.

34 Rosen, *Miracle Cure*, 302.

35 "Inappropriate Antibiotic Prescribing for Adults Comes With Increased Risks," Pew Charitable Trusts, January 27, 2023, https://www.pewtrusts.org/en/research-and-analysis/fact-sheets/2023/01/inappropriate-antibiotic-prescribing-for-adults-comes-with-increased-risks.

36 Rosen, *Miracle Cure*, 231.

37 A. Hollis and Z. Ahmed, "Preserving antibiotics, rationally," *The New England Journal of Medicine* 369, no. 26 (2013): 2474–2476, https://doi.org/10.1056/NEJMp1311479; K. Tiseo, L. Huber, M. Gilbert, et al., "Global Trends in Antimicrobial Use in Food Animals from 2017 to 2030," *Antibiotics (Basel, Switzerland)* 9, no. 12 (2020): 918, https://doi.org/10.3390/antibiotics9120918.

38 Rosen, *Miracle Cure*, 236-237.

39 F. Rajer and L. Sandegren, "The Role of Antibiotic Resistance Genes in the Fitness Cost of Multiresistance Plasmids," *mBio* 13, no. 1 (2022): e0355221, https://doi.org/10.1128/mbio.03552-21.

40 Ibid.

41 Richard E. Dixon, "Control of Health-Care-Associated Infections, 1961–2011," *Morbidity and Mortality Weekly Report* 60, no. 04 (October 7, 2011): 58–63, https://www.cdc.gov/mmwr/preview/mmwrhtml/su6004a10.htm.

42 K. Hillier, "Babies and bacteria: phage typing, bacteriologists, and the birth of infection control," *Bulletin of the History of Medicine* 80, no. 4 (2006): 733–761, https://doi.org/10.1353/bhm.2006.0130.

43 Ibid.; F. Torriani and R. Taplitz, "History of infection prevention and control," *Infectious Diseases* (2010): 76–85, https://doi.org/10.1016/B978-0-323-04579-7.00006-X.

44 F. D. Lowy, "Antimicrobial resistance: the example of *Staphylococcus aureus*," *The Journal of Clinical Investigation* 111, no. 9 (2003): 1265–1273, https://doi.org/10.1172/JCI18535.

45 M. Vestergaard, D. Frees, and H. Ingmer, "Antibiotic Resistance and the MRSA Problem," *Microbiology Spectrum* 7, no. 2 (2019), 10.1128/microbiolspec.GPP3-0057-2018, https://doi.org/10.1128/microbiolspec.GPP3-0057-2018.

46 Dixon, "Control of Health-Care-Associated Infections, 1961–2011."

47 Centers for Disease Control and Prevention, "Public Health Focus: Surveillance, Prevention, and Control of Nosocomial Infections," *Morbidity and Mortality Weekly Report* 41, no. 42 (October 23, 1992): 783787, https://www.cdc.gov/mmwr/preview/mmwrhtml/00017800.htm.

48 E. Charani and A. Holmes, "Antibiotic Stewardship—Twenty Years in the Making," *Antibiotics (Basel, Switzerland)* 8, no. 1 (2019): 7, https://doi.org/10.3390/antibiotics8010007.

49 "CMS Final Rule on Antibiotic Stewardship Programs," American Society for Microbiology, October 18, 2019, https://asm.org/articles/policy/2019/cms-final-rule-on-antibiotic-stewardship-programs.

50 "COVID-19: U.S. impact on antimicrobial resistance, special report 2022," National Center for Emerging and Zoonotic Infectious Disease (U.S.) Division of Healthcare Quality Promotion, June 2022, https://stacks.cdc.gov/view/cdc/119025.

51 Rogers, "The changing pattern of life-threatening microbial disease."

52 Ibid.

53 Martin Blaser, interview, October 28, 2023.

54 Ibid.; see also this footnote reference: A. R. Omran, "The epidemiologic transition: a theory of the epidemiology of population change. 1971," *The Milbank Quarterly* 83, no. 4 (2005): 731–757, https://doi.org/10.1111/j.1468-0009.2005.00398.x.

55 Rogers, "The changing pattern of life-threatening microbial disease."

56 A. L. Cogen, V. Nizet, and R. L. Gallo, "Skin microbiota: a source of disease or defence?" *The British Journal of Dermatology* 158, no. 3 (2008): 442–455, https://doi.org/10.1111/j.1365-2133.2008.08437.x.

57 "2019 Antibiotic Resistance Threats Report," Centers for Disease Control and Prevention.

58 P. Feuerstadt, N. Theriault, and G. Tillotson, "The burden of CDI in the United States: a multifactorial challenge," *BMC Infectious Diseases* 23, no. 1 (2023): 132, https://doi.org/10.1186/s12879-023-08096-0.

59 L. Heinlen and J. D. Ballard, "*Clostridium difficile* infection," *The American Journal of the Medical Sciences* 340, no. 3 (2010): 247–252, https://doi.org/10.1097/MAJ.0b013e3181e939d8.

60 Pierre-Joseph van Beneden, *Animal Parasites and Messmates* (Appleton and Company, 1876), 1, 83.

61 Blaser interview.

62 Sehgal and Khanna, "Gut microbiome and *Clostridioides difficile* infection: a closer look at the microscopic interface," *Therapeutic Advances in Gastroenterology* 14 (2021): 1756284821994736, https://doi.org/10.1177/1756284821994736.

63 Blaser interview.

64 Martin J. Blaser, *Missing Microbes* (Picador, 2014), 187; C. M. Pike and C. M. Theriot, "Mechanisms of Colonization Resistance Against *Clostridioides difficile*," *The Journal of Infectious Diseases* 223, no. 12, supplement 2 (2021): S194–S200, https://doi.org/10.1093/infdis/jiaa408.

65 K. Sehgal and S. Khanna, "Gut microbiome and *Clostridioides difficile* infection: a closer look at the microscopic interface."

66 Blaser, *Missing Microbes*, 187.

67 McCabe and Jackson, "Gram-Negative Bacteremia: I. Etiology and Ecology"; T. van der Poll, M. Shankar-Hari, and W. J. Wiersinga, "The immunology of sepsis," *Immunity* 54, no. 11 (2021): 2450–2464, https://doi.org/10.1016/j.immuni.2021.10.012.

68 K. E., Rudd, S. C. Johnson, K. M. Agesa, et al., "Global, regional, and national sepsis incidence and mortality, 1990-2017: analysis for the Global Burden of Disease Study," *The Lancet* 395, no. 10219 (2020): 200–211, doi: 10.1016/S0140-6736(19)32989-7, PMID: 31954465, PMCID: PMC6970225; "Global Report on the Epidemiology and Burden of Sepsis," World Health Organization, September 9, 2020, https://www.who.int/publications/i/item/9789240010789.

69 D. C. Angus, W. T. Linde-Zwirble, J. Lidicker, et al., "Epidemiology of severe sepsis in the United States: analysis of incidence, outcome, and associated costs of care," *Critical Care Medicine* 29, no. 7 (2001): 1303–1310, https://doi.org/10.1097/00003246-200107000-00002.

70 "About Chronic Diseases," Centers for Disease Control and Prevention, October 4, 2024, https://www.cdc.gov/chronic-disease/about/index.html.

71 Seymour and Wiersinga, eds., *Handbook of Sepsis*, 18.

72 Ibid.; Angus, Linde-Zwirble, Lidicker, et al., "Epidemiology of severe sepsis in the United States: analysis of incidence, outcome, and associated costs of care."

73 Seymour and Wiersinga, eds., *Handbook of Sepsis*, 19.

74 Agency for Healthcare Research and Quality, "Health Care-Associated Infections," Patient Safety Network, June 15, 2024, https://psnet.ahrq.gov/primer/health-care-associated-infections.

75 "Global Report on Infection Prevention and Control," World Health Organization, May 23, 2022, https://www.who.int/publications/i/item/9789240051164.

Chapter Six: "It's Our Response That Makes the Disease"

1   R. C. Bone, "Why sepsis trials fail," *JAMA* 276, no. 7 (1996): 565–566.

2   W. R. McCabe and G. G. Jackson, "Gram-Negative Bacteremia: II. Clinical, Laboratory, and Therapeutic Observations," *Archives of Internal Medicine* 110, no. 6 (1962): 856–864, doi:10.1001/archinte.1962.03620240038007; David Gilbert, interview, April 1, 2024; D. N. Gilbert, J. A. Barnett, and J. P. Sanford, "*Escherichia coli* bacteremia in the squirrel monkey. I. Effect of cobra venom factor treatment," *The Journal of Clinical Investigation* 52, no. 2 (1973): 406–413.

3   McCabe and Jackson, "Gram-Negative Bacteremia."

4   Ibid.; J. A. Barnett and J. P. Sanford, "Bacterial Shock," *JAMA* 209, no. 10 (1969): 1514–1517, doi:10.1001/jama.1969.03160230048012.

5   Mukherjee, *The Song of the Cell*, 177.

6   Y. C. Martins, F. L. Ribeiro-Gomes, and C. T. Daniel-Ribeiro, "A short history of innate immunity," *Memorias do Instituto Oswaldo Cruz* 118 (2023): e230023, https://doi.org/10.1590/0074-02760230023.

7   Mukherjee, *The Song of the Cell*, 173–175.

8   I. L. Bennett Jr., and P. B. Beeson, "Studies on the pathogenesis of fever. I. The effect of injection of extracts and suspensions of uninfected rabbit tissues upon the body temperature of normal rabbits," *The Journal of Experimental Medicine* 98, no. 5 (1953): 477–492, https://doi.org/10.1084/jem.98.5.477.

9   Ibid.; Valy Menkin, "Biochemical Mechanisms in Inflammation," *British Medical Journal* 1, no. 5185 (May 21, 1960): 1521–1528, https://doi.org/10.1136/bmj.1.5185.1521.

10 C. A. Dinarello, N. P. Goldin, and S. M. Wolff, "Demonstration and characterization of two distinct human leukocytic pyrogens," *The Journal of Experimental Medicine* 139, no. 6 (1974): 1369–1381, https://doi.org/10.1084/jem.139.6.1369.

11 W. Joost Wiersinga, conversation, February 4, 2025.

12 L. Thomas, "Notes of a Biology-Watcher: Germs," *The New England Journal of Medicine* 287, no. 11 (1972): 553–555.

13 "The History Behind the Discovery of Toll-Like Receptors," *Yale Medicine Magazine*, archived at Internet Archive, capture date October 25, 2022, https://web.archive.org/web/20250614162850/https://medicine.yale.edu/news/yale-medicine-magazine/article/the-history-behind-the-discovery-of-toll-like-receptors/.

14 Bennett, Dolin, and Blaser, *Mandell, Douglas, and Bennett's Principles and Practice of Infectious Diseases*, 997.

15 Seymour and Wiersinga, eds., *Handbook of Sepsis*, 33.

16 Van der Poll, Shankar-Hari, and Wiersinga, "The immunology of sepsis"; S. Y. Seong and P. Matzinger, "Hydrophobicity: an ancient damage-associated molecular pattern that initiates innate immune responses," *Nature Reviews Immunology* 4, no. 6 (2004): 469–478, https://doi.org/10.1038/nri1372.

17 Bennett, Dolin, and Blaser, *Mandell, Douglas, and Bennett's Principles and Practice of Infectious Diseases*, 9th ed., 997.

18 Ibid., 998.

19 Ibid.

20 Thomas, "Notes of a Biology-Watcher: Germs."

21 Bennett, Dolin, and Blaser, *Mandell, Douglas, and Bennett's Principles and Practice of Infectious Diseases*, 9th ed., 998.

22 J. L. Vincent, Y. Sakr, M. Singer, et al., "Prevalence and Outcomes of Infection Among Patients in Intensive Care Units in 2017," *JAMA* 323, no. 15 (2020): 1478–1487, https://doi.org/10.1001/jama.2020.2717; Blaser, Cohen, and Holland, *Mandell, Douglas, and Bennett's Principles and Practice of Infectious Diseases*, 10th ed., 936.

23 Bennett, Dolin, and Blaser, *Mandell, Douglas, and Bennett's Principles and Practice of Infectious Diseases*, 998.

24 "Understanding Influenza (Flu) Infection: An Influenza Virus Binds to a Respiratory Tract Cell," CDC Seasonal Influenza Resource Center, accessed May 15, 2024, https://www.cdc.gov/flu-resources/php/resources/index.html.

25 R. Balk, "Roger C. Bone, MD and the evolving paradigms of sepsis," *Contributions to Microbiology* 17 (2011): 1–11, https://doi.org/10.1159/000323970.

26 Seymour and Wiersinga, eds., *Handbook of Sepsis*, 7.

27 Mukherjee, *The Song of the Cell*, 164.

28 G. A. Cortes, M. J. Moore, and S. El-Nakeep, "Physiology, Von Willebrand Factor," in *StatPearls*, StatPearls Publishing, last update February 20, 2023, https://www.ncbi.nlm.nih.gov/books/NBK559062/.

29 Mukherjee, *The Song of the Cell*, 166.

30 Funk, Parrillo, and Kumar, "Sepsis and septic shock: a history."

31 Seymour and Wiersinga, eds., *Handbook of Sepsis*, 9.

32 S. F. Fujimura, "Purple Death: The Great Flu of 1918," *Perspectives in Health* 8, no. 3 (2003), https://www.paho.org/en/who-we-are/history-paho/purple-death-great-flu-1918

33 Edwin Kiester Jr., "Purple Death: When the 1918 Flu Pandemic Came to Pittsburgh," *Pitt Med*, last updated 2020 https://www.pittmed.health.pitt.edu/story/purple-death.

34 D. M. Morens, J. K. Taubenberger, and A. S. Fauci, "Predominant role of bacterial pneumonia as a cause of death in pandemic influenza: implications for pandemic influenza preparedness," *The Journal of Infectious Diseases* 198, no. 7 (2008): 962–970, https://doi.org/10.1086/591708.

35 R. Sender, Y. M. Bar-On, S. Gleizer, and R. Milo, "The total number and mass of SARS-CoV-2 virions," *medRxiv* 118, no. 25 (2021): e2024815118, https://doi.org/10.1101/2020.11.16.20232009.

36 S. Montazersaheb, S. M. H. Khatibi, M. S. Hejazi, et al., "COVID-19 infection: an overview on cytokine storm and related interventions," *Virology Journal* 19, no. 1 (2022): 92, https://doi.org/10.1186/s12985-022-01814-1; W. Joost Wiersinga, conversation, February 4, 2025.

37 "About Zoonotic Diseases," Centers for Disease Control and Prevention, April 7, 2025, https://www.cdc.gov/one-health/about/about-zoonotic-diseases.html.

38 "Climate change may have driven the emergency of SARS-CoV-2," University of Cambridge, February 5, 2021, https://www.cam.ac.uk/research/news/climate-change-may-have-driven-the-emergence-of-sars-cov-2.

39 M. Gilbert, J. Slingenbergh, and X. Xiao, "Climate change and avian influenza," *Revue Scientifique et Technique (International Office of Epizootics)* 27, no. 2 (2008): 459–466.

40 C. J. Carlson, G. F. Albery, C. Merow, et al., "Climate change increases cross-species viral transmission risk," *Nature* 607 (2022): 555–562, https://doi.org/10.1038/s41586-022-04788-w.

Chapter Seven: Trials and Tribulations

1   J. C. Marshall, "Why have clinical trials in sepsis failed?" *Trends in Molecular Medicine* 20, no. 4 (2014): 195–203, https://doi.org/10.1016/j.molmed.2014.01.007.

2   "Anecdotal evidence," Wikipedia, last edited October 4, 2025, https://en.wikipedia.org/w/index.php?title=Anecdotal_evidence&oldid=1235409632.

3   S. Tibi, "Al-Razi and Islamic medicine in the 9th century," *Journal of the Royal Society of Medicine* 99, no. 4 (2006): 206–207, https://doi.org/10.1177/014107680609900425.

4   Stephanie Nicola, "What to Know About the History of Bloodletting," WebMD, April 20, 2022, https://www.webmd.com/a-to-z-guides/what-to-know-history-bloodletting.

5   Tibi, "Al-Razi and Islamic medicine in the 9th century."

6   Ibid.

7   Ibid.

8   Mukherjee, *The Emperor of All Maladies*, 131.

9   Ibid.

10 P. Armitage, "Fisher, Bradford Hill, and randomization," *International Journal of Epidemiology* 32, no. 6 (2003): 925–948, https://doi.org/10.1093/ije/dyg286.

11 Mukherjee, *The Emperor of All Maladies*, 131.

12 P. Armitage, "Fisher, Bradford Hill, and randomization."

13 John Marshall, interview, October 25, 2024.

14 Ibid.

15 S. van Haren Noman, H. Visser, A. F. Muller, and G. J. Limonard, "Addison's Disease Caused by Tuberculosis: Diagnostic and Therapeutic Difficulties," *European Journal of Case Reports in Internal Medicine* 5, no. 8 (2018): 000911, https://doi.org/10.12890/2018_000911.

16 G. Arthur, "Epinephrine: a short history," *The Lancet Respiratory Medicine* 3, no. 5 (2015): 350–351, https://doi.org/10.1016/S2213-2600(15)00087-9.

17 Marta Zaraska, "The Anxious History of Understanding Cortisol," *Medscape Medical News: Features*, May 11, 2021, https://www.medscape.com/viewarticle/950930.

18 Kevin Rodolfo, "What is Homeostasis?" *Scientific American*, January 3, 2000, https://www.scientificamerican.com/article/what-is-homeostasis; S. Libretti and Y. Puckett, "Physiology, Homeostasis," in *StatPearls*, last updated May 1, 2023, StatPearls Publishing, 2025–, https://www.ncbi.nlm.nih.gov/books/NBK559138.

19 L. N. Csonka and A. D. Hanson, "Prokaryotic osmoregulation: genetics and physiology," *Annual Review of Microbiology* 45 (1991): 569–606, https://doi.org/10.1146/annurev.mi.45.100191.003033.

20 Edward Kendall, "The development of cortisone as a therapeutic agent," Nobel Lecture, December 11, 1950, https://www.nobelprize.org/uploads/2018/06/kendall-lecture.pdf; E. W. Boland, "The effects of cortisone and adrenocorticotropic hormone (ACTH) on certain rheumatic diseases," *California Medicine* 72, no. 6 (1950): 405–414.

21 J. M. Pearce, "Thomas Addison (1793–1860)," *Journal of the Royal Society of Medicine* 97, no. 6 (2004): 297–300, https://doi.org/10.1177/014107680409700615.

22 S. Weitzman and S. Berger, "Clinical trial design in studies of corticosteroids for bacterial infections," *Annals of Internal Medicine* 81, no. 1 (1974): 36–42, https://doi.org/10.7326/0003-4819-81-1-36.

23 John Marshall, interview, October 25, 2024.

24 Weitzman and Berger, "Clinical trial design in studies of corticosteroids for bacterial infections"; R. C. Bone, C. J. Fisher Jr., T. P. Clemmer, et al., "A controlled clinical trial of high-dose methylprednisolone in the treatment of severe sepsis and septic shock," *The New England Journal of Medicine* 317, no. 11 (1987): 653–658, https://doi.org/10.1056/NEJM198709103171101.

25 R. C. Bone, W. J. Sibbald, and C. L. Sprung, "The ACCP-SCCM consensus conference on sepsis and organ failure," *Chest* 101, no. 6 (1992): 1481–1483, https://doi.org/10.1378/chest.101.6.1481; Marshall, "Why have clinical trials in sepsis failed?"

26 Marshall, "Why have clinical trials in sepsis failed?"

27 Ibid.

28 Ibid.

29 Ibid.

30 R. C. Bone, "A critical evaluation of new agents for the treatment of sepsis," *JAMA* 266, no. 12 (1991): 1686–1691.

31 Ibid.

32 J. C. Hurley, "Towards clinical applications of anti-endotoxin antibodies; a re-appraisal of the disconnect," *Toxins* 5, no. 12 (2013): 2589–2620, https://doi.org/10.3390/toxins5122589.

33 Bone, "A critical evaluation of new agents for the treatment of sepsis."

34 Hurley, "Towards clinical applications of anti-endotoxin antibodies; a re-appraisal of the disconnect"; John Marshall, interview, October 25, 2024.

35 P. Q. Eichacker, C. Parent, A. Kalil, et al., "Risk and the efficacy of anti-inflammatory agents: retrospective and confirmatory studies of sepsis," *American Journal of Respiratory and Critical Care Medicine* 166, no. 9 (2002): 1197–1205, https://doi.org/10.1164/rccm.200204-302OC; Kevin Tracey, remarks during End Sepsis National Sepsis Forum, Washington, DC, September 13, 2023.

36 Eichacker, Parent, Kalil, et al., "Risk and the efficacy of anti-inflammatory agents: retrospective and confirmatory studies of sepsis."

37 Marshall, "Why have clinical trials in sepsis failed?"

38 S. M. Wolff and J. V. Bennett, "Gram-Negative-Rod Bacteremia," *The New England Journal of Medicine* 291, no. 14 (1974): 733–734.

39 M. M. Parker and J. E. Parrillo, "Septic shock. Hemodynamics and pathogenesis," *JAMA* 250, no. 24 (1983): 3324–3327.

40 Wolff and Bennett, "Gram-Negative-Rod Bacteremia."

41 Eichacker, Parent, Kalil, et al., "Risk and the efficacy of anti-inflammatory agents: retrospective and confirmatory studies of sepsis."

42 David Gilbert, interview, April 1, 2024.

43 Marshall, "Why have clinical trials in sepsis failed?"

44 Ibid.; David Gilbert, interview, April 1, 2024.

45 Seymour and Wiersinga, eds., *Handbook of Sepsis*, 220. Blaser, Cohen, and Holland, *Mandell, Douglas, and Bennett's Principles and Practice of Infectious Diseases*, 10th ed., 941.

46 C. L. Sprung, D. Annane, D. Keh, et al., "Hydrocortisone therapy for patients with septic shock," *The New England Journal of Medicine* 358, no. 2 (2008): 111–124, https://doi.org/10.1056/NEJMoa071366.

47 Derek Angus, interview, September 21, 2022.

48 B. Shakoory, J. A. Carcillo, W. W. Chatham, et al., "Interleukin-1 Receptor Blockade Is Associated With Reduced Mortality in Sepsis Patients With Features of Macrophage Activation Syndrome: Reanalysis of a Prior Phase III Trial," *Critical Care Medicine* 44, no. 2 (2016): 275–281, https://doi.org/10.1097/CCM.0000000000001402.

49 H. Shubin and M. H. Weil, "Bacterial Shock," *JAMA* 235, no. 4 (1976): 421–424, doi:10.1001/jama.1976.03260300045034.

50 Centers for Disease Control and Prevention, "Current Trends Increase in National Hospital Discharge Survey Rates for Septicemia – United States, 1979–1987," *Morbidity and Mortality Weekly Report* 39, no. 2 (January 19, 1990): 31–34, https://www.cdc.gov/mmwr/preview/mmwrhtml/00001539.htm.

51 Ibid.; G. L. Armstrong, L. A. Conn, and R. W. Pinner, "Trends in infectious disease mortality in the United States during the 20th century," *JAMA* 281, no. 1 (1999): 61–66, https://doi.org/10.1001/jama.281.1.61.

52 A. Tomasz, "Multiple-Antibiotic-Resistant Pathogenic Bacteria – A Report on the Rockefeller University Workshop," *The New England Journal of Medicine* 330, no. 17 (1994): 1247–51.

53 A. G. Mainous III, V. A. Diaz, E. M. Matheson, et al., "Trends in hospitalizations with antibiotic-resistant infections: U.S., 1997–2006," *Public Health Reports* 126, no. 3 (2011): 354–360, https://doi.org/10.1177/003335491112600309.

54 Tomasz, "Multiple-Antibiotic-Resistant Pathogenic Bacteria – A Report on the Rockefeller University Workshop."

55 Ibid.; R. F. Breiman, J. C. Butler, F. C. Tenover, et al., "Emergence of drug-resistant pneumococcal infections in the United States," *JAMA* 271, no. 23 (1994): 1831–1835; Centers for Disease Control and Prevention, "Antibiotic-Resistant *Streptococcus pneumoniae*," December 17, 2024, https://www.cdc.gov/pneumococcal/php/drug-resistance/index.html.

56 Balk, "Roger C. Bone, MD and the evolving paradigms of sepsis."

57 Centers for Disease Control and Prevention, "Varying Estimates of Sepsis Mortality Using Death Certificates and Administrative Codes – United States, 1999–2014," *Morbidity and Mortality Weekly Report* 65, no. 13, (April 8, 2016): 342–45, https://www.cdc.gov/mmwr/volumes/65/wr/mm6513a2.htm; R. C. Bone, "Gram-negative sepsis: a dilemma of modern medicine," *Clinical Microbiology Reviews* 6, no. 1 (1993): 57–68, https://doi.org/10.1128/CMR.6.1.57; Centers for Disease Control and Prevention, "Varying Estimates of Sepsis Mortality Using Death Certificates and Administrative Codes"; Armstrong, Conn, and Pinner, "Trends in infectious disease mortality in the United States during the 20th century."

58 Armstrong, Conn, and Pinner, "Trends in infectious disease mortality in the United States during the 20th century."

59 Bone, Fisher Jr., Clemmer, et al., "A controlled clinical trial of high-dose methylprednisolone in the treatment of severe sepsis and septic shock."

60 Balk, "Roger C. Bone, MD and the evolving paradigms of sepsis."

61 Marshall, "Why have clinical trials in sepsis failed?"

62 Ibid.

63 Ibid.

64 Ibid.; Bone, Fisher Jr., Clemmer, et al., "A controlled clinical trial of high-dose methylprednisolone in the treatment of severe sepsis and septic shock."

65 Bone, Fisher. Jr., Clemmer, et al., "A controlled clinical trial of high-dose methylprednisolone in the treatment of severe sepsis and septic shock."

66 Ibid.

67 Ibid.; Wolff and Bennett, "Gram-Negative-Rod Bacteremia."

68 Bone, Fisher Jr., Clemmer, et al., "A controlled clinical trial of high-dose methylprednisolone in the treatment of severe sepsis and septic shock."

69 Emanuel Rivers, "Early Goal Directed Therapy in Severe Sepsis and Septic Shock: 20 Years Later," IMPEC Masterclass Sepsis presentation, March 31–April 1, 2022, Marseille, France. Video presentation provided by expert on September 19, 2022.

70 Bone, Fisher Jr., Clemmer, et al., "A controlled clinical trial of high-dose methylprednisolone in the treatment of severe sepsis and septic shock"; P. B. Lockhart, M. T. Brennan, H. C. Sasser, et al., "Bacteremia associated with toothbrushing and dental extraction," *Circulation* 117, no. 24 (2008): 3118–3125, https://doi.org/10.1161/CIRCULATIONAHA.107.758524.

71 Bone, Fisher Jr., Clemmer, et al., "A controlled clinical trial of high-dose methylprednisolone in the treatment of severe sepsis and septic shock."

72 John Marshall, interview, October 25, 2024.

73 Ibid.

74 Ibid.

Chapter Eight: SIRS

1 R. C. Bone, "Let's agree on terminology: definitions of sepsis," *Critical Care Medicine* 19, no. 7 (1991): 973–976, https://doi.org/10.1097/00003246-199107000-00024.

2 Ibid.; R. C. Bone, "Sepsis, the sepsis syndrome, multi-organ failure: a plea for comparable definitions," *Annals of Internal Medicine* 114, no. 4 (1991): 332–333, https://doi.org/10.7326/0003-4819-114-4-332.

3 R. C. Bone, R. A. Balk, F. B. Cerra, et al., "Definitions for sepsis and organ failure and guidelines for the use of innovative therapies in sepsis," *Chest* 101, no. 6 (1992): 1644–1655, https://doi.org/10.1378/chest.101.6.1644; R. C. Bone, W. J. Sibbald, and C. L. Sprung, "The ACCP-SCCM consensus conference on sepsis and organ failure," *Chest* 101, no. 6 (1992): 1481–1483, https://doi.org/10.1378/chest.101.6.1481.

4 John Marshall, email correspondence, May 25, 2025.

5 Ibid.

6 Ibid.

7 Bone, Balk, Cerra, et al., "Definitions for sepsis and organ failure and guidelines for the use of innovative therapies in sepsis."

8 Ibid.

9 Ibid.

10 Ibid.

11 Vincent, "Dear SIRS, I'm Sorry to Say That I Don't Like You," *Critical Care Medicine* 25, no. 2 (1997): 372–374; John Marshall, email correspondence, May 25, 2025.

12 David Gilbert, interview, April 1, 2024.

13 Ibid.

14 K. Rawat, S. Syeda, and A. Shrivastava, "Neutrophil-derived granule cargoes: paving the way for tumor growth and progression," *Cancer Metastasis Reviews* 40, no. 1 (2021): 221–244, https://doi.org/10.1007/s10555-020-09951-1.

15 Seymour and Wiersinga, eds., *Handbook of Sepsis*, 37.

16 E. McKenna, A. U. Mhaonaigh, R. Wubben, et al., "Neutrophils: Need for Standardized Nomenclature," *Frontiers in Immunology* 12 (2021): 602963; Mukherjee, *The Song of the Cell*, 175.

17 C. Rosales, "Neutrophil: A Cell with Many Roles in Inflammation or Several Cell Types?" *Frontiers in Physiology* 9 (2018): 113, https://doi.org/10.3389/fphys.2018.00113.

18 W. M. Nauseef and N. Borregaard, "Neutrophils at work," *Nature Immunology* 15, no. 7 (2014): 602–611, https://doi.org/10.1038/ni.2921.

19 Mukherjee, *The Song of the Cell*, 176; Meyer and Prescott, "Sepsis and Septic Shock."

20 R. Cavallazzi, C. L. Bennin, A. Hirani, et al., "Is the band count useful in the diagnosis of infection? An accuracy study in critically ill patients," *Journal of Intensive Care Medicine* 25, no. 6 (2010): 353–357, https://doi.org/10.1177/0885066610377980.

21 D. J. Wallace and J. M. Kahn, "Florence Nightingale and the Conundrum of Counting ICU Beds," *Critical Care Medicine* 43, no. 11 (2015): 2517–2518, https://doi.org/10.1097/CCM.0000000000001290.

22 P. Young, V. Hortis De Smith, M. C. Chambi, and B. C. Finn, "Florence Nightingale (1820-1910), a 101 años de su fallecimiento [Florence Nightingale (1820-1910), 101 years after her death]," *Revista Médica de Chile* 139, no. 6 (2011): 807–13, PMID: 22051764.

23 F. E. Kelly, K. Fong, N. Hirsch, and J. P. Nolan, "Intensive care medicine is 60 years old: the history and future of the intensive care unit," *Clinical Medicine* 14, no. 4 (2014): 376–379, https://doi.org/10.7861/clinmedicine.14-4-376.

24 "Dr. Peter Safar, 79; Pioneer of CPR Helped Set Up Intensive Care Units," *Los Angeles Times* via Associated Press, August 7, 2003, https://www.latimes.com/archives/la-xpm-2003-aug-07-me-safar7-story.html.

25 "A Tradition of Firsts: A Brief History of the Department of Critical Care Medicine," University of Pittsburgh School of Medicine, Department of Critical Care Medicine, accessed May 21, 2024, https://www.ccm.pitt.edu/about-us/tradition-firsts-brief-history-department-critical-care-medicine.

26 N. A. Halpern, S. M. Pastores, and R. J. Greenstein, "Critical care medicine in the United States 1985-2000: an analysis of bed numbers, use, and costs," *Critical Care Medicine* 32, no. 6 (2004): 1254–1259, https://doi.org/10.1097/01.ccm.0000128577.31689.4c.

27 W. A. Knaus, "APACHE 1978–2001: The Development of a Quality Assurance System Based on Prognosis: Milestones and Personal Reflections," *Archives of Surgery* 137, no. 1 (2002): 37–41, https://doi.org/10.1001/archsurg.137.1.37.

28 Ibid.

29 William Knaus, "APACHE II Score," MDCALC+, accessed May 21, 2024. https://www.mdcalc.com/calc/1868/apache-ii-score.

30 "Design and development of the Diagnosis Related Group," Centers for Medicare and Medicaid Services Online, October 2024, https://www.cms.gov/icd10m/fy2025-version42.0-fullcode-cms/fullcode_cms/Design_and_Development_of_the_Diagnosis_Related_Group_(DRGs).pdf.

31 Knaus, "APACHE 1978–2001."

32 Knaus, "APACHE II Score."

33 W. A. Knaus, E. A. Draper, D. P. Wagner, and J. E. Zimmerman, "APACHE II: a severity of disease classification system," *Critical Care Medicine* 13, no. 10 (1985): 818–829.

34 Ibid.

35 W. A. Knaus, E. A. Draper, D. P. Wagner, and J. E. Zimmerman, "An evaluation of outcome from intensive care in major medical centers," *Annals of Internal Medicine* 104, no. 3 (1986): 410–418, https://doi.org/10.7326/0003-4819-104-3-410.

36 Ibid.

37 Ibid.

38 Knaus, Draper, Wagner, and Zimmerman, "APACHE II: a severity of disease classification system."

39 David Schmidt, email correspondence, October 5, 2023.

40 William Knaus, interview, November 9, 2023.

41 Knaus, "APACHE 1978-2001: The Development of a Quality Assurance System Based on Prognosis: Milestones and Personal Reflections."

42 David Schmidt, email correspondence, October 5, 2023.

43 M. E. Charlson, F. L. Sax, C. R. MacKenzie, et al., "Assessing illness severity: does clinical judgment work?" *Journal of Chronic Diseases* 39, no. 6 (1986): 439–452, https://doi.org/10.1016/0021-9681(86)90111-6.

44 Ibid.

45 J. A. Kruse, M. C. Thill-Baharozian, and R. W. Carlson, "Comparison of clinical assessment with APACHE II for predicting mortality risk in patients admitted to a medical intensive care unit," *JAMA* 260, no. 12 (1988): 1739–1742.

46 W. Schumer, "Steroids in the treatment of clinical septic shock," *Annals of Surgery* 184, no. 3 (1976): 333–341, https://doi.org/10.1097/00000658-197609000-00011.

47 Bone, Sibbald, and Sprung, "The ACCP-SCCM consensus conference on sepsis and organ failure," *Chest* 101, no. 6 (1992): 1481–1483, https://doi.org/10.1378/chest.101.6.1481.

48 Bone, "Gram-negative sepsis: a dilemma of modern medicine."

49 Bone, Sibbald, and Sprung, "The ACCP-SCCM consensus conference on sepsis and organ failure."

50 W. A. Knaus, X. Sun, O. Nystrom, and D. P. Wagner, "Evaluation of definitions for sepsis," *Chest* 101, no. 6 (1992): 1656–1662, https://doi.org/10.1378/chest.101.6.1656.

51 Adapted from Bone, Balk, Cerra, et al., "Definitions for sepsis and organ failure and guidelines for the use of innovative therapies in sepsis."

52 Bone, Balk, Cerra, et al., "Definitions for sepsis and organ failure and guidelines for the use of innovative therapies in sepsis."

53 Ibid., John Marshall, email correspondence, May 25, 2025.

54 Bone, Balk, Cerra, et al., "Definitions for sepsis and organ failure and guidelines for the use of innovative therapies in sepsis."

55 John Marshall, interview, October 25, 2024.

56 John Marshall, email correspondence, May 25, 2025.

Chapter Nine: The Golden Hour

1 A. Q. Alarhayem, J. G. Myers, D. Dent, et al., "Time is the enemy: Mortality in trauma patients with hemorrhage from torso injury occurs long before the 'golden hour,'" *American Journal of Surgery* 212, no. 6 (2016): 1101–1105, https://doi.org/10.1016/j.amjsurg.2016.08.018.

2 A. Roguin, "Rene Theophile Hyacinthe Laënnec (1781-1826): the man behind the stethoscope," *Clinical Medicine & Research* 4, no. 3 (2006): 230–235, https://doi.org/10.3121/cmr.4.3.230; René-Théophile-Hyacinthe Laennec, *De l'Auscultation Médiate, ou Traité du Diagnostic des Maladies des Poumons et du Cœur*, vol. 1 (J.-A. Brosson et J.-S. Chaudé, 1819), 174.

3 R. M. Hardaway, "Wound shock: a history of its study and treatment by military surgeons," *Military Medicine* 169, no. 4 (2004): 265–269.

4   A. R. Hunter, "Old Unhappy Far Off Things: Some reflections on the significance of the early work on shock," Joseph Clover Lecture, March 16 1966, https://www.ncbi.nlm.nih.gov/pmc/articles/PMC2312102/pdf/annrcse00238-0003.pdf; A. Blalock, "Shock and Hemorrhage," *Bulletin of the New York Academy of Medicine* 12, no. 11 (1936): 610–622.

5   Blalock, "Shock and Hemorrhage."

6   Funk, Parrillo, and Kumar, "Sepsis and septic shock: a history"; American College of Cardiology, "Just One More, Vivien Thomas: Remembering a Pioneering Legend," *Cardiology Magazine*, February 4, 2021, https://www.acc.org/Latest-in-Cardiology/Articles/2021/02/01/01/42/Just-One-More-Vivien-Thomas-Remembering-a-Pioneering-Legend.

7   R. Chaudhry, J. H. Miao, and A. Rehman, "Physiology, Cardiovascular," in *StatPearls*, StatPearls Publishing, last update October 16, 2022, https://www.ncbi.nlm.nih.gov/books/NBK493197/.

8   B. M. Pluim, A. H. Zwinderman, A. van der Laarse, and E. E. van der Wall, "The athlete's heart. A meta-analysis of cardiac structure and function," *Circulation* 101, no. 3 (2000): 336–344, https://doi.org/10.1161/01.cir.101.3.336.

9   Hardaway, "Wound shock: a history of its study and treatment by military surgeons"; Constantinos Koutserimpas, Kalliopi Alpantaki, and George Samonis, "Trauma Management in Homer's *Iliad*," *International Wound Journal* 14, no. 4 (2017): 682–684, https://doi.org/10.1111/iwj.12672.

10 R. Zarychanski, R. E. Ariano, B. Paunovic, and D. D. Bell, "Historical perspectives in critical care medicine: blood transfusion, intravenous fluids, inotropes/vasopressors, and antibiotics," *Critical Care Clinics* 25, no. 1 (2009): 201–220, https://doi.org/10.1016/j.ccc.2008.10.003.

11 Ibid.; Neil Turner, "Thomas Latta and the Invention of IV Fluid Therapy," Edinburgh Medicine Timeline, University of Edinburgh, July 4, 2022, https://blogs.ed.ac.uk/edmed-timeline/thomas-latta-and-the-invention-of-iv-fluid-therapy/.

12 Zarychanski, Ariano, Paunovic, and Bell, "Historical perspectives in critical care medicine: blood transfusion, intravenous fluids, inotropes/vasopressors, and antibiotics."

13 Hardaway, "Wound shock: a history of its study and treatment by military surgeons."

14 Ibid.

15 "The History of IV Therapy," ivWatch, accessed May 22, 2024, https://www.ivwatch.com/2020/11/10/the-history-of-iv-therapy/.

16 M. H. Weil and W. W. Spink, "The Shock Syndrome Associated with Bacteremia Due to Gram-Negative Bacilli," *Archives of Internal Medicine* 101, no. 2 (1958): 184–193, doi:10.1001/archinte.1958.00260140016004.

17 Zarychanski, Ariano, Paunovic, and Bell, "Historical perspectives in critical care medicine"; Hardaway, "Wound shock."

18 Zarychanski, Ariano, Paunovic, and Bell, "Historial perspectives in critical care medicine"; Weil and Spink, "The Shock Syndrome Associated with Bacteremia Due to Gram-Negative Bacilli."

19 D. Skinner and C. S. Keefer, "Significance of Bacteremia caused by *Staphylococcus aureus*: A study of one hundred and twenty-two cases and a review of the literature concerned with experimental infection in animals," *Archives of Internal Medicine* 68, no. 5 (1941): 851–875, doi:10.1001/archinte.1941.00200110003001.

20 Ibid.

21 M. R. Marchick, J. A. Kline, and A. E. Jones, "The significance of non-sustained hypotension in emergency department patients with sepsis," *Intensive Care Medicine* 35, no. 7 (2009): 1261–1264, https://doi.org/10.1007/s00134-009-1448-x.

22 E. J. Kompanje, T. C. Jansen, B. van der Hoven, and J. Bakker, "The first demonstration of lactic acid in human blood in shock by Johann Joseph Scherer (1814–1869) in January 1843," *Intensive Care Medicine* 33, no. 11 (2007): 1967–1971, https://doi.org/10.1007/s00134-007-0788-7.

23 A. Philp, A. L. Macdonald, and P. W. Watt, "Lactate—a signal coordinating cell and systemic function," *The Journal of Experimental Biology* 208, no. 24 (2005): 4561–4575, https://doi.org/10.1242/jeb.01961.

24 Kompanje, Jansen, van der Hoven, and Bakker, "The first demonstration of lactic acid in human blood in shock by Johann Joseph Scherer (1814–1869) in January 1843."

25 D. F. Wilson, "Oxidative phosphorylation: regulation and role in cellular and tissue metabolism," *The Journal of Physiology* 595, no. 23 (2017): 7023–7038, https://doi.org/10.1113/JP273839.

26 L. W. Andersen, J. Mackenhauer, J. C. Roberts, et al., "Etiology and therapeutic approach to elevated lactate levels," *Mayo Clinic Proceedings* 88, no. 10 (2013): 1127–1140, https://doi.org/10.1016/j.mayocp.2013.06.012.

27 F. E. Kelly, K. Fong, N. Hirsch, and J. P. Nolan, "Intensive care medicine is 60 years old: the history and future of the intensive care unit," *Clinical Medicine* 14, no. 4 (2014): 376–379, https://doi.org/10.7861/clinmedicine.14-4-376.

28 Josh Farkas, "Understanding Lactate in Sepsis & Using it to Our Advantage," PulmCrit(EMCrit), July 5, 2015, https://emcrit.org/pulmcrit/understanding-lactate-in-sepsis-using-it-to-our-advantage.

29 Funk, Parrillo, and Kumar, "Sepsis and septic shock: a history."

30 S. Lambden, "Bench to bedside review: therapeutic modulation of nitric oxide in sepsis-an update," *Intensive Care Medicine Experimental* 7, no. 1 (2019): 64, https://doi.org/10.1186/s40635-019-0274-x.

31 M. Hossain, S. M. Qadri, and L. Liu, "Inhibition of nitric oxide synthesis enhances leukocyte rolling and adhesion in human microvasculature," *Journal of Inflammation* 9, no. 28 (2012), https://doi.org/10.1186/1476-9255-9-28; C. Hierholzer and T. R. Billiar, "Nitric oxide in trauma and sepsis," in *Surgical Treatment: Evidence-Based and Problem-Oriented*, eds. R. G. Holzheimer and J. A. Mannick (Zuckschwerdt, 2001).

32 E. D. Frank, "Septic shock. 1964," *International Anesthesiology Clinics* 37, no. 1 (1999), 129–136, https://doi.org/10.1097/00004311-199903710-00007.

33 W. C. Shoemaker, K. J. Printen, J. J. Amato, et al., "Hemodynamic patterns after acute anesthetized and unanesthetized trauma. Evaluation of the sequence of changes in cardiac output and derived calculations," *Archives of Surgery* 95, no. 3 (1967): 492–499, https://doi.org/10.1001/archsurg.1967.01330150168021.

34 Ibid.

35 W. C. Shoemaker, E. S. Montgomery, E. Kaplan, and D. H. Elwyn, "Physiologic Patterns in Surviving and Nonsurviving Shock Patients: Use of Sequential Cardiorespiratory Variables in Defining Criteria for Therapeutic Goals and Early Warning of Death," *Archives of Surgery* 106, no. 5 (1973): 630–636, doi:10.1001/archsurg.1973.01350170004003.

36 Shoemaker, Printen, Amato, et al., "Hemodynamic patterns after acute anesthetized and unanesthetized trauma. Evaluation of the sequence of changes in cardiac output and derived calculations."

37 "History of the Shock Trauma Center," University of Maryland Medical Center, accessed May 24, 2024, https://www.umms.org/ummc/health-services/shock-trauma/about/history.

38 Shoemaker, Montgomery, Kaplan, and Elwyn, "Physiologic Patterns in Surviving and Non-surviving Shock Patients: Use of Sequential Cardiorespiratory Variables in Defining Criteria for Therapeutic Goals and Early Warning of Death."

39 E. Rivers, B. Nguyen, S. Havstad, et al., "Early goal-directed therapy in the treatment of severe sepsis and septic shock," *The New England Journal of Medicine* 345, no. 19 (2001): 1368–1377, https://doi.org/10.1056/NEJMoa010307.

40 L. Gattinoni, L. Brazzi, P. Pelosi, et al., "A trial of goal-oriented hemodynamic therapy in critically ill patients. SvO2 Collaborative Group," *The New England Journal of Medicine* 333, no. 16 (1995): 1025–1032, https://www.nejm.org/doi/full/10.1056/NEJM199510193331601.

Chapter Ten: The Rips

1 Institute of Medicine, *Hospital-Based Emergency Care: At the Breaking Point* (National Academies Press, 2007), https://doi.org/10.17226/11621, xi.

2 A. B. Frakt, "How much do hospitals cost shift? A review of the evidence," *The Milbank Quarterly* 89, no. 1 (2011): 90–130, https://doi.org/10.1111/j.1468-0009.2011.00621.x; Institute of Medicine, *Hospital-Based Emergency Care*, 30.

3 Institute of Medicine, *Hospital-Based Emergency Care*, xiii, xiv, 20.

4 D. B. Chalfin, S. Trzeciak, A. Likourezos, et al., "Impact of delayed transfer of critically ill patients from the emergency department to the intensive care unit," *Critical Care Medicine* 35, no. 6 (2007): 1477–1483, https://doi.org/10.1097/01.CCM.0000266585.74905.5A.

5 Institute of Medicine, *Hospital-Based Emergency Care*, 3.

6 Ibid., 12.

7 Ibid., xv.

8 E. Rivers, "Early Goal-Directed Therapy in Severe Sepsis and Septic Shock: 20 Years Later," IMPEC Masterclass Sepsis Presentation, March 31–April 1, 2022, Marseille, France, video presentation provided by expert on September 19, 2022.

9 Ibid.

10 J. S. Lundberg, T. M. Perl, T. Wiblin, et al., "Septic shock: an analysis of outcomes for patients with onset on hospital wards versus intensive care units," *Critical Care Medicine* 26, no. 6 (1998): 1020–1024, https://doi.org/10.1097/00003246-199806000-00019.

11 R. M. Klevens, J. R. Edwards, C. L. Richards, et al., "Estimating health care-associated infections and deaths in U.S. hospitals, 2002," *Public Health Reports* 122, no. 2 (2007): 160–166, https://doi.org/10.1177/003335490712200205.

12 Peter Attia and Bill Gifford, *Outlive: The Science and Art of Longevity* (Harmony Books, 2023), 16.

13 "History of Lifeguards in the United States: Lifeguards in the Beginning," Watermen, accessed July 28, 2024, https://www.originalwatermen.com/history-lifeguards-united-states.

14 US Lifesaving Association, "United States Lifesaving Association (USLA) History," accessed July 28, 2024, https://www.usla.org/page/HISTORY/United-States-Lifesaving-Association-USLA-History.htm.

15 Paige Austin, "Drowning in California: It Doesn't Look Like You Think It Does," *Pacific Palisades, Community Corner*, July 3, 2019, https://patch.com/california/pacificpalisades/drowning-california-it-doesn-t-look-you-think-it-does.

16 Justin McHenry, interview, August 9, 2022.

17 Ibid.

18 Ibid.; Jeanne Fratello, "Lifeguards Protected 5.8 Million Beachgoers in Manhattan Beach in 2021," MB News, January 6, 2022, https://www.thembnews.com/2022/01/06/383556/lifeguards-protected-5-8-million-beachgoers-in-manhattan-beach-in-2021.

19 Marissa Martinelli, "A Real-Life Lifeguard Assesses the Lifeguarding in *Baywatch*," *Slate*, June 1, 2017, https://slate.com/culture/2017/06/a-real-lifeguard-assesses-baywatch-s-depiction-of-lifeguarding.html.

20 US Lifesaving Association, "American Lifeguard Rescue and Drowning Statistics for Beaches," accessed July 24, 2023, https://www.usla.org/page/statistics.

21 Gawande, *The Checklist Manifesto*.

22 R. P. Dellinger, A. Rhodes, L. Evans, et al., "Surviving Sepsis Campaign," *Critical Care Medicine* 51, no. 4 (2023): 431–444, https://doi.org/10.1097/CCM.0000000000005804.

23 Ofri, *When We Do Harm*, 8.

24 M. R. Chassin and W. Galvin, "The urgent need to improve health care quality. Institute of Medicine National Roundtable on Health Care Quality," *JAMA* 280, no. 11 (1998): 1000–1005.

25 Institute of Medicine (US) Committee on Quality of Health Care in America, L. T. Kohn, J. M. Corrigan, and M. S. Donaldson, eds., *To Err is Human: Building a Safer Health System* (National Academies Press, 2000).

26 Ofri, *When We Do Harm*, 6–7; R. Wachter and P. Pronovost, "The 100,000 Lives Campaign: A Scientific and Policy Review," *Joint Commission Journal on Quality and Patient Safety* 32, no. 11 (2006): 621–27, https://doi.org/10.1016/S1553-7250(06)32080-6.

27 Institute of Medicine (US) Committee on Quality of Health Care in America, Kohn, Corrigan, and Donaldson, eds., *To Err is Human*, ix.

28 Institute of Medicine (US) Committee on Quality of Health Care in America, *Crossing the Quality Chasm: A New Health System for the 21st Century* (National Academies Press, 2000).

29 Ibid.; A. Sura and N. R. Shah, "Pay-for-Performance Initiatives: Modest Benefits for Improving Healthcare Quality," *American Health & Drug Benefits* 3, no. 2 (2010): 135–142.

30 E. A. McGlynn, S. M. Asch, J. Adams, et al., "The quality of health care delivered to adults in the United States," *The New England Journal of Medicine* 348, no. 26 (2003): 2635–2645, https://doi.org/10.1056/NEJMsa022615.

31 K. W. Kizer, "The National Quality Forum Seeks to Improve Health Care," *Academic Medicine* 75, no. 4 (2000): 320–321; "NQF's History," National Quality Forum, accessed May 24, 2024, https://www.qualityforum.org/about_nqf/history.

32 "Consensus Development Process," National Quality Forum, accessed May 24, 2024, archived at Internet Archive, capture date July 11, 2009, https://web.archive.org/web/20090711154254/https://www.qualityforum.org/Measuring_Performance/Consensus_Development_Process.aspx.

33 "Pre-Rule making and Measures Under Consideration 2022 Frequently Asked Questions," Centers for Medicare and Medicaid Services, January 28, 2022, archived at Internet Archive, capture date November 4, 2023, https://web.archive.org/web/20250626035844/https://www.cms.gov/files/document/pre-rulemaking-faq-2022-01102022-508.pdf; Sean Townsend, interview, March 27, 2024.

34 N. West and T. Eng, "Monitoring and reporting hospital-acquired conditions: a federalist approach," *Medicare & Medicaid Research Review* 4, no. 4 (2014), https://doi.org/10.5600/mmrr.004.04.a04.

35 Ibid.

36 Ibid.; "Records of the Agency for Health Care Policy and Research," National Archives, accessed November 12, 2025, https://www.archives.gov/research/guide-fed-records/groups/510.html; Robert Valdez, remarks during End Sepsis National Sepsis Forum, September 13, 2023.

37 West and Eng, "Monitoring and reporting hospital-acquired conditions: a federalist approach."

38 Joelle Baehrend, "100,000 Lives Campaign: Ten Years Later," Institute for Healthcare Improvement, June 17, 2016, https://www.ihi.org/insights/100000-lives-campaign-ten-years-later.

39 "History," Institute for Healthcare Improvement, accessed May 24, 2024, https://www.ihi.org/about/history.

40 Baehrend, "100,000 Lives Campaign: Ten Years Later."

41 "What Is a Bundle," Institute for Healthcare Improvement, March 1, 2012, https://www.ihi.org/insights/what-is-a-bundle.

42 AHRQ, "Rapid Response Systems," Patient Safety Network, July 18, 2024, https://psnet.ahrq.gov/primer/rapid-response-systems.

43 P. S. Chan, R. Jain, B. K. Nallmothu, R. A. Berg, and C. Sasson, "Rapid Response Teams: A Systematic Review and Meta-Analysis," *Archives of Internal Medicine* 170, no. 1 (2010): 18–26, https://pubmed.ncbi.nlm.nih.gov/20065195.

44 Baehrend, "100,000 Lives Campaign: Ten Years Later"; Wachter and Pronovost, "The 100,000 Lives Campaign: A scientific and policy review."

45 Elaine Rinicker, interview, December 6, 2022.

46 Ibid.; The International Symposium on Intensive Care & Emergency Medicine, "Home," accessed November 12, 2025, https://www.isicem.org.

47 R. C. Bone, "Sepsis clinical trials. Don Quixote revisited," *Chest* 107, no. 2 (1995): 298–299, https://doi.org/10.1378/chest.107.2.298.

48 Elaine Rinicker, interview, December 6, 2022.

49 Ibid.

50 W. A. Knaus, E. A. Draper, D. P. Wagner, and J. E. Zimmerman, "An evaluation of outcome from intensive care in major medical centers," *Annals of Internal Medicine* 104, no. 3 (1986): 410–418, https://doi.org/10.7326/0003-4819-104-3-410.

51 Elaine Rinicker, email correspondence, December 7, 2022.

52 Ibid.

53 M. Poeze, G. Ramsay, H. Gerlach, et al., "An international sepsis survey: a study of doctors' knowledge and perception about sepsis," *Critical Care* 8, no. 6 (2004): R409–R413, https://doi.org/10.1186/cc2959.

54 M. M. Levy, M. P. Fink, J. C. Marshall, et al., "2001 SCCM/ESICM/ACCP/ATS/SIS International Sepsis Definitions Conference," *Critical Care Medicine* 31, no. 4 (2003): 1250–1256, https://doi.org/10.1097/01.CCM.0000050454.01978.3B.

55 Ibid.

56 Carl Flatley, "Erin Flatley," Sepsis Alliance, accessed May 27, 2025, https://www.sepsis.org/faces/erin-flatley/.

57 Jamie Thompson, "Making a difference out of her memory," *Tampa Bay Times*, September 12, 2005, https://www.tampabay.com/archive/2005/08/21/making-a-difference-out-of-her-memory/.

58 Ibid.

59 "Florida father on a mission to raise awareness of disease that took his daughter's life," Fox 4 Southwest Florida, September 8, 2022, https://www.yahoo.com/news/florida-father-mission-raise-awareness-005022779.html?guccounter=1.

60 Thompson, "Making a difference out of her memory."

61 Elaine Rinicker, interview, December 6, 2022.

62 Mitchell Levy, interview, December 8, 2022; Dellinger, Rhodes, Evans, et al., "Surviving Sepsis Campaign."

63 Dellinger, Rhodes, Evans, et al., "Surviving Sepsis Campaign."

64 "European Societies Unite Against Severe Sepsis: The Barcelona Declaration," *Medscape Medical News*, September 17, 2002, https://www.medscape.com/viewarticle/442395.

Chapter Eleven: Bending the World

1 Simon Sinek (@simonsinek), X, September 23, 2022.

2 Rivers, "Early Goal Directed Therapy in Severe Sepsis and Septic Shock: 20 Years Later."

3 Rivers, Nguyen, Havstad, et al., "Early goal-directed therapy in the treatment of severe sepsis and septic shock."

4 Ibid.

5 M. McKenna, "Controversy swirls around early goal-directed therapy in sepsis: pioneer defends ground-breaking approach to deadly disease," *Annals of Emergency Medicine* 52, no. 6 (2008): 651–654, https://doi.org/10.1016/j.annemergmed.2008.10.013.

6 Rivers, Nguyen, Havstad, et al., "Early goal-directed therapy in the treatment of severe sepsis and septic shock."

7 Ibid.

8 Sean Townsend, interview, March 27, 2024.

9 Alex Yartsev, "Critique of early goal-directed therapy protocol for sepsis," Deranged Physiology, last updated September 8, 2016, https://derangedphysiology.com/main/required-reading/infectious-diseases-antibiotics-and-sepsis/Chapter%201.1.3/critique-early-goal-directed-therapy-protocol-sepsis.

10 Donald Yealy, interview, September 19, 2022.

11 Derek Angus, interview, September 21, 2022.

12 H. Weiler and W. Ruf, "Activated protein C in sepsis: the promise of nonanticoagulant activated protein C," *Current Opinion in Hematology* 15, no. 5 (2008): 487–493, https://doi.org/10.1097/MOH.0b013e32830abdf4.

13 S. Danese, S. Vetrano, L. Zhang, et al., "The protein C pathway in tissue inflammation and injury: pathogenic role and therapeutic implications," *Blood* 115, no. 6 (2010): 1121–30, doi: 10.1182/blood-2009-09-201616, epub, PMID: 20018912, PMCID: PMC2920225.

14 G. R. Bernard, J. L. Vincent, P. F. Laterre, et al., "Efficacy and safety of recombinant human activated protein C for severe sepsis," *The New England Journal of Medicine* 344, no. 10 (2001): 699–709, https://doi.org/10.1056/NEJM200103083441001.

15 J. P. Siegel, "Assessing the use of activated protein C in the treatment of severe sepsis," *The New England Journal of Medicine* 347, no. 13 (2002): 1030–1034, https://doi.org/10.1056/NEJMsb021512.

16 Bernard, Vincent, Laterre, et al., "Efficacy and safety of recombinant human activated protein C for severe sepsis."

17 Ibid.

18 Ibid.; D. C. Angus, "Drotrecogin alfa (activated) . . . a sad final fizzle to a roller-coaster party," *Critical Care* 16, no. 1 (2012): 107, https://doi.org/10.1186/cc11152.

19 H. S. Warren, A. F. Suffredini, P. Q. Eichacker, and R. S. Munford, "Risks and benefits of activated protein C treatment for severe sepsis," *The New England Journal of Medicine* 347, no. 13 (2002): 1027–1030, https://doi.org/10.1056/NEJMsb020574.

20 Siegel, "Assessing the use of activated protein C in the treatment of severe sepsis."

21 C. Lösch and M. Neuhäuser, "The statistical analysis of a clinical trial when a protocol amendment changed the inclusion criteria," *BMC Medical Research Methodology* 8, no. 16 (2008), https://doi.org/10.1186/1471-2288-8-16.

22 Siegel, "Assessing the use of activated protein C in the treatment of severe sepsis."

23 Ibid.; Warren, Suffredini, Eichacker, and Munford, "Risks and benefits of activated protein C treatment for severe sepsis."

24 Warren, Suffredini, Eichacker, and Munford, "Risks and benefits of activated protein C treatment for severe sepsis."

25 Ibid.; Naomi O'Grady, interview, May 16, 2024; Siegel, "Assessing the use of activated protein C in the treatment of severe sepsis."

26 Antonio Regalado, "To sell pricey drug, Lilly fuels a debate over rationing," *Wall Street Journal*, September 18, 2003, https://shorturl.at/TtPYp.

27 Warren, Suffredini, Eichacker, and Munford, "Risks and benefits of activated protein C treatment for severe sepsis."

28 Ibid.

29 Siegel, "Assessing the use of activated protein C in the treatment of severe sepsis."

30 P. Q. Eichacker, C. Parent, A. Kalil, et al., "Risk and the efficacy of antiinflammatory agents: retrospective and confirmatory studies of sepsis," *American Journal of Respiratory and Critical Care Medicine* 166, no. 9 (2002): 1197–1205, https://doi.org/10.1164/rccm.200204-302OC.

31 Warren, Suffredini, Eichacker, and Munford, "Risks and benefits of activated protein C treatment for severe sepsis"; Naomi O'Grady, interview, May 16, 2024.

32 Siegel, "Assessing the use of activated protein C in the treatment of severe sepsis."

33 D. A. Sweeney, R. L. Danner, P. Q. Eichacker, and C. Natanson, "Once is not enough: clinical trials in sepsis," *Intensive Care Medicine* 34, no. 11 (2008): 1955–1960, https://doi.org/10.1007/s00134-008-1274-6; Warren, Suffredini, Eichacker, and Munford, "Risks and benefits of activated protein C treatment for severe sepsis."

34 Ibid.; Siegel, "Assessing the use of activated protein C in the treatment of severe sepsis."

35 C. G. Durbin Jr., "Is industry guiding the sepsis guidelines? A perspective," *Critical Care Medicine* 35, no. 3 (2007): 689–691, https://doi.org/10.1097/01.CCM.0000257723.46818.F3; M. H. Hassan, "Clinical Practice Guidelines: A Primer on Development and Dissemination," *Mayo Clinic Proceedings* 92, no. 3 (2017): 423–433, https://doi.org/10.1016/j.mayocp.2017.01.001.

36 Ibid.

37 "European Societies Unite Against Severe Sepsis: The Barcelona Declaration," *Medscape Medical News*.

38 Durbin Jr., "Is industry guiding the sepsis guidelines? A perspective."

39 Mitchell Levy, email correspondence, March 17, 2025.

40 R. P. Dellinger, J. M. Carlet, H. Masur, et al., "Surviving Sepsis Campaign guidelines for management of severe sepsis and septic shock," *Critical Care Medicine* 32, no. 3 (2004): 858–873, https://doi.org/10.1097/01.ccm.0000117317.18092.e4.

41 Ibid.

42 Elaine Rinicker, interview, December 6, 2022.

43 Dellinger, Carlet, Masur, et al., "Surviving Sepsis Campaign guidelines for management of severe sepsis and septic shock."

44 Ibid.; Acute Respiratory Distress Syndrome Network, R. G. Brower, M. M. Matthay, et al., "Ventilation with lower tidal volumes as compared with traditional tidal volumes for acute lung injury and the acute respiratory distress syndrome," *The New England Journal of Medicine* 342, no. 18 (2000): 1301–1308, https://doi.org/10.1056/NEJM200005043421801.

45 R. P. Dellinger, A. Rhodes, L. Evans, et al., "Surviving Sepsis Campaign," *Critical Care Medicine* 51, no. 4 (2023): 431–444, https://doi.org/10.1097/CCM.0000000000005804.

46 M. M. Levy, P. J. Pronovost, R. P. Dellinger, et al., "Sepsis change bundles: converting guidelines into meaningful change in behavior and clinical outcome," *Critical Care Medicine* 32, no. 11 (2004): S595–S597, https://doi.org/10.1097/01.ccm.0000147016.53607.c4.

47 Ibid.

48 Sean Townsend, interview, March 27, 2024.

49 Ibid.

50 Ibid.

51 Ibid.

52 Dellinger, Rhodes, Evans, et al., "Surviving Sepsis Campaign."

53 R. P. Dellinger and J. L. Vincent, "The Surviving Sepsis Campaign sepsis change bundles and clinical practice," *Critical Care* 9, no. 6 (2005): 653–654, https://doi.org/10.1186/cc3952.

54 Erkan Hassan, "Evolution and Current Status of Sepsis Bundles," Sepsis Program Optimization, accessed July 6, 2024, https://sepsisprogramoptimization.com/spo-bundles.

55 Liz Ryan, "'If You Can't Measure It, You Can't Manage It': Not True," *Forbes*, February 10, 2014, https://www.forbes.com/sites/lizryan/2014/02/10/if-you-cant-measure-it-you-cant-manage-it-is-bs/?sh=68868a727b8b.

56 Sean Townsend, interview, March 27, 2024.

57 Dellinger, Rhodes, Evans, et al., "Surviving Sepsis Campaign."

58 Ibid.

59 Ibid.

60 A. V. Barochia, X. Cui, D. Vitberg, et al., "Bundled care for septic shock: an analysis of clinical trials," *Critical Care Medicine* 38, no. 2 (2010): 668–678, https://doi.org/10.1097/CCM.0b013e3181cb0ddf.

61 Dellinger, Rhodes, Evans, et al., "Surviving Sepsis Campaign."

62 This concept is well-known, but I first heard reference to the "multiplier effect" of sepsis bundles from Kevin Tracey's remarks during the 2023 End Sepsis National Sepsis Forum, September 13, 2023.

63 P. Q. Eichacker, C. Natanson, and R. L. Danner, "Surviving sepsis—practice guidelines, marketing campaigns, and Eli Lilly," *The New England Journal of Medicine 355*, no. 16 (2006): 1640–1642, https://doi.org/10.1056/NEJMp068197.

64 P. Q. Eichacker, C. Natanson, and R. L. Danner, "Separating practice guidelines from pharmaceutical marketing," *Critical Care Medicine 35*, no. 12 (2007): 2878–2880; P. R. Dellinger and C. G. Durbin Jr., "Reply," *Critical Care Medicine 35*, no. 11 (2007): 2878–2880, https://doi.org/10.1097/01.CCM.0000290379.47485.D2.

65 Eichacker, Natanson, and Danner, "Surviving sepsis—practice guidelines, marketing campaigns, and Eli Lilly"; Durbin Jr., "Is industry guiding the sepsis guidelines? A perspective."

66 Eichacker, Natanson, and Danner, "Surviving sepsis—practice guidelines, marketing campaigns, and Eli Lilly."

67 Ibid.

68 Eichacker, Natanson, and Danner, "Separating practice guidelines from pharmaceutical marketing."

69 Eichacker, Natanson, and Danner, "Surviving sepsis—practice guidelines, marketing campaigns, and Eli Lilly"; Regalado, "To sell pricey drug, Lilly fuels a debate over rationing"; Richard Knox, "Report: Lilly Promoted Drug Under False Pretenses," NPR: All Things Considered, October 8, 2006, https://www.npr.org/2006/10/18/6298643/report-lilly-promoted-drug-under-false-pretenses.

70 Knox, "Report: Lilly Promoted Drug Under False Pretenses."

71 Regalado, "To sell pricey drug, Lilly fuels a debate over rationing."

72 Ibid.; Staff, "FDA Committee Split on Lilly's Xigris," *Forbes*, October 17, 2001, https://www.forbes.com/2001/10/17/1016xigris.html.

73 Staff, "FDA Committee Split on Lilly's Xigris."

74 Regalado, "To sell pricey drug, Lilly fuels a debate over rationing."

75 Ibid.

76 Ibid.

77 Ibid.; N. S. Ward and M. M. Levy, "Rationing and critical care medicine," *Critical care medicine 35*, no. 2 (2007): S102–S105, https://doi.org/10.1097/01.CCM.0000252922.55244.FB.

78 Regalado, "To sell pricey drug, Lilly fuels a debate over rationing."

79 Ibid.

80 Ibid.

81 Ibid.

82 US Centers for Disease Control and Prevention ICD-9-CM Coordination and Maintenance Committee Meeting, November 1–2, 2001, https://www.cdc.gov/nchs/data/icd/icdp1101.pdf.

83 Regalado, "To sell pricey drug, Lilly fuels a debate over rationing."

84 R. Dellinger and C. G. Durbin, "Separating practice guidelines from pharmaceutical marketing – Reply," Critical Care Medicine 35 no. 12 (2007): 2878-2880, doi: 10.1097/01.CCM.0000290379.47485.D2.

85 Ibid.; Dellinger, Carlet, Masur et al., "Surviving Sepsis Campaign guidelines for management of severe sepsis and septic shock."

86 Ibid.

87 Ibid.

88 D. Blumenthal, "Doctors and drug companies," *The New England Journal of Medicine 351*, no. 18 (2004): 1885–1890, https://doi.org/10.1056/NEJMhpr042734.

89 Knox, "Report: Lilly Promoted Drug Under False Pretenses."

90 Durbin Jr., "Is industry guiding the sepsis guidelines? A perspective."

91 Mitchell Levy, interview, December 8, 2022.

92 Bono, "My wish: Three actions for Africa," TED2005, https://www.ted.com/talks/bono_my_wish_three_actions_for_africa/transcript.

93 Thompson, "Making a difference out of her memory."

94 Ibid.

95 Sean Townsend, interview, March 27, 2024.

96 Ibid.

Chapter Twelve: Surviving Sepsis

1   Ruth Brentari, "Using Kaiser Permanente HealthConnect to Transform Primary Care Delivery," Health Informatics New Zealand, November 17, 2007, https://www.slideshare.net/slideshow/using-kaiser-permanente-healthconnect-to-transform-primary-care-delivery/170745.

2   Alan Whippy, letter from Alan Whippy to Nancy Schlichting, Detroit, Michigan, December 1, 2011.

3   "2010 CMS Statistics," Department of Health and Human Services, last modified September 10, 2024, https://www.cms.gov/Research-Statistics-Data-and-Systems/Statistics-Trends-and-Reports/CMS-Statistics-Reference-Booklet/Downloads/CMS_Stats_2010.pdf.

4   Ibid.

5   "Hospital Quality Alliance: Improving Care Through Information," Centers for Medicare and Medicaid Services, accessed July 6, 2024, https://www.cms.gov/Medicare/Quality-Initiatives-Patient-Assessment-Instruments/HospitalQualityInits/downloads/hospitalhqa-factsheet200512.pdf.

6   "Hospital Quality Initiative Public Reporting: Hospital Care Compare and Provider Data Catalog," Centers for Medicare and Medicaid Service, accessed July 6, 2024, https://www.cms.gov/medicare/quality/initiatives/hospital-quality-initiative/hospital-compare.

7   A. Sura and N. R. Shah, "Pay-for-Performance Initiatives: Modest Benefits for Improving Healthcare Quality," *American Health & Drug Benefits* 3, no. 2 (2010): 135–142; "Ernest A. Codman, MD, FACS, 1869–1940," American College of Surgeons, accessed July 6, 2024, https://www.facs.org/about-acs/archives/past-highlights/codmanhighlight; "The Joint Commission History Timeline: Beginnings: 1910–1986," The Joint Commission, accessed July 6, https://digitalassets.jointcommission.org/api/public/content/fa21761405c44eac8bf95637fc450598?v=441260d1; K. Hines, N. Mouchtouris, J. J. Knightly, and J. Harrop, "A Brief History of Quality Improvement in Health Care and Spinal Surgery," *Global Spine Journal* 10, no. 1 (2020): 5S–9S, https://doi.org/10.1177/2192568219853529; "Redefine Quality in Hospital Care," The Joint Commission, accessed July 6, 2024, https://www.jointcommission.org/what-we-offer/accreditation/health-care-settings/hospital/.

8   J. S. Faust and S. D. Weingart, "The Past, Present, and Future of the Centers for Medicare and Medicaid Services Quality Measure SEP-1: The Early Management Bundle for Severe Sepsis/Septic Shock," *Emergency Medicine Clinics of North America* 35, no. 1 (2017): 219–231, https://doi.org/10.1016/j.emc.2016.09.006.

9   "NQF #0500. Severe sepsis and septic shock: management bundle," National Quality Forum.

10 "Infectious Disease Consensus Standards Endorsement Maintenance 2012, Workgroup D Conference Call Transcript," National Quality Forum, August 23, 2012.

11 Sean Townsend, interview, March 27, 2024.

12 Alan Whippy, letter to Nancy Schlichting.

13 R. P. Dellinger, M. M. Levy, J. M. Carlet, et al., "Surviving Sepsis Campaign: international guidelines for management of severe sepsis and septic shock: 2008," *Intensive Care Medicine* 34, no. 1 (2008): 17–60, https://doi.org/10.1007/s00134-007-0934-2.

14 "What is GRADE?" BMJ Best Practice, accessed July 6, 2024, https://bestpractice-bmj-com.bibliotheek.ehb.be/info/evidence/learn-ebm/what-is-grade/#:~:text=GRADE%20(Grading%20of%20Recommendations%2C%20Assessment,for%20making%20clinical%20practice%20recommendations.

15 Dellinger, Levy, Carlet, et al., "Surviving Sepsis Campaign: international guidelines for management of severe sepsis and septic shock: 2008."

16 Thomas M Burton, "New Therapy for Sepsis Infections Raises Hope but Many Questions," *The Wall Street Journal*, August 14, 2008, https://www.wsj.com/articles/SB121867179036438865; "Rivers and Henry Ford Hospital issued a response: Henry Ford Health System. Letter to the Editor," *The Wall Street Journal*, August 19, 2008, https://emcrit.org/wp-content/uploads/Henry-Ford-Hospital-Reply-to-WSJ-10.27.2008.pdf.

17 University of Pittsburgh, "NIH Grants Pitt's Medical School $8.4 M to Determine Best Treatments for Sepsis," *PittChronicle*, October 9, 2006, https://www.chronicle.pitt.edu/story/nih-grants-pitt's-medical-school-84-m-determine-best-treatments-sepsis.

18 E. Abraham, P. F. Laterre, R. Garg, et al., "Drotrecogin alfa (activated) for adults with severe sepsis and a low risk of death," *The New England Journal of Medicine 353*, no. 13 (2005): 1332–1341, https://doi.org/10.1056/NEJMoa050935.

19 Dellinger, Levy, Carlet, et al., "Surviving Sepsis Campaign: international guidelines for management of severe sepsis and septic shock: 2008."

20 E. Damiani, A. Donati, G. Serafini, et al., "Effect of performance improvement programs on compliance with sepsis bundles and mortality: a systematic review and meta-analysis of observational studies," *PloS One* 10, no. 5 (2015): e0125827, https://doi.org/10.1371/journal.pone.0125827.

21 P. Dellinger, "Straight talk with . . . Phillip Dellinger [Interviewed by Roxanne Khamsi]," *Nature Medicine* 18, no. 7 (2012): 1002, https://doi.org/10.1038/nm0712-1002.

22 R. P. Dellinger, A. Rhodes, L. Evans, et al., "Surviving Sepsis Campaign," *Critical Care Medicine*, 51 no. 4 (2023): 431–444. https://doi.org/10.1097/CCM.0000000000005804.

23 A. Kumar, D. Roberts, K. E. Wood, et al., "Duration of hypotension before initiation of effective antimicrobial therapy is the critical determinant of survival in human septic shock," *Critical Care Medicine* 34, no. 6 (2006): 1589–1596, https://doi.org/10.1097/01.CCM.0000217961.75225.E9.

24 Dellinger, Levy, Carlet, et al., "Surviving Sepsis Campaign: international guidelines for management of severe sepsis and septic shock: 2008."

25 Internal Northwest Kaiser Permanente Quality Improvement Data, 2010.

26 G. E. Carr, T. C. Yuen, J. F. McConville, et al., "Early cardiac arrest in patients hospitalized with pneumonia: a report from the American Heart Association's Get With the Guidelines-Resuscitation Program," *Chest* 141, no. 6 (2012): 1528–1536, https://doi.org/10.1378/chest.11-1547.

27 Ibid.

28 A. A. Quartin, R. M. Schein, D. H. Kett, and P. N. Peduzzi, "Magnitude and duration of the effect of sepsis on survival. Department of Veterans Affairs Systemic Sepsis Cooperative Studies Group," *JAMA* 277, no. 3 (1997): 1058–1063.

29 Rivers, Nguyen, Havstad, et al., "Early goal-directed therapy in the treatment of severe sepsis and septic shock."

30 T. J. Iwashyna, E. W. Ely, D. M. Smith, and K. M. Langa, "Long-term cognitive impairment and functional disability among survivors of severe sepsis," *JAMA* 304, no. 16 (2010): 1787–1794, https://doi.org/10.1001/jama.2010.1553.

31 D. C. Angus, "The lingering consequences of sepsis: a hidden public health disaster?" *JAMA* 304, no. 16 (2010): 1833–1834. https://doi.org/10.1001/jama.2010.1546.

32 Iwashyna, Ely, Smith, and Langa, "Long-term cognitive impairment and functional disability among survivors of severe sepsis."

33 Angus, "The lingering consequences of sepsis: a hidden public health disaster?"

34 Laura Evans, interview, October 10, 2022.

35 Levy, Fink, Marshall, et al., "2001 SCCM/ESICM/ACCP/ATS/SIS International Sepsis Definitions Conference."

36 Mitchell Levy, interview, December 8, 2022.

37 V. Liu, J. W. Morehouse, J. Soule, et al., "Fluid volume, lactate values, and mortality in sepsis patients with intermediate lactate values," *Annals of the American Thoracic Society* 10, no. 5 (2013): 466–473, https://doi.org/10.1513/AnnalsATS.201304-099OC.

38 This notion of greater responsibility was solidified through discussions with sepsis expert Nirav Shah during an interview on November 30, 2022.

39 A. E. Jones, N. I. Shapiro, and M. Roshon, "Implementing early goal-directed therapy in the emergency setting: the challenges and experiences of translating research innovations into clinical reality in academic and community settings," *Academic Emergency Medicine* 14, no. 11 (2007): 1072–1078, https://doi.org/10.1197/j.aem.2007.04.014.

40 David Schmidt, interview, October 25, 2022.

Chapter Thirteen: Rory's Lessons

1 Dwyer, "An Infection, Unnoticed, Turns Unstoppable"; "Rory Staunton," End Sepsis: The Legacy of Rory Staunton, October 11, 2025, https://www.endsepsis.org/about-rory-staunton/#:~:text=Rory%20Staunton%20%2D%20End%20Sepsis,sorry%20but%20Rory%20was%20dead.

2 Dwyer, "An Infection, Unnoticed, Turns Unstoppable."

3 V. X. Liu, G. J. Escobar, R. Chaudhary, and H. C. Prescott, "Healthcare Utilization and Infection in the Week Prior to Sepsis Hospitalization," *Critical Care Medicine* 46, no. 4 (2018): 513–516, https://doi.org/10.1097/CCM.0000000000002960.

4 A. H. Flannery, C. M. Venn, A. Gusovsky, et al., "Frequency and Types of Healthcare Encounters in the Week Preceding a Sepsis Hospitalization: A Systematic Review," *Critical Care Explorations* 4, no. 2 (2022): e0635, https://doi.org/10.1097/CCE.0000000000000635.

5 M. M. Levy, A. Rhodes, G. S. Phillips, et al., "Surviving Sepsis Campaign: association between performance metrics and outcomes in a 7.5-year study," *Critical Care Medicine* 43, no. 1 (2015): 3–12, https://doi.org/10.1097/CCM.0000000000000723.

6 Ibid.

7   P. E. Marik, J. D. Farkas, R. Spiegel, et al., "POINT: Should the Surviving Sepsis Campaign Guidelines Be Retired? Yes," *Chest* 155, no. 1 (2019): 12–14, https://doi.org/10.1016/j.chest.2018.10.008; David Talan, "Opinion: How the Surviving Sepsis Campaign Got Almost Everything Wrong," ACEP Now, March 13, 2018, https://www.acepnow.com/article/opinion-surviving-sepsis-campaign-got-almost-everything-wrong/.

8   David Schmidt, interview, October 25, 2022.

9   R. P. Dellinger, M. M. Levy, A. Rhodes, et al., "Surviving sepsis campaign: international guidelines for management of severe sepsis and septic shock: 2012," *Critical Care Medicine* 41, no. 2 (2013): 580–637, https://doi.org/10.1097/CCM.0b013e31827e83af.

10 K. Kaukonen, M. Bailey, S. Suzuki, et al., "Mortality Related to Severe Sepsis and Septic Shock Among Critically Ill Patients in Australia and New Zealand, 2000–2012," *JAMA* 311, no. 13 (2014): 1308–1316, doi:10.1001/jama.2014.2637.

11 S. K. Gohil, C. Cao, M. Phelan, et al., "Impact of Policies on the Rise in Sepsis Incidence, 2000–2010," *Clinical Infectious Diseases* 62, no. 6 (2016): 695–703, https://doi.org/10.1093/cid/civ1019.

12 M. P. Sormani, "The Will Rogers phenomenon: the effect of different diagnostic criteria," *Journal of Neurological Science* 287, Suppl 1 (2009): S46–S49, doi: 10.1016/S0022-510X(09)713000, PMID: 20106348.

13 Dellinger, Levy, Rhodes, et al., "Surviving Sepsis Campaign: international guidelines for management of severe sepsis and septic shock: 2012."

14 Levy, Rhodes, Phillips, et al., "Surviving Sepsis Campaign: association between performance metrics and outcomes in a 7.5-year study."

15 Internal sepsis data, Kaiser Permanente Northern California.

16 B. Freedman, "Equipoise and the ethics of clinical research," *The New England Journal of Medicine* 317, no. 3 (1987): 141–145, https://doi.org/10.1056/NEJM198707163170304.

17 Derek Angus, interview, April 3, 2024.

18 Dwyer, "An Infection, Unnoticed, Turns Unstoppable."

19 Ibid.

20 Orlaith Staunton, email correspondence, October 16, 2024; "Medical Documents in Sepsis Death," *The New York Times*, July 11, 2012, https://archive.nytimes.com/www.nytimes.com/interactive/2012/07/11/nyregion/medical-documents-in-depsis-death.jpg.

21 Orlaith Staunton, email correspondence, October 16, 2024.

22 Dwyer, "An Infection, Unnoticed, Turns Unstoppable."

23 Dwyer, "Death of a Boy Prompts New Medical Efforts Nationwide"; "Medical Documents in Sepsis Death," *The New York Times.*

24 Orlaith Staunton, interview, May 5, 2025.

25 Dwyer, "Death of a Boy Prompts New Medical Efforts Nationwide"; "Medical Documents in Sepsis Death," *The New York Times.*

26 Dellinger, Levy, Rhodes, et al., "Surviving Sepsis Campaign: international guidelines for management of severe sepsis and septic shock: 2012."

27 N. I. Shapiro, M. D. Howell, D. Talmor, et al., "Serum lactate as a predictor of mortality in emergency department patients with infection," *Annals of Emergency Medicine* 45, no. 5 (2005): 524–528, https://doi.org/10.1016/j.annemergmed.2004.12.006.

28 M. E. Mikkelsen, A. N. Miltiades, D. F. Gaieski, et al., "Serum lactate is associated with mortality in severe sepsis independent of organ failure and shock," *Critical Care Medicine* 37, no. 5 (2009): 1670–1677, https://doi.org/10.1097/CCM.0b013e31819fcf68.

29 Shapiro, Howell, Talmor, et al., "Serum lactate as a predictor of mortality in emergency department patients with infection."

30 Kaiser Permanente internal data.

31 Dwyer, "An Infection, Unnoticed, Turns Unstoppable."

32 Eric Roth, conversation with colleague, 2017.

33 L. J. Schlapbach, R. S. Watson, L. R. Sorce, et al., "International Consensus Criteria for Pediatric Sepsis and Septic Shock," *JAMA* 331, no. 8 (2024): 665–674, https://doi.org/10.1001/jama.2024.0179.

34 K. E., Rudd, S. C. Johnson, K. M. Agesa, et al., "Global, regional, and national sepsis incidence and mortality, 1990-2017: analysis for the Global Burden of Disease Study," *The Lancet* 395, no. 10219 (2020): 200–211, doi: 10.1016/S0140-6736(19)32989-7, PMID: 31954465, PMCID: PMC6970225.

35 Scott Weiss, interview, October 4, 2022.

36 E. F. Carlton, M. A. Perry-Eaddy, and H. C. Prescott, "Context and Implications of the New Pediatric Sepsis Criteria," *JAMA* 331, no. 8 (2024): 646–649, https://doi.org/10.1001/jama.2023.27979.

37 Scott Weiss, interview, October 4, 2022.

38 Ibid.

39 F. Balamuth, E. R. Alpern, M. K. Abbadessa, et al., "Improving Recognition of Pediatric Severe Sepsis in the Emergency Department: Contributions of a Vital Sign-Based Electronic Alert and Bedside Clinician Identification," *Annals of Emergency Medicine* 70, no. 6 (2017): 759–768.e2, https://doi.org/10.1016/j.annemergmed.2017.03.019.

40 Ibid.

41 Ibid.

42 Ibid.

43 V. M. Ranieri, B. T. Thompson, P. S. Barie, et al., "Drotrecogin alfa (activated) in adults with septic shock," *The New England Journal of Medicine* 366, no. 22 (2012): 2055–2064, https://doi.org/10.1056/NEJMoa1202290.

44 Judy Stone, "Lilly's Shocker, or the Post-Marketing Blues," *Scientific American*, November 2, 2011, https://www.scientificamerican.com/blog/guest-blog/lillys-shocker-or-the-post-marketing-blues/.

45 Mitchell Levy, interview, April 3, 2023.

46 P. S. Lai and B. T. Thompson, "Why activated protein C was not successful in severe sepsis and septic shock: are we still tilting at windmills?" *Current Infectious Disease Reports* 15, no. 5 (2013): 407–412, https://doi.org/10.1007/s11908-013-0358-9.

47 John Marshall, interview, October 25, 2024.

48 Mitchell Levy, interview, April 3, 2023.

49 Lai and Thompson, "Why activated protein C was not successful in severe sepsis and septic shock: are we still tilting at windmills?"; Stone, "Lilly's Shocker, or the Post-Marketing Blues," *Scientific American* Online. Last updated November 2, 2011, https://www.scientificamerican.com/blog/guest-blog/lillys-shocker-or-the-post-marketing-blues/.

50 Bernard, Vincent, and Laterre, "Efficacy and safety of recombinant human activated protein C for severe sepsis"; Ranieri, Thompson, Barie, et al., "Drotrecogin alfa (activated) in adults with septic shock"; Lai and Thompson, "Why activated protein C was not successful in severe sepsis and septic shock: are we still tilting at windmills?"

51 Ranieri, Thompson, Barie, et al., "Drotrecogin alfa (activated) in adults with septic shock."

52 Stone, "Lilly's Shocker, or the Post-Marketing Blues"; Ranieri, Thompson, Barie, et al., "Drotrecogin alfa (activated) in adults with septic shock."

53 Mitchell Levy, interview, April 3, 2023.

54 Dellinger, Levy, Rhodes, et al., "Surviving Sepsis Campaign: international guidelines for management of severe sepsis and septic shock: 2012."

Chapter Fourteen: Regulations and Regression

1 "Harkin Marks World Sepsis Day, Announces Upcoming Hearing on Efforts to Reduce Healthcare-Associated Infections," U.S. Senate Committee on Health, Education, Labor and Pensions, September 13, 2013, https://www.help.senate.gov/ranking/newsroom/press/harkin-marks-world-sepsis-day-announces-upcoming-hearing-on-efforts-to-reduce-healthcare-associated-infections.

2 Orlaith and Ciaran Staunton, interview, October 7, 2022.

3 Ibid.

4 "Testimony of Ciaran Staunton," United States Senate Committee on Health, Education, Labor and Pensions, September 24, 2013, https://www.help.senate.gov/imo/media/doc/Staunton.pdf.

5 Orlaith and Ciaran Staunton, interview, October 7, 2022.

6 Dwyer, "An Infection, Unnoticed, Turns Unstoppable"; Sunday with Miriam, "Ciaran and Orlaith Staunton," RTE Radio 1, November 6, 2022, https://www.rte.ie/radio/radio1/clips/22167937/.

7 Dwyer, "Death of a Boy Prompts New Medical Efforts Nationwide," *The New York Times*, October 25, 2012, https://www.nytimes.com/2012/10/26/nyregion/tale-of-rory-stauntons-death-prompts-new-medical-efforts-nationwide.html.

8 Sunday with Miriam, "Ciaran and Orlaith Staunton."

9 Ciaran Staunton, email correspondence, October 16, 2024.

10 Nirav Shah, interview, November 30, 2022.

11 Nirav Shah, remarks during 2023 End Sepsis National Sepsis Forum, September 13, 2023.

12 Nirav Shah, interview, November 30, 2022; New York State Department of Health, *Sepsis Care Improvement Initiative: Report to the Governor and Legislature 2015* (New York State Department of Health, 2015), https://www.health.ny.gov/press/reports/docs/2015_sepsis_care_improvement_initiative.pdf.

13 Nirav Shah, interview, November 30, 2022.

14 Ibid.

15 Ciaran Staunton, email correspondence, October 16, 2024.

16 Teresa Dumain, "Sepsis: The biggest threat you've never heard of," Northwell Health, Feinstein Institutes for Medical Research, August 3, 2023, https://feinstein.northwell.edu/news/insights/sepsis-the-biggest-threat-youve-never-heard-of.

17 Ibid.

18 Nirav Shah, interview, November 30, 2022.

19 Dumain, "Sepsis: The biggest threat you've never heard of"; Dwyer, "Death of a Boy Prompts New Medical Efforts Nationwide."

20 Nirav Shah, interview, November 30, 2022.

21 2023 End Sepsis National Sepsis Forum, September 13, 2023.

22 Nirav Shah, interview, November 30, 2022.

23 Dwyer, "Death of a Boy Prompts New Medical Efforts Nationwide."

24 Nirav Shah, interview, November 30, 2022.

25 Ibid.

26 K. H. Gigli, K. J. Rak, T. B. Hershey, et al., "A Roadmap for Successful State Sepsis Regulations: Lessons From New York," *Critical Care Explorations* 3, no. 9 (2021): e0521, https://doi.org/10.1097/CCE.0000000000000521.

27 Nirav Shah, interview, November 30, 2022.

28 Ibid.

29 "About End Sepsis," End Sepsis, accessed July 7, 2024, https://www.endsepsis.org/about/.

30 M. M. Levy, F. C. Gesten, G. S. Phillips, et al., "Mortality Changes Associated with Mandated Public Reporting for Sepsis: The Results of the New York State Initiative," *American Journal of Respiratory and Critical Care Medicine* 198, no. 11 (2018): 1406–1412, https://doi.org/10.1164/rccm.201712-2545OC.

31 I. V. R. Evans, G. S. Phillips, and E. R. Alpern, "Association Between the New York Sepsis Care Mandate and In-Hospital Mortality for Pediatric Sepsis," *JAMA* 320, no. 4 (2018): 358–367, https://doi.org/10.1001/jama.2018.9071.

32 Sunday with Miriam, "Ciaran and Orlaith Staunton."

33 Orlaith and Ciaran Staunton, letter to Thomas R. Frieden, director, US Centers for Disease Control and Prevention, January 24, 2014.

34 Ibid.

35 Orlaith and Ciaran Staunton, interview, January 30, 2025.

36 Ibid.

37 Sean Townsend, interview, March 27, 2024.

38 "Quality Measures: How They Are Developed, Used, & Maintained," US Centers for Medicare and Medicaid Services, September 2021, https://mmshub.cms.gov/sites/default/files/Guide-Quality-Measures-How-They-Are-Developed-Used-Maintained.pdf.

39 "Consensus Development Process," National Quality Forum; "Infectious Disease Endorsement Maintenance Steering Committee," National Quality Forum, Final Steering Committee Roster, September 2012 (document reviewed via contemporaneous print copy; original NQF webpage no longer publicly accessible).

40 "Consensus Standards Approval Committee Amendment to the National Voluntary Consensus Standards: Infectious Disease Endorsement Maintenance 2012, Addendum Report Member Voting Results," National Quality Forum, February 12, 2013.

41 A. E. Jones, N. I. Shapiro, and M. Roshon, "Implementing early goal-directed therapy in the emergency setting: the challenges and experiences of translating research innovations into clinical reality in academic and community settings."

42 Sean Townsend, interview, March 27, 2024.

43 Ibid.; Andrew E. Sama, letter to Steven Brotman and Edward Septimus (co-chairs, Infectious Disease Endorsement Maintenance Steering Committee) and Reva Winkler (senior director, Performance Measures), National Quality Forum, November 19, 2012.

44 Mitchell Levy, interview, December 8, 2022.

45 Sean Townsend, interview, March 27, 2024.

46 Hardaway, "Wound shock: a history of its study and treatment by military surgeons."

47 Ibid.

48 W. A. Altemeier and W. R. Cole, "Nature and treatment of septic shock," *A.M.A. Archives of Surgery* 77, no. 4 (1958): 498–507, https://doi.org/10.1001/archsurg.1958.04370010030004.

49 J. A. Carcillo, A. L. Davis, and A. Zaritsky, "Role of early fluid resuscitation in pediatric septic shock," *JAMA* 266, no. 9 (1991): 1242–1245; Leon Chameides, *Pediatric Advanced Life Support* (American Heart Association, 1988).

50 Derek Angus, interview, April 3, 2024.

51 Dellinger, Levy, Rhodes, "Surviving Sepsis Campaign: international guidelines for management of severe sepsis and septic shock: 2012."

52 T. G. Cherpanath, A. Hirsh, B. F. Geerts, et al., "Predicting Fluid Responsiveness by Passive Leg Raising: A Systematic Review and Meta-Analysis of 23 Clinical Trials," *Critical Care Medicine* 44, no. 5 (2016): 981–991, https://doi.org/10.1097/CCM.0000000000001556.

53 B. Andrews, L. Muchemwa, P. Kelly, et al., "Simplified severe sepsis protocol: a randomized controlled trial of modified early goal-directed therapy in Zambia," *Critical Care Medicine* 42, no. 11 (2014): 2315–2324, https://doi.org/10.1097/CCM.0000000000000541; K. Maitland, S. Kiguli, R. O. Opoka, et al., "Mortality after fluid bolus in African children with severe infection," *The New England Journal of Medicine* 364, no. 26 (2011): 2483–2495, https://doi.org/10.1056/NEJMoa1101549.

54 P. E. Marik and M. L. N. G. Malbrain, "The SEP-1 quality mandate may be harmful: How to drown a patient with 30 mL per kg fluid!" *Anaesthesiology Intensive Therapy* 49, no. 5 (2017): 323–328, https://doi.org/10.5603/AIT.a2017.0056.

55 Dellinger, Levy, Rhodes, et al., "Surviving Sepsis Campaign: international guidelines for management of severe sepsis and septic shock: 2012."

56 Darcy Marciniuk, et al., letter from the American College of Chest Physicians, American Association of Critical-Care Nurses, Greater New York Hospital Association, Midwest Critical Care Collaborative, National Association for Medical Direction of Respiratory Care, Society for Academic Emergency Medicine, and Society of Hospital Medicine to the National Quality Forum Board of Directors, April 4, 2013.

57 A. E. Jones, N. I. Shapiro, S. Trzeciak, et al., "Lactate clearance vs central venous oxygen saturation as goals of early sepsis therapy: a randomized clinical trial," *JAMA* 303, no. 8 (2010): 739–746, https://doi.org/10.1001/jama.2010.158.

58 D. C. McGee and M. K. Gould, "Preventing complications of central venous catheterization," *The New England Journal of Medicine* 348, no. 12 (2003): 1123–1133, https://doi.org/10.1056/NEJMra011883.

59 D. S. Jaswal, C. Natanson, and P. Q. Eichacker, "Endorsing performance measures is a matter of trust," *BMJ* 360 (2018): k703, https://doi.org/10.1136/bmj.k703; "Infectious Disease Endorsement Maintenance Steering Committee," National Quality Forum.

60 "Correction and Clarification," *British Medical Journal* 364 (2019): l215, doi:10.1136/bmj.l215BMJ; Jaswal, Natanson, and Eichacker, "Endorsing performance measures is a matter of trust."

61 Ibid.

62 "Disclosure of Interest Policy for Steering Committees and Technical Advisory Panels," National Quality Forum, January 14, 2010, archived at Internet Archive, capture date June 14, 2024, https://web.archive.org/web/20240921213911/https://www.qualityforum.org/Setting_Priorities/Partnership/Coordinating_Committee/Disclosure_of_Interest_policy_and_form.aspx.

63 Steven Brotman, remarks during National Quality Forum Infectious Disease Endorsement Maintenance Steering Committee Meeting, August 28, 2012.

64 Tiffany Osborn, remarks during National Quality Forum Infectious Disease Endorsement Maintenance Steering Committee Meeting, August 28, 2012.

65 "NQF Endorses Additional Infectious Disease Measures," National Quality Forum (press release), March 6, 2013, archived at Internet Archive, capture date May 2, 2014, https://web.archive.org/web/20140502211919/https://www.qualityforum.org/News_And_Resources/Press_Releases/2013/NQF_Endorses_Additional_Infectious_Disease_Measures.aspx; Reva Winkler and Alexis Morgan, memo to Consensus Standards Approval Committee (CSAC), RE: An Amendment to the National Voluntary Consensus Standards: Infectious Disease Endorsement Maintenance 2012, Addendum Report Member Voting Results, February 12, 2013.

66 Darcy Marciniuk, et al., letter from the American College of Chest Physicians, et al.

67 "About Our Work," Global Sepsis Alliance, accessed July 8, 2024, https://globalsepsisalliance.org/about.

68 Interview with Stauntons, January 30, 2025, October 16, 2024, and March 12, 2024.

69 "Harkin Marks World Sepsis Day, Announces Upcoming Hearing on Efforts to Reduce Healthcare Associated Infections," U.S. Senate Committee on Health, Education, Labor, and Pensions.

70 Ibid.

71 Sean Townsend, interview, March 27, 2024; "Testimony of Ciaran Staunton," United States Senate Committee on Health, Education, Labor and Pensions.

72 Faust and Weingart, "The Past, Present, and Future of the Centers for Medicare and Medicaid Services Quality Measure SEP-1: The Early Management Bundle for Severe Sepsis/Septic Shock."

73 Ciaran Staunton, email correspondence, October 16, 2024; "About End Sepsis," End Sepsis.

74 ProCESS Investigators, "A randomized trial of protocol-based care for early septic shock," *The New England Journal of Medicine* 370, no. 18 (2014): 1683–1693, https://doi.org/10.1056/NEJMoa1401602.

75 Ibid.

76 P. R. Mouncey, T. M. Osborn, G. S. Power, et al., "Trial of early, goal-directed resuscitation for septic shock," *The New England Journal of Medicine* 372, no. 14 (2015): 1301–1311, https://doi.org/10.1056/NEJMoa1500896; ARISE Investigators and ANZICS Clinical Trials Group, S. L. Peake, et al., "Goal-directed resuscitation for patients with early septic shock," *The New England Journal of Medicine* 371, no. 16 (2014): 1496–1506, https://doi.org/10.1056/NEJMoa1404380.

77 Sean Townsend, interview, March 27, 2024; S. Sharif, J. J. Owen, and S. Upadhye, "The end of early-goal directed therapy?" *The American Journal of Emergency Medicine* 34, no. 2 (2016): 292–294, https://doi.org/10.1016/j.ajem.2015.10.039; P. E. Marik, "The demise of early goal-directed therapy for severe sepsis and septic shock," *Acta Anaesthesiologica Scandinavica* 59, no. 5 (2015): 561–567, https://doi.org/10.1111/aas.12479; A. M. Dell'Anna and F. S. Taccone, "Early-goal directed therapy for septic shock: is it the end?" *Minerva Anestesiologica* 81, no. 10 (2015): 1138–1143; C. M. Lilly, "The ProCESS Trial—A New Era of Sepsis Management," *The New England Journal of Medicine* 370, no. 18 (2014): 1750–1751, https://doi.org/10.1056/NEJMe1402564.

78 Talan, "Opinion: How the Surviving Sepsis Campaign Got Almost Everything Wrong."

79 Rivers, Nguyen, Havstad, et al., "Early goal-directed therapy in the treatment of severe sepsis and septic shock"; ProCESS Investigators, "A Randomized Trial of Protocol-Based Care for Early Septic Shock."

80 PRISM Investigators, "Early, Goal-Directed Therapy for Septic Shock—A Patient-Level Meta-Analysis," *The New England Journal of Medicine* 376, no. 23 (2017): 2223–2234, https://doi.org/10.1056/NEJMoa1701380.

81 ProCESS Investigators, "A randomized trial of protocol-based care for early septic shock"; Mouncey, Osborn, Power, et al., "Trial of early, goal-directed resuscitation for septic shock"; ARISE Investigators and ANZICS Clinical Trials Group, S. L. Peake, et al., "Goal-directed resuscitation for patients with early septic shock."

82 Derek Angus, interview, April 3, 2024.

83 Ibid.

84 Ibid.

85 Ibid.; A. F. Shah, V. B. Talisa, C-C. H. Chang, et al., "Heterogeneity in the Effect of Early Goal-Directed Therapy for Septic Shock: A Secondary Analysis of Two Multicenter International Trials," *Critical Care Medicine* 53, no. 1 (2025): e4–e14, doi: 10.1097/CCM.0000000000006463.

86 PRISM Investigators, "Early, Goal-Directed Therapy for Septic Shock—a Patient-Level Meta-Analysis."

87 Talan, "Opinion: How the Surviving Sepsis Campaign Got Almost Everything Wrong"; Justin Morgenstern, "Petition to retract the 2018 surviving sepsis campaign guidelines," First 10EM, updated February 14, 2019, https://first10em.com/petition-to-retire-the-surviving-sepsis-campaign-guidelines/.

88 "Voting Draft Report: NQF Endorsed Measure for Patient Safety," NQF Staff, memo to Patient Safety Standing Committee, September 12, 2014.

89 Henry Ford Health Systems and the measure steward, memo to NQF's Patient Safety Standing Committee and NQF Consensus Standards Approval Committee (CSAC), June 26, 2014.

90 Josh Farkas, "Petition to retire the surviving sepsis campaign guidelines," PulmCrit (EMCrit), May 2, 2018, https://emcrit.org/pulmcrit/ssc-petition/.

91 Marik and Malbrain, "The SEP-1 quality mandate may be harmful: How to drown a patient with 30 mL per kg fluid!"; P. E. Marik, "Iatrogenic salt water drowning and the hazards of a high central venous pressure," *Annals of Intensive Care* 4, no. 21 (2014), https://doi.org/10.1186/s13613-014-0021-0; Morgenstern, "Petition to retire the surviving sepsis campaign guidelines."

92 Faust and Weingart, "The Past, Present, and Future of the Centers for Medicare and Medicaid Services Quality Measure SEP-1."

93 Lilly, "The ProCESS trial—a new era of sepsis management."

94 "Measure Submission and Evaluation Worksheet, NQF #0500 Severe Sepsis and Septic Shock Management Bundle," National Quality Forum, last updated October 5, 2012.

95 Levy, Gesten, Phillips, et al., "Mortality Changes Associated with Mandated Public Reporting for Sepsis."

96 C. W. Seymour, F. Gesten, H. C. Prescott, et al., "Time to Treatment and Mortality during Mandated Emergency Care for Sepsis," *The New England Journal of Medicine* 376, no. 23 (2017): 2235–2244, https://doi.org/10.1056/NEJMoa1703058.

97 Evans, Phillips, and Alpern, "Association Between the New York Sepsis Care Mandate and In-Hospital Mortality for Pediatric Sepsis."

98 Nirav Shah, interview, November 30, 2022.

99 Ibid.

100 Foster Gesten, email conversation, August 15, 2024.

101 Nirav Shah, interview, November 30, 2022.

Chapter Fifteen: Mickey

1   "Mickey," interview, September 15, 2022. Mickey is a pseudonym, though he authorized the full release of his story and medical information.

2   A. J. Walkey and P. K. Lindenauer, "Keeping It Simple in Sepsis Measures," *Journal of Hospital Medicine* 12, no. 12 (2017): 1019–1020, https://doi.org/10.12788/jhm.2873; E. J. Septimus, C. M. Coopersmith, J. Whittle, et al., "Sepsis National Hospital Inpatient Quality Measure (SEP-1): Multistakeholder Work Group Recommendations for Appropriate Antibiotics for the Treatment of Sepsis," *Clinical Infectious Diseases* 65, no. 9 (2017): 1565–1569, https://doi.org/10.1093/cid/cix603; A. K. Venkatesh, T. Slesinger, J. Whittle, et al., "Preliminary Performance on the New CMS Sepsis-1 National Quality Measure: Early Insights from the Emergency Quality Network (E-QUAL)," *Annals of Emergency Medicine* 71, no. 1 (2018): 10–15.e1, https://doi.org/10.1016/j.annemergmed.2017.06.032; J. S. Faust, "Moving Beyond the Centers for Medicare and Medicaid Services' 'Severe Sepsis and Septic Shock Early Management Bundle' Core Quality Measure," *Annals of Emergency Medicine* 78, no. 1 (2021): 20–26, https://doi.org/10.1016/j.annemergmed.2021.03.003; Faust and Weingart, "The Past, Present, and Future of the Centers for Medicare and Medicaid Services Quality Measure SEP-1: The Early Management Bundle for Severe Sepsis/Septic Shock."

3   "Quality Measurement and Quality Improvement," Centers for Medicare & Medicaid Services, accessed July 11, 2024, https://www.cms.gov/medicare/quality-initiatives-patient-assessment-instruments/mms/quality-measure-and-quality-improvement-.

4   Faust and Weingart, "The Past, Present, and Future of the Centers for Medicare and Medicaid Services Quality Measure SEP-1: The Early Management Bundle for Severe Sepsis/Septic Shock."

5   Scott Weingart, "We are Complicit – A glimpse into the current state of Severe Sepsis/Septic Shock Quality Measures," EMCrit RACC, accessed July 11, 2024, https://emcrit.org/emcrit/current-state-of-severe-sepsis-quality-measures; Marik and Malbrain, "The SEP-1 quality mandate may be harmful: How to drown a patient with 30 mL per kg fluid!"

6   Josh Farkas, "Petition to Retire the Surviving Sepsis Campaign Guidelines."

7   M. Singer, C. S. Deustchman, C. W. Seymour, et al., "The Third International Consensus Definitions for Sepsis and Septic Shock (Sepsis-3)," *JAMA* 315, no. 8 (2016): 801–810, https://doi.org/10.1001/jama.2016.0287.

8   David Gilbert, interview, April 1, 2024.

9   W. A. Knaus, X. Sun, O. Nystrom, and D. P. Wagner, "Evaluation of definitions for sepsis," *Chest* 101, no. 6 (1992): 1656–1662, https://doi.org/10.1378/chest.101.6.1656.

10   Rahul Awati, Robert Sheldon, and John Burke, "What is signal-to-noise ratio and how is it measured?" TechTarget, accessed July 11, 2024, https://www.techtarget.com/searchnetworking/definition/signal-to-noise-ratio.

11   M. M. Levy, M. P. Fink, J. C. Marshall, et al., "2001 SCCM/ESICM/ACCP/ATS/SIS International Sepsis Definitions Conference," *Intensive Care Medicine* 29, no. 4 (2003): 530–538, https://doi.org/10.1007/s00134-003-1662-x.

12   Derek Angus, interview, September 21, 2022.

13   Singer, Deutschman, Seymour, et al., "The Third International Consensus Definitions for Sepsis and Septic Shock (Sepsis-3)," JAMA 315, no. 8 (2016): 801–810, https://doi.org/10.1001/jama.2016.0287.

14   Ibid.

15   Ibid.

16 J-L. Vincent, "Sequential Organ Failure Assessment (SOFA) Score," MDCalc, accessed November 13, 2025, https://www.mdcalc.com/calc/691/sequential-organ-failure-assessment-sofa-score.

17 Singer, Deutschman, Seymour, et al., "The Third International Consensus Definitions for Sepsis and Septic Shock (Sepsis-3)," JAMA 315, no. 8 (2016): 801–810, https://doi.org/10.1001/jama.2016.0287.

18 C. W. Seymour, V. X. Liu, T. J. Iwashyna, et al., "Assessment of Clinical Criteria for Sepsis: For the Third International Consensus Definitions for Sepsis and Septic Shock (Sepsis-3)," JAMA 315, no. 8 (2016): 762–774, https://doi.org/10.1001/jama.2016.0288.

19 X. Wang, Z. Guo, Y, Chai, et al., "Application Prospect of the SOFA Score and Related Modification Research Progress in Sepsis," *Journal of Clinical Medicine* 12, no. 10 (2023): 3493, https://doi.org/10.3390/jcm12103493.

20 Derek Angus, interview, September 21, 2022.

21 Vincent Liu, email correspondence, September 15, 2024.

22 S. A. Sterling, M. A. Puskarich, A. F. Glass, F. Guirgis, and A. E. Jones, "The Impact of the Sepsis-3 Septic Shock Definition on Previously Defined Septic Shock Patients," *Critical Care Medicine* 45, no. 9 (2017), 1436–1442, https://doi.org/10.1097/CCM.0000000000002512.

23 Laura Evans, interview, October 10, 2022.

24 Ibid.

25 Office of the Medical Director and Office of Quality and Patient Safety, "New York State Report on Sepsis Care Improvement Initiative: Hospital Quality Performance," New York State Department of Health, April 2019, https://www.health.ny.gov/press/reports/docs/2017_sepsis_care_improvement_initiative.pdf.

26 Derek Angus, interview, September 21, 2022.

27 Ibid.

28 Ibid.

29 "Amy Watts," interview, September 22, 2022.

30 Ibid.

31 Derek Angus, interview, April 3, 2024; J. A. Kellum, L. Kong, M. P. Fink, et al., "Understanding the inflammatory cytokine response in pneumonia and sepsis: results of the Genetic and Inflammatory Markers of Sepsis (GenIMS) Study," *Archives of Internal Medicine* 167, no. 15 (2007): 1655–1663, https://doi.org/10.1001/archinte.167.15.1655.

32 V. X. Liu, G. J. Escobar, R. Chaudhary, and H. C. Prescott, "Healthcare Utilization and Infection in the Week Prior to Sepsis Hospitalization," *Critical Care Medicine* 46, no. 4 (2018): 513–516, https://doi.org/10.1097/CCM.0000000000002960.

33 Derek Angus, interview, April 3, 2024.

34 Mitchell Levy, interview, December 8, 2022.

35 C. Rhee, K. Chiotos, S. E. Cosgrove, et al., "Infectious Diseases Society of America Position Paper: Recommended Revisions to the National Severe Sepsis and Septic Shock Early Management Bundle (SEP-1) Sepsis Quality Measure," *Clinical Infectious Diseases* 72, no. 4 (2021): 541–552, https://doi.org/10.1093/cid/ciaa059.

36 R. M. Wachter, S. A. Flanders, C. Fee, "Public reporting of antibiotic timing in patients with pneumonia: lessons from a flawed performance measure," *Annals of Internal Medicine* 149, no. 1 (2008): 29–32, https://doi.org/10.7326/0003-4819-149-1-200807010-00007.

37 Ibid.; Rhee, Chiotos, Cosgrove, et al., "Infectious Diseases Society of America Position Paper."

38 Ibid.

39 Ibid.

40 Ibid.

41 P. M. C. Klein Klouwenberg, O. L. Cremer, L. A. van Vught, et al., "Likelihood of infection in patients with presumed sepsis at the time of intensive care unit admission: a cohort study," *Critical Care* 19, no. 1 (2015): 319, https://doi.org/10.1186/s13054-015-1035-1.

42 A. E. Jones, A. C. Heffner, J. M. Horton, and M. R. Marchick, "Etiology of illness in patients with severe sepsis admitted to the hospital from the emergency department," *Clinical Infectious Diseases* 50, no. 6 (2010): 814–820, https://doi.org/10.1086/650580.

43 V. X. Liu, V. Fielding-Singh, J. D. Green, et al., "The Timing of Early Antibiotics and Hospital Mortality in Sepsis," *American Journal of Respiratory and Critical Care Medicine* 196, no. 7 (2017): 856–863, https://doi.org/10.1164/rccm.201609-1848OC.

44 "Amy Watts," interview, September 22, 2022.

45 Ibid.

46 R. M. Ratwani, A. Fong, J. S. Puthumana, and A. Z. Hettinger, "Emergency Physician Use of Cognitive Strategies to Manage Interruptions," *Annals of Emergency Medicine* 70, no. 5 (2017): 683–687, https://doi.org/10.1016/j.annemergmed.2017.04.036.

47 J. I. Westbrook, E. Coiera, W. T. M. Dunsmuir, et al., "The impact of interruptions on clinical task completion," *Quality & Safety in Health Care* 19, no. 4 (2010): 284–289, https://doi.org/10.1136/qshc.2009.039255.

48 R. M. Wynn, J. L. Howe, L. C. Kelahan, A. Fong, R. W. Filice, and R. M. Ratwani, "The Impact of Interruptions on Chest Radiograph Interpretation: Effects on Reading Time and Accuracy," *Academic Radiology* 25, no. 12 (2018): 1515–1520, https://doi.org/10.1016/j.acra.2018.03.016.

49 "Amy Watts," interview, September 22, 2022.

50 E. Relihan, V. O'Brien, S. O'Hara, and B. Silke, "The impact of a set of interventions to reduce interruptions and distractions to nurses during medication administration," *Quality & Safety in Health Care* 19, no. 5 (2010): e52, https://doi.org/10.1136/qshc.2009.036871.

51 J. I. Westbrook, A. Woods, M. I. Rob, et al., Association of interruptions with an increased risk and severity of medication administration errors," *Archives of Internal Medicine* 170, no. 8 (2010): 683–690, https://doi.org/10.1001/archinternmed.2010.65.

52 B. J. Drew, P. Harris, J. K. Zègre-Hemsey, et al., "Insights into the problem of alarm fatigue with physiologic monitor devices: a comprehensive observational study of consecutive intensive care unit patients," *PloS One* 9, no. 10 (2014): e110274, https://doi.org/10.1371/journal.pone.0110274.

53 Melissa Denny, interview, October 5, 2022.

54 Blaser, Cohen, and Holland, *Mandell, Douglas, and Bennett's Principles and Practice of Infectious Diseases*, 10th ed., 934.

55 "Mickey," interview, September 15, 2022.

Chapter Sixteen: The Pandemic

1 "Impact of the COVID-19 Pandemic on the Hospital and Outpatient Clinician Workforce: Challenges and Policy Responses," Assistant Secretary for Planning and Evaluation Office of Health Policy, May 3, 2022, https://aspe.hhs.gov/sites/default/files/documents/d00f83e424d58c535273ec21906b199e/aspe-covid-workforce-report.pdf.

2   Noelle Crombie, "Hector Calderon, Oregon's first COVID-19 patient, feared the worst: 'It was like a truck running over me,'" *The Oregonian*, June 23, 2021, https://www.oregonlive.com/news/2021/06/hector-calderon-oregons-first-covid-19-patient-feared-the-worst-it-was-like-a-truck-running-over-me.html.

3   Maggie Vespa, "'Such a great victory': One year later, an update on Oregon's first COVID patient," KGW8, February 27, 2021, https://www.kgw.com/article/news/health/coronavirus/one-year-later-an-update-on-oregons-first-covid-patient/283-2f98a350-0515-4c09-998c-f883e761326e#longform_chapter_2.

4   "CDC Museum COVID-19 timeline," accessed July 13, 2024, https://www.cdc.gov/museum/timeline/covid19.html.

5   "WHO COVID-19 dashboard," World Health Organization, accessed July 13, 2024, https://data.who.int/dashboards/covid19/deaths?n=o.

6   "WHO Chief Declares End to COVID-19 as a Global Health Emergency," UN News, May 5, 2023, https://news.un.org/en/story/2023/05/1136367.

7   "Chapter 1. The economic impacts of the COVID-19 crisis," World Development Report 2022, World Bank Group, accessed July 13, 2024, https://www.worldbank.org/en/publication/wdr2022/brief/chapter-1-introduction-the-economic-impacts-of-the-covid-19-crisis.

8   C. N. Shappell, M. Klompas, C. Chan, et al., "Use of Electronic Clinical Data to Track Incidence and Mortality for SARS-CoV-2-Associated Sepsis," *JAMA Network Open* 6, no. 9 (2023): e2335728, https://doi.org/10.1001/jamanetworkopen.2023.35728.

9   Mary Van Beusekom, "WHO updates COVID treatment guidelines, risk estimates for hospitalization," University of Minnesota, Center for Infectious Disease Research and Policy (CIDRAP), November 10, 2023, https://www.cidrap.umn.edu/covid-19/who-updates-covid-treatment-guidelines-risk-estimates-hospitalization.

10 A. Liu, Y. Li, Z. Wan, et al., "Seropositive Prevalence of Antibodies Against SARS-CoV-2 in Wuhan, China," *JAMA Network Open* 3, no. 10 (2020): e2025717.

11 "COVID-19 – a global pandemic: What do we know about SARS-CoV-2 and COVID-19?" World Health Organization, June 5, 2020, https://www.who.int/docs/default-source/coronaviruse/risk-comms-updates/update-28-covid-19-what-we-know-may-2020.pdf?sfvrsn=ed6e286c_2.

12 "Mortality Analyses," Johns Hopkins Coronavirus Resource Center, accessed July 13, 2024, https://coronavirus.jhu.edu/data/mortality; "Estimating Mortality from COVID-19," World Health Organization, August 4, 2020, https://www.who.int/news-room/commentaries/detail/estimating-mortality-from-covid-19.

13 "Fast Facts on U.S. Hospitals, 2024," American Hospital Association, accessed July 13, 2024, https://www.aha.org/statistics/fast-facts-us-hospitals.

14 P. Sandhu, A. B. Shah, F. B. Ahmad, et al., "Emergency Department and Intensive Care Unit Overcrowding and Ventilator Shortages in US Hospitals During the COVID-19 Pandemic, 2020–2021," *Public Health Reports* 137, no. 4 (2022): 796–802, https://doi.org/10.1177/00333549221091781.

15 M. G. Findling, R. J. Blendon, and J. M. Benson, "Delayed Care with Harmful Health Consequences—Reported Experiences from National Surveys During Coronavirus Disease 2019," *JAMA Health Forum* 12, no. 1 (2020): e201463, https://doi.org/10.1001/jamahealthforum.2020.1463; Chanu Rhee, email correspondence, July 17, 2024.

16 "COVID-19: U.S. Impact on Antimicrobial Resistance, Special Report 2022," National Center for Emerging and Zoonotic Infectious Diseases (U.S.), Division of Healthcare Quality Promotion, June 2022, https://stacks.cdc.gov/view/cdc/119025; "WHO reports widespread overuse of antibiotics in patients hospitalized with COVID-19," World Health Organization, April 26, 2024, https://www.who.int/news/item/26-04-2024-who-reports-widespread-overuse-of-antibiotics-in-patients--hospitalized-with-covid-19.

17 D-Y. Lin, Y. Gu, B. Wheeler, et al., "Effectiveness of Covid-19 Vaccines over a 9-Month Period in North Carolina," *The New England Journal of Medicine* 386, no. 10 (2022): 933–941, https://doi.org/10.1056/NEJMoa2117128.

18 Y. Xie, T. Choi, and Z. Al-Aly, "Postacute Sequelae of SARS-CoV-2 Infection in the Pre-Delta, Delta, and Omicron Eras," *The New England Journal of Medicine* 391, no. 6 (2024): 515–525, https://doi.org/10.1056/NEJMoa2403211; Paul Offit, "Asking the Uncomfortable Questions About Vaccines: Doctor Mike," YouTube, December 18, 2024, https://www.youtube.com/watch?v=A27ameSqcQs.

19 O. J. Watson, G. Barnsley, J. Toor, et al., "Global impact of the first year of COVID-19 vaccination: a mathematical modelling study," *The Lancet Infectious Diseases* 22, no. 9 (2022): 1293–1302, https://doi.org/10.1016/S1473-3099(22)00320-6.

20 "Coronavirus Disease 2019 (COVID-19) Vaccine Safety," Centers for Disease Control and Prevention, November 3, 2023, https://www.cdc.gov/coronavirus/2019-ncov/vaccines/safety/safety-of-vaccines.html; "Contraindications and Precautions to mRNA COVID-19 vaccination," Centers for Disease Control and Prevention, accessed July 13, 2024, https://dsh.ca.gov/COVID-19/docs/Vaccination/COVID-19_Vaccines_Update_on_Allergic_Reactions_Contraindications_and_Precautions.pdf.

21 "COVID-19 Infection Poses Higher Risk for Myocarditis than Vaccines," American Heart Association News, August 22, 2022, https://www.heart.org/en/news/2022/08/22/covid-19-infection-poses-higher-risk-for-myocarditis-than-vaccines.

22 Offit, "Asking the Uncomfortable Questions About Vaccines."

23 Kristen Panthagani, "Science, Policy, and Values," Your Local Epidemiologist, October 9, 2024, https://substack.com/home/post/p-149820583.

24 Ibid.

25 "Transcript: Dr. Scott Gottlieb on *Face the Nation* with Margaret Brennan," CBS News, August 26, 2024, https://www.cbsnews.com/news/scott-gottlieb-former-fda-commissioner-face-the-nation-transcript-08-25-2024/.

26 Panthagani, "Science, Policy, and Values."

27 Ibid.

28 T. D. Shanafelt, C. P. West, L. N. Dyrbye, et al., "Changes in Burnout and Satisfaction With Work-Life Integration in Physicians During the First 2 Years of the COVID-19 Pandemic," *Mayo Clinic Proceedings* 97, no. 12 (2022): 2248–2258, https://doi.org/10.1016/j.mayocp.2022.09.002.

29 C. J. Li, Y. B. Shah, E. D. Harness, et al., "Physician Burnout and Medical Errors: Exploring the Relationship, Cost, and Solutions," *American Journal of Medical Quality* 38, no. 4 (2023): 196–202, https://doi.org/10.1097/JMQ.0000000000000131.

30 Sara Berg, "Physician burnout rate drops below 50% for first time in 4 years," American Medical Association News Wire, July 2, 2024, https://www.ama-assn.org/practice-management/physician-health/physician-burnout-rate-drops-below-50-first-time-4-years.

31 K. Shen, J. C. P. Eddelbuettel, and M. D. Eisenberg, "Job Flows Into and Out of Health Care Before and After the COVID-19 Pandemic," *JAMA Health Forum* 5, no. 1 (2024): e234964, https://doi.org/10.1001/jamahealthforum.2023.4964.

32 T. Burki, "Platform trials: the future of medical research?" *The Lancet Respiratory Medicine* 11, no. 3 (2023): 232–233, https://doi.org/10.1016/S2213-2600(23)00052-8.

33 John Marshall, interview, October 25, 2024.

34 Chanu Rhee, email correspondence, July 17, 2024.

35 Vespa, "'Such a great victory.'"

36 Eduardo Antonio Hernandez, "First Oregon Man Diagnosed with COVID Blessed to Have a Second Chance," KOMO News, updated March 2, 2022, https://komonews.com/news/local/first-oregon-man-diagnosed-with-covid-blessed-to-have-second-chance.

37 Brian Kennedy and Alec Tyson, "Americans' Trust in Scientists, Positive Views of Science Continue to Decline," Pew Research Center, November 14, 2023, https://www.pewresearch.org/science/2023/11/14/americans-trust-in-scientists-positive-views-of-science-continue-to-decline/.

38 Institute of Medicine, *Hospital-Based Emergency Care*, xiii, xv-xvi, 263–264.

39 "WHO Chief Declares End to COVID-19 as a Global Health Emergency," UN News; "End of the Federal COVID-19 Public Health Emergency (PHE) Declaration," Centers for Disease Control and Prevention Archives, accessed July 13, 2024, https://archive.cdc.gov/#/details?url=https://www.cdc.gov/coronavirus/2019-ncov/your-health/end-of-phe.html.

40 Offit, "Asking the Uncomfortable Questions About Vaccines."

41 M. S. Sinha, W. E. Parmet, and G. S. Gonsalves, "Déjà Vu All Over Again - Refusing to Learn the Lessons of Covid-19," *The New England Journal of Medicine* 391, no. 6 (2024): 481–483, https://doi.org/10.1056/NEJMp2406427.

42 Naomi O'Grady, interview, May 16, 2024.

43 Sinha, Parmet, and Gonsalves, "Déjà Vu All Over Again."

44 Apoorva Mandavilli, "'A Dangerous Virus': Bird Flu Enters a New Phase," *The New York Times*, January 29, 2025, https://www.nytimes.com/2025/01/27/health/bird-flu-h5n1.html

45 "First H5 Bird Flu Death Reported in United States," Centers for Disease Control and Prevention, January 6, 2025, https://www.cdc.gov/media/releases/2025/m0106-h5-birdflu-death.html.

46 Mandavilli, "'A Dangerous Virus.'"

47 Ibid.

48 Panthagani, "Science, Policy, and Values."

Chapter Seventeen: What Really Matters

1 Daniel H. Pink, *Drive: The Surprising Truth About What Motivates Us* (Riverhead, 2009).

2 "Amy Watts," interview, September 22, 2022.

3 Ibid.

4 "CMS Hospital Compare," Medicare.gov, accessed May 2021, https://www.medicare.gov/care-compare/?redirect=true&providerType=Hospital.

5 Rhee, Dantes, Epstein, et al., "Incidence and Trends of Sepsis in US Hospitals Using Clinical vs Claims Data, 2009-2014."

6   S. R. Townsend, G. S. Phillips, R. Duseja, et al., "Effects of Compliance With the Early Management Bundle (SEP-1) on Mortality Changes Among Medicare Beneficiaries With Sepsis: A Propensity Score Matched Cohort Study," *Chest* 161, no. 2 (2022): 392–406, https://doi.org/10.1016/j.chest.2021.07.2167.

7   K. E., Rudd, S. C. Johnson, K. M. Agesa, et al., "Global, regional, and national sepsis incidence and mortality, 1990-2017: analysis for the Global Burden of Disease Study," *The Lancet* 395, no. 10219 (2020): 200–211, doi: 10.1016/S0140-6736(19)32989-7, PMID: 31954465, PMCID: PMC6970225.

8   A. E. Barnato, S. L. Alexander, W. T. Linde-Zwirble, et al., "Racial variation in the incidence, care, and outcomes of severe sepsis: analysis of population, patient, and hospital characteristics," *American Journal of Respiratory and Critical Care Medicine* 177, no. 3 (2008): 279–284, https://doi.org/10.1164/rccm.200703-480OC.

9   Seymour and Wiersinga, eds., *Handbook of Sepsis*, 19.

10 Ibid., 19.

11 N. R. Henry, A. C. Hanson, P. J. Schulte, et al., "Disparities in Hypoxemia Detection by Pulse Oximetry Across Self-Identified Racial Groups and Associations with Clinical Outcomes," *Critical Care Medicine* 50, no. 2 (2022): 204–211, https://doi.org/10.1097/CCM.0000000000005394.

12 Tenon, *Memoirs on Paris Hospitals*, vii.

13 "Maternal Sepsis," World Health Organization, accessed July 13, 2024, https://www.who.int/teams/sexual-and-reproductive-health-and-research-(srh)/areas-of-work/maternal-and-perinatal-health/maternal-sepsis.

14 "California Pregnancy-Associated Mortality Review (CA-PAMR)," California Department of Public Health, last updated July 9, 2024, https://www.cdph.ca.gov/Programs/CFH/DMCAH/Pages/PAMR.aspx.

15 C. Padilla and A. Palanisamy, "Managing Maternal Sepsis: Early Warning Criteria to ECMO," *Clinical Obstetrics and Gynecology* 60, no. 2 (2017): 418–424, https://doi.org/10.1097/GRF.0000000000000269.

16 "Maternal Sepsis Campaign," End Sepsis, accessed November 14, 2025, https://www.end-sepsis.org/mothers/.

17 "Overturning Roe v. Wade: Health Consequences for Pregnant People Likely to Include an Increase in Maternal Sepsis," Sepsis Alliance, June 24, 2022, https://www.sepsis.org/news/overturning-roe-v-wade-health-consequences-for-pregnant-people-likely-to-include-an-increase-in-maternal-sepsis/.

18 "More Pregnant Women Face Life-Threatening Sepsis in Wake of Strict Abortion Laws," PBS News, February 27, 2025, https://www.pbs.org/newshour/show/more-pregnant-women-face-life-threatening-sepsis-in-wake-of-strict-abortion-laws.

19 "Statement on Maternal Sepsis," World Health Organization, May 31, 2017, https://iris.who.int/bitstream/handle/10665/254608/WHO-RHR-17.02-eng.pdf?sequence=1.

20 "Patient Safety Measure Evaluation Web Meeting, Spring 2021 Cycle," National Quality Forum, June 24, 2021.

21 "Patient Safety Post-Comment Web Meeting," National Quality Forum, October 13, 2021.

22 "Patient Safety Measure Evaluation Web Meeting, Spring 2021 Cycle," National Quality Forum.

23 "Patient Safety, Spring 2021 Cycle: Public and Member Comments," National Quality Forum, Spring 2021.

24 "Patient Safety, Spring 2021, Measure Review Cycle, Post-Comment Standing Committee Meeting," National Quality Forum, October 13, 2021.

25 "NQF Releases Statement Detailing Appeals Board Decision on SEP-1 Endorsement Status," National Quality Forum, archived at Internet Archive, capture date May 6, 2022, https://web.archive.org/web/20250613123008/https://www.qualityforum.org/News_And_Resources/Press_Releases/2022/NQF_Releases_Statement_Detailing_Appeals_Board_Decision_on_SEP-1_Endorsement_Status.aspx.

26 "Patient Safety, Spring 2021, Measure Review Cycle, Post-Comment Standing Committee Meeting," National Quality Forum.

27 Mukherjee, *The Laws of Medicine*, 59.

28 Nirav Shah, remarks during 2023 National Forum on Sepsis, End Sepsis, Washington, DC, September 13, 2023

Chapter Eighteen: Getting It Right

1 Jessi Hempel, "Transcript: Episode 101: Brené Brown on getting it right," LinkedIn News, March 22, 2021, https://www.linkedin.com/pulse/transcript-episode-101-brené-brown-getting-right-jessi-hempel.

2 Eric Walter, interview, December 2, 2022.

3 Laura Evans, interview, October 10, 2022.

4 "U.S. adults are lacking knowledge about infection and sepsis prevention," Sepsis Alliance, September 13, 2024, https://www.sepsis.org/news/sepsis-awareness-reaches-69-while-misconceptions-about-sepsis-and-infections-exist/.

5 "Hospital Care Compare," Medicare.gov, accessed November 14, 2025, https://www.medicare.gov/care-compare/?providerType=Hospital.

6 I. J. Barbash, B. S. Davis, J. G. Yabes, et al., "Treatment Patterns and Clinical Outcomes After the Introduction of the Medicare Sepsis Performance Measure (SEP-1)," *Annals of Internal Medicine* 174, no. 7 (2021): 927–935, https://doi.org/10.7326/M20-5043; S. R. Townsend, G. S. Phillips, R. Duseja, et al., "Effects of Compliance With the Early Management Bundle (SEP-1) on Mortality Changes Among Medicare Beneficiaries With Sepsis: A Propensity Score Matched Cohort Study," *Chest* 161, no. 2 (2022): 392–406, https://doi.org/10.1016/j.chest.2021.07.2167.

7 Kevin Tracey, remarks during 2023 End Sepsis National Sepsis Forum, September 13, 2023.

8 Laura Evans, interview, October 10, 2022.

9 Kedar Mate, remarks during 2023 End Sepsis National Sepsis Forum, September 13, 2023.

10 Ronald Kline, interview, August 16, 2024.

11 Townsend, Phillips, Duseja, et al., "Effects of Compliance With the Early Management Bundle (SEP-1) on Mortality Changes Among Medicare Beneficiaries With Sepsis."

12 Rhee, Chiotos, Cosgrove, et al., "Infectious Diseases Society of America Position Paper: Recommended Revisions to the National Severe Sepsis and Septic Shock Early Management Bundle (SEP-1) Sepsis Quality Measure."

13 Sean Townsend, interview, March 27, 2024.

14 H. Ueyama and S. Kiyonaka, "Predicting the Need for Fluid Therapy: Does Fluid Responsiveness Work?" *Journal of Intensive Care* 5, no. 34 (2017): https://doi.org/10.1186/s40560-017-0210-7; F. Michard and J. L. Teboul, "Predicting fluid responsiveness in ICU patients: a critical analysis of the evidence," *Chest* 121, no. 6 (2002): 2000–2008, https://doi.org/10.1378/chest.121.6.2000.

15 K. Maitland, S. Kiguli, R. O. Opoka, et al., "Mortality after fluid bolus in African children with severe infection," *The New England Journal of Medicine* 364, no. 26 (2011): 2483–2495, https://doi.org/10.1056/NEJMoa1101549; Andrews, Muchemwa, Kelly, et al., "Simplified severe sepsis protocol: a randomized controlled trial of modified early goal-directed therapy in Zambia"; B. Andrews, M. W. Semler, L. Muchemwa, et al., "Effect of an Early Resuscitation Protocol on In-hospital Mortality Among Adults With Sepsis and Hypotension: A Randomized Clinical Trial," *JAMA* 318, no. 13 (2017): 1233–1240, https://doi.org/10.1001/jama.2017.10913; Hallie Prescott, email correspondence, September 10, 2025.

16 Seymour, Gesten, Prescott, et al., "Time to Treatment and Mortality during Mandated Emergency Care for Sepsis."

17 Evans, Rhodes, Alhazzani, et al., "Surviving sepsis campaign: international guidelines for management of sepsis and septic shock 2021."

18 C. Rhee, J. R. Strich, K. Chiotos, et al., "Improving Sepsis Outcomes in the Era of Pay-for-Performance and Electronic Quality Measures: A Joint IDSA/ACEP/PIDS/SHEA/SHM/SIDP Position Paper," *Clinical Infectious Diseases* 78, no. 3 (2024): 505–513, https://doi.org/10.1093/cid/ciad447.

19 Ibid.

20 A. L. Pakyz, C. M. Orndahl, A. Johns, et al., "Impact of the Centers for Medicare and Medicaid Services Sepsis Core Measure on Antibiotic Use," *Clinical Infectious Diseases* 72, no. 4 (2021): 556–565, https://doi.org/10.1093/cid/ciaa456.

21 H. C. Prescott, S. Seelye, X. Q. Wang, et al., "Temporal Trends in Antimicrobial Prescribing During Hospitalization for Potential Infection and Sepsis," *JAMA Internal Medicine* 182, no. 8 (2022): 805–813, https://doi.org/10.1001/jamainternmed.2022.2291.

22 Rhee, Strich, Chiotos, et al., "Improving Sepsis Outcomes in the Era of Pay-for-Performance and Electronic Quality Measures."

23 I. C. Gyssens, P. J. van den Broek, B. J. Kullberg, et al., "Optimizing antimicrobial therapy. A method for antimicrobial drug use evaluation," *The Journal of Antimicrobial Chemotherapy* 30, no. 5 (1992): 724–727, https://doi.org/10.1093/jac/30.5.724.

24 "Core Elements of Hospital Antibiotic Stewardship Programs," Centers for Disease Control and Prevention, March 14, 2024, https://www.cdc.gov/antibiotic-use/hcp/core-elements/hospital.html?CDC_AAref_Val=https://www.cdc.gov/antibiotic-use/core-elements/hospital.html.

25 "National Action Plan for Combating Antibiotic-Resistance Bacteria, 2020–2025," Office of the Assistant Secretary for Planning and Evaluation, October 8, 2020, https://aspe.hhs.gov/reports/national-action-plan-combating-antibiotic-resistant-bacteria-2020-2025.

26 "Core Elements of Hospital Antibiotic Stewardship Programs," Centers for Disease Control and Prevention.

27 "Four Moments of Antibiotic Decision Making," Agency for Healthcare Research and Quality, accessed July 14, 2024, https://www.ahrq.gov/antibiotic-use/acute-care/four-moments/index.html.

28 Pakyz, Orndahl, Johns, et al., "Impact of the Centers for Medicare and Medicaid Services Sepsis Core Measure on Antibiotic Use."

29 J. A. Jernigan, K. M. Hatfield, H. Wolford, et al., "Multidrug-resistant bacterial infections in US hospitalized patients, 2012–2017," *The New England Journal of Medicine* 382, no. 14 (2020): 1309–1319; T. M. Pham, Y. Zhang, M. Nevers, et al., "Trends in infection incidence and antimicrobial resistance in the US Veterans Affairs Healthcare System: a nationwide retrospective cohort study (2007–22)," *The Lancet Infectious Diseases* 24, no. 12 (2024): 1333–1346, https://doi.org/10.1016/S1473-3099(24)00416-X.

30 "Outpatient Antibiotic Prescribing in the United States, Annual Report," Centers for Disease Control and Prevention, September 15, 2025, https://www.cdc.gov/antibiotic-use/hcp/data-research/antibiotic-prescribing.html.

31 European Union, "Key messages for hospital prescribers," European Antibiotic Awareness Day: A European Health Initiative, October 7, 2021, https://antibiotic.ecdc.europa.eu/en/get-informed/key-messages/hospital-prescribers.

32 "Outpatient Antibiotic Prescribing in the United States, Annual Report," Centers for Disease Control and Prevention.

33 A. Hollis and Z. Ahmed, "Preserving antibiotics, rationally," *The New England Journal of Medicine* 369, no. 26 (2013): 2474–2476, https://www.nejm.org/doi/full/10.1056/NEJMp1311479.

34 Ronald Kline, remarks during 2023 End Sepsis National Sepsis Forum, September 13, 2023.

35 Rhee, Strich, Chiotos, et al., "Improving Sepsis Outcomes in the Era of Pay-for-Performance and Electronic Quality Measures."

36 J. S. Ford, J. C. Morrison, M. Kyaw, et al., "The Effect of Severe Sepsis and Septic Shock Management Bundle (SEP-1) Compliance and Implementation on Mortality Among Patients With Sepsis: A Systematic Review," *Annals of Internal Medicine* 178, no. 4 (2025): 543–557, https://doi.org/10.7326/ANNALS-24-02426.

37 James Ford, email correspondence, February 26, 2025.

38 Derek Angus, interview, April 3, 2024.

39 "Public Comment Summary Report: Community-Onset Sepsis: 30-day Mortality," US Centers for Medicare & Medicaid Services, June 10, 2022, https://mmshub.cms.gov/sites/default/files/Sepsis-Blueprint-PubComSum-508.pdf; Raymond Dantes, "New Developments in Sepsis Quality Measurement (CE Session)," Sepsis Alliance Institute, Sepsis Alliance Summit, accessed October 14, 2025, https://learn.sepsis.org/products/new-developments-in-sepsis-quality-measurement-ce-session.

40 Rhee, Strich, Chiotos, et al., "Improving Sepsis Outcomes in the Era of Pay-for-Performance and Electronic Quality Measures."

41 M. W. Sjoding, T. J. Iwashyna, J. B. Dimick, et al., "Gaming hospital-level pneumonia 30-day mortality and readmission measures by legitimate changes to diagnostic coding," *Critical Care Medicine* 43, no. 5 (2015): 989–995, https://doi.org/10.1097/CCM.0000000000000862.

42 Raymund Dantes, interview, October 31, 2022; C. W. Seymour, C. M. Coopersmith, C. S. Deutschman, et al., "Application of a Framework to Assess the Usefulness of Alternative Sepsis Criteria," *Critical Care Medicine* 44, no. 3 (2016): e122–e130, https://doi.org/10.1097/CCM.0000000000001724.

43 Rhee, Strich, Chiotos, et al., "Improving Sepsis Outcomes in the Era of Pay-for-Performance and Electronic Quality Measures."

44 Ronald Kline, remarks during 2023 End Sepsis National Sepsis Forum, September 13, 2023.

45 C. Rhee, R. Wang, Y. Song, et al., "Risk Adjustment for Sepsis Mortality to Facilitate Hospital Comparisons Using Centers for Disease Control and Prevention's Adult Sepsis Event Criteria and Routine Electronic Clinical Data," *Critical Care Explorations* 1, no. 10 (2019): e0049, https://doi.org/10.1097/CCE.0000000000000049.

46 William Knaus, interview, November 9, 2022.

47 Raymund Dantes, interview, October 31, 2023, and follow-up email correspondence September 9, 2024; Kristina Betz, "Sepsis Quality Measures coming to the National Healthcare Safety Network," Sepsis Alliance Institute, Sepsis Alliance Summit, accessed October 14, 2025, https://learn.sepsis.org/products/new-developments-in-sepsis-quality-measurement-ce-session.

48 Laura Evans, interview, October 10, 2022.

49 Ibid.

50 Jonny Wilkinson. "ENCOMPASS—STAR Programme in Sepsis Survivors," *CRITICALCARE NORTHAMPTON: Reviewing Critical Care, Journals & FOAMed*, last updated June 12, 2025, https://criticalcarenorthampton.com/2025/06/12/encompass/.

51 Colonel Ian Stewart, remarks during 2023 End Sepsis National Sepsis Forum, September 13, 2023.

52 Derek Angus, interview, April 3, 2024.

53 "Summary of Technical Expert Panel (TEP): Sepsis Readmission Measure," CMS Measures Management System, Centers for Medicare & Medicaid Services, accessed September 9, 2025, https://mmshub.cms.gov/get-involved/technical-expert-panel/updates.

54 L. J. Schlapbach, R. S. Watson, L. R. Sorce, et al., "International Consensus Criteria for Pediatric Sepsis and Septic Shock," *JAMA* 331, no. 8 (2024): 665–674, https://doi.org/10.1001/jama.2024.0179; S. L. Weiss, M. J. Peters, W. Alhazzani, et al., "Surviving sepsis campaign international guidelines for the management of septic shock and sepsis-associated organ dysfunction in children," *Intensive Care Medicine* 46 Suppl 1 (2020): 10–67, https://doi.org/10.1007/s00134-019-05878-6.

55 R. Paul, M. Niedner, R. Riggs, et al., "Bundled Care to Reduce Sepsis Mortality: The Improving Pediatric Sepsis Outcomes (IPSO) Collaborative," *Pediatrics* 152, no. 2 (2023): e2022059938, https://doi.org/10.1542/peds.2022-059938.

56 Scott Weiss, interview, October 4, 2022.

57 Kedar Mate, remarks during 2023 End Sepsis National Sepsis Forum, September 13, 2023.

58 H. C. Prescott, P. J. Posa, and R. Dantes, "The Centers for Disease Control and Prevention's Hospital Sepsis Program Core Elements," *JAMA* 330, no. 17 (2023): 1617–1618, https://doi.org/10.1001/jama.2023.16693.

59 Denise Cardo, remarks during 2023 End Sepsis National Sepsis Forum, September 13, 2023.

60 Ibid.

61 "Measures Under Consideration (MUC) Lists: Pre-Rulemaking MUC Lists and Recommendation Reports," Centers for Medicare and Medicaid Services, accessed December 15, 2025, https://mmshub.cms.gov/measure-lifecycle/measure-implementation/pre-rulemaking/lists-and-reports/overview.

62 Laura Evans, interview, October 10, 2022.

63 NYS Sepsis Care Improvement Initiative and NYS Regulations, New York State Department of Health, September 2025, https://www.health.ny.gov/diseases/conditions/sepsis/care_improvement_initiative.htm.

64 Kevin Tracey, remarks during 2023 End Sepsis National Sepsis Forum, September 13, 2023.

Chapter Nineteen: Hereafter

1   "'Heroes' Single Is Forty Years Old Today," DavidBowie.com, September 23, 2017, https://www.davidbowie.com/blog/2017/9/23/heroes-single-is-forty-years-old-today.

2   C. W. Seymour, J. N. Kennedy, S. Wang, et al., "Derivation, Validation, and Potential Treatment Implications of Novel Clinical Phenotypes for Sepsis," *JAMA* 321, no. 20 (2019): 2003–2017, https://doi.org/10.1001/jama.2019.5791

3   "Sepsis Alliance Reinforces Call for National Sepsis Action Plan as Awareness of the Term Sepsis Dips to 63%," Sepsis Alliance, September 13, 2023, https://www.sepsis.org/news/sepsis-alliance-reinforces-call-for-national-sepsis-action-plan-as-awareness-of-the-term-sepsis-dips-to-63.

4   "Education," End Sepsis, accessed November 14, 2025, https://www.endsepsis.org/work/education/.

5   Orlaith Staunton, email conversation, October 16, 2024.

6   "About Get Ahead of Sepsis," Centers for Disease Control and Prevention, September 25, 2025, https://www.cdc.gov/sepsis/get-ahead-of-sepsis/index.html.

7   Robert Pearl, *Mistreated: Why We Think We're Getting Good Health Care and Why We're Usually Wrong* (Public Affairs, 2017), 34.

8   Laura Evans, interview, October 10, 2023.

9   Ibid.

10   "Congress Approves Sepsis Funding and Issues Sepsis Directives in the FY23 Budget in Historic First," End Sepsis, January 25, 2023, https://www.prnewswire.com/news-releases/congress-approves-sepsis-funding-and-issues-sepsis-directives-in-the-fy23-budget-in-historic-first-301729624.html.

11   "Lulu's Law," Sepsis Alliance, accessed July 15, 2023, https://www.sepsis.org/sepsis-alliance-voices/lulus-law/; United States Congress, "H.R. 8865, LuLu's Law: 117th Congress (2021–2022)," Congress.gov, accessed October 14, 2025, https://www.congress.gov/bill/117th-congress/house-bill/8865.

12   "Senators Introduce the SEPSIS Act," American Hospital Association, September 12, 2024, https://www.aha.org/news/headline/2024-09-12-senators-introduce-sepsis-act; United States Congress, "S. 1929, SEPSIS Act: 119th Congress (2025)," Congress.gov, accessed October 14, 2025, https://www.congress.gov/bill/119th-congress/senate-bill/1929/text.

13   M. M. Levy, L. E. Evans, and A. Rhodes, "The Surviving Sepsis Campaign Bundle: 2018 Update," *Intensive Care Medicine* 44, no. 6 (2018): 925–928, https://doi.org/10.1007/s00134-018-5085-0.

14   "Surviving Sepsis Campaign: Retract the SSC 2018 Guidelines," Care2 Petitions, accessed November 14, 2025, https://www.thepetitionsite.com/772/830/097/surviving-sepsis-campaign-sccm-esicm/.

15   H. E. Frank, L. Evans, G. Phillips, et al., "Assessment of implementation methods in sepsis: study protocol for a cluster-randomized hybrid type 2 trial," *Trials* 24, no. 1 (2023): 620, https://doi.org/10.1186/s13063-023-07644-y; "Cluster Randomized Trials," National Institutes of Health Pragmatic Trials Collaboratory, accessed July 15, 2024, https://rethinkingclinicaltrials.org/chapters/design/experimental-designs-and-randomization-schemes/cluster-randomized-trials/.

16   David Gilbert, interview, April 1, 2024.

17   Ibid.

18   Ibid.

19 Laura Evans, interview, October 10, 2022.

20 Y-N. Liu, Y-F. Zhang, Q. Xu, et al., "Infection and co-infection patterns of community-acquired pneumonia in patients of different ages in China from 2009 to 2020: a national surveillance study," *The Lancet Microbe* 4, no. 5 (2023): e330–e339, https://doi.org/10.1016/S2666-5247(23)00031-9.

21 Evans, Rhodes, Alhazzani, et al., "Surviving sepsis campaign: international guidelines for management of sepsis and septic shock 2021."

22 Laura Evans, interview, October 10, 2022; Blaser, Cohen, and Holland, *Mandell, Douglas, and Bennett's Principles and Practice of Infectious Diseases*, 10th ed., 942.

23 Blaser, Cohen, and Holland, *Mandell, Douglas, and Bennett's Principles and Practice of Infectious Diseases*, 10th ed., 943.

24 Abimbola Farinde, "Procalcitonin (PCT)," Medscape, updated November 6, 2025, https://emedicine.medscape.com/article/2096589-overview#a5.

25 Evans, Rhodes, Alhazzani, et al., "Surviving sepsis campaign: international guidelines for management of sepsis and septic shock: 2021."

26 Ibid.

27 "Prenosis Announces FDA De Novo Marketing Authorization of the Sepsis ImmunoScore," Prenosis, April 3, 2024, https://prenosis.com/news/prenosis-announces-fda-de-novo-marketing-authorization-of-immunoscore/; "De Novo Classification Request for Prenosis Sepsis ImmunoScore (DEN230036)," US Food and Drug Administration, April 2, 2024, https://www.accessdata.fda.gov/cdrh_docs/pdf23/DEN230036.pdf.

28 "First-of-Its-Kind Technology Using Deformability Cytometry to Detect Sepsis," Cytovale, accessed June 15, 2025, https://cytovale.com/our-solution/our-science/.

29 R. Haas and S. C. McGill, "Artificial Intelligence for the Prediction of Sepsis in Adults," CADTH Horizon Scan, March 2022, https://www.ncbi.nlm.nih.gov/books/NBK596676.

30 M. E. Matheny, D. Whicher, and S. Thadaney Israni, "Artificial Intelligence in Health Care: A Report from the National Academy of Medicine," *JAMA* 323, no. 6 (2020): 509–510, https://doi.org/10.1001/jama.2019.21579.

31 F. Cabitza, R. Rasoini, and G. F. Gensini, "Unintended Consequences of Machine Learning in Medicine," *JAMA* 318, no. 6 (2017): 517–518, https://doi.org/10.1001/jama.2017.7797.

32 Derek Angus, interview, April 3, 2024.

33 Ibid.

34 "Wearables and AI to Predict and Prevent Sepsis Outside the Hospital," Sepsis Scout, accessed November 14, 2025, https://www.ycombinator.com/companies/sepsis-scout.

35 Derek Angus, interview, April 3, 2024.

36 Ibid.

37 "Bacterial Vaccines in Clinical and Preclinical Development 2021," World Health Organization, July 12, 2022, https://www.who.int/publications/i/item/9789240052451.

38 "BARDA support protects against drug-resistant threats," BARDA, archived at Internet Archive, capture date May 6, 2023, https://web.archive.org/web/20230506042657/https://medicalcountermeasures.gov/stories/amr/.

39 "Power the AMRevolution," Sepsis Alliance, accessed July 15, 2024, https://www.sepsis.org/power-the-amrevolution/; U.S. Congress, *Pioneering Antimicrobial Subscriptions to End Upsurging Resistance (PASTEUR) Act of 2023*, S.1355, 118th Congress, 1st session, introduced April 27, 2023, https://www.congress.gov/bill/118th-congress/senate-bill/1355.

40 M. Naghavi, S. E. Vollset, K. S. Ikuta, et al., "Global burden of bacterial antimicrobial resistance 1990-2021: a systematic analysis with forecasts to 2050," *The Lancet* 404, no. 10459 (2024): 1199–1226,

41 Richard Besser, Mandy K. Cohen, William Foege, et al., "We Ran the C.D.C.: Kennedy Is Endangering Every American's Health," *The New York Times*, September 1, 2025, https://www.nytimes.com/2025/09/01/opinion/cdc-leaders-kennedy.html.

42 Ibid.; Madeline Halpert, "RFK Jr Cancels $500m in Funding for mRNA Vaccines for Diseases Like Covid," BBC News, August 5, 2025, https://www.bbc.com/news/articles/c74dzdddvmjo; Will Stone, "Panel Picked by RFK Jr. Will Scrutinize the Vaccine Schedule for Kids," NPR, June 25, 2025, https://www.npr.org/sections/shots-health-news/2025/06/25/nx-s1-5445254/cdc-review-vaccine-schedule-children.

43 Gavi Staff, "New Data Shows Vaccines Have Saved 154 Million Lives in the Past 50 Years: An Analysis of the Impact of 50 Years of the Global Vaccine Programme Shows the Extraordinary Value of Vaccination," VaccinesWork, April 24, 2024, https://www.gavi.org/vaccineswork/new-data-shows-vaccines-have-saved-154-million-lives-past-50-years.

44 K. E. Rudd, S. C. Johnson, K. M. Agesa, et al., "Global, regional, and national sepsis incidence and mortality, 1990–2017: analysis for the Global Burden of Disease Study," *The Lancet* 395, no. 10219 (2020): 200–211, https://doi.org/10.1016/S0140-6736(19)32989-7.

45 Alison Fox-Robichaud, remarks during Sepsis Forum 2023, June 21, 2023.

46 Nirav Shah, remarks during 2023 End Sepsis National Sepsis Forum, September 13, 2023.

47 David Gilbert, interview, February 11, 2025.

Epilogue: Save a Life, Save the World

1 H. Steven Moffic, "Save a Life and You Save the World," *Psychiatric Times*, October 24, 2023, https://www.psychiatrictimes.com/view/save-a-life-and-you-save-the-world.

2 Justin McHenry, interview, August 9, 2022.

3 "USLA National Lifeguard Championship Results 2000," United States Lifesaving Association, accessed November 12, 2025, https://www.usla.org/page/2000Results.

4 Fred Swegles, "The BEST on the beach," *The Orange County Register*, August 29, 2007, https://www.ocregister.com/2007/08/29/the-best-on-the-beach/.

5 Michael S. Bartlett, "Lifeguard Legend Retires from Teaching and Coaching," *American Lifeguard Magazine*, Spring 2004, 20–21.

6 Elisabeth Ward, interview, December 13, 2022.

7 Ibid.

8 Ibid.

9 Orlaith Staunton, remarks at 2023 End Sepsis National Sepsis Forum, Washington, DC, September 13, 2023.

Index

Note: Page numbers in *italics* indicate figures, **bold** indicate tables in the text, and references following "n" refer to the notes.

#

100,000 Lives Campaign, 167, 168, 183, 185, 213

A

abdominal sepsis, 34–35
Abraham, E. P., 69
acetyl-CoA, 146
activated protein C (APC), 176–77. *See also* Xigris (drotrecogin alfa)
Acute Physiology and Chronic Health Evaluation Score (APACHE / APACHE II), 126–31, 169, 179–80, 197–98, 220, 257, 310
acute respiratory distress syndrome (ARDS), 61, 83, 95–96, 182, 202, 330
Addison, Thomas, 102
adrenal glands, 102–4
    cortex, 103–4
adrenaline, 102, 102n, 103, 122, 143
    noradrenaline, 103
Adult Sepsis Event (ASE), 309, 309n
AdvaMed, 240n
advanced cardiovascular life support (ACLS), 141
Affordable Care Act, 195n, 242
afterload, 138n. *See also* heart
age, 79–80

Agency for Healthcare Research and Quality (AHRQ), 126, 166, 166n, 181–82, 304, 320
agglutination, 56, 56n
AIMS. *See* Assessment of Implementation Methods in Sepsis and Respiratory Failure
aldosterone, 104
alert system, 261–63
    false alarms, 218–19, 261, 267, 268
al-Razi, Abu Bakr, 100–101
Amenhotep IV, 23, 24
American College of Chest Physicians, 118
American College of Emergency Physicians (ACEP), 292
American College of Surgeons, 195n
American Federation of Teachers, 319
American Heart Association, 141, 239n
American Sepsis Alliance. *See* Sepsis Alliance
Angus, Derek, 203–4, 245–46, 261, 263–64, 311, 324–26
animalcules, 30
animalia minuta, 26
Animal Parasites and Messmates (van Beneden), 77–78n
Annals of Internal Medicine, 104, 305
anthrax, 43
antibiotics, 47–49, 51–52, 62, 67–69, 302–5

antistreptococcal, 57
bacteriostatic, 62, 62n
broad-spectrum, 78, 133, 174, 288,
 302–3, 327
complexities of selection in sepsis (Tom's
 case), 53–54, 60–65
livestock use, 73
microbiome and, 78
overprescription, 72–73, 121, 253,
 298, 303
and pneumonia treatment, 57–58, 62
rapid administration requirement, 199,
 212–13, 264–66, 302–3, 322–23
resistance *see* antimicrobial
 resistance (AMR)
stewardship programs (ASP), 75, 303–4,
 304n, 313
sulfa, 62
viral infections, 302
antibodies, 55–56
anti-endotoxin, 106
monoclonal, 106
Anti-Infective Drugs Advisory Committee
 (AIDAC), 178
antimicrobial resistance (AMR), 14–15,
 67–71, 111–12, 302–5, 313
antibiotic stewardship, 75, 303–4,
 304n, 313
CDC on, 160
COVID-19, 274
deaths from, 71, 80–81
hospital infections through history, 35–41
human contribution to, 72–73
infection control programs, 73–75
microbiome and, 78
new therapies to reduce, 327
opportunistic infections, 75–78
prevention, 80–82
spread and mechanisms, 70–72
antiserum therapy, 55–57
Archives of Internal Medicine, 144
ARDSNet study, 182n
ARISE study, 198, 244, 244n.
Aristotle, 25, 36, 41
arsphenamine, 51
artificial intelligence (AI) tools, 126,
 319, 323–25
ASE. *See* Adult Sepsis Event

Assessment of Implementation Methods in
 Sepsis and Respiratory Failure (AIMS),
 321, 321n, 325
Association for Professionals in Infection
 Control and Epidemiology (APIC), 74
ATP, 146
Attia, Peter, 162
autolysis, 20
Avicenna, 28, 41n, 51n (footnote),

B
bacteremia, 4, 8, 69, 104–5, 112, 113, 115
bacteriocins, 77n
balancing measures, 313
bands, 119, 123
Barcelona Declaration, 172, 182, 298
Barnett, Jack A., 85n
Bayer, 168–69
Bayesian inference, 6–7
Beecham Group, 69
Behring, Emil von, 55
Belsito, Marybeth, 187
Belsito & Co., 186–89
Bennett, Ivan, 86
Berlin Society for Physiology, 43
Berwick, Donald, 167, 183
Berzelius, Jacob, 145–46
Biden, Joe, 320
biomarkers, 322–23
Biomedical Advanced Research and
 Development Authority (BARDA),
 319, 327
Bizzozero, Giulio, 92
Blalock, Alfred, 4, 137
Blaser, Martin, 76, 80
blood coagulation, 92–94, 176–77
bloodletting, 100
blood pressure, 4n, 139
intravenous fluid boluses, 238, 239
low, 4, 12, 114, 131, 136, 142, 145
normal, 4n, 207n, 222
blood transfusion, 142
blood vessels, 137, 139–40
capillaries, 60
cholesterol plaque, 93
dilation, 148
endothelial cells, 92
endothelium, 148
nitric oxide, 148

blood volume, 137–43, 151, 197. *See also* cardiovascular system
Blumenthal, David, 189
Blundell, James, 142
B lymphocytes (B cells), 55, 106
Bone, Roger, 113–15, 118, 119, 131, 168–69, 246, 253
Book of Prognostics, The (Hippocrates), 26
Borgognoni, Theodoric, 28
Bottomly, H. Kim, 87
botulinum toxin, 10–11
botulism, 10
Bumstead, John, 47, 48
Byington, Cara, 230
Byington, Nate, 230

C
Calderon, Hector, 271, 279
California Maternal Quality Care Collaborative (CMQCC), 291
Candida albicans, 76
Cannon, Walter, 103
Canon of Medicine (Avicenna), 28
capillaries, 60
    fluid leakage from, 140, 140n
    See also blood vessels
Carcillo, Joseph, 238–39
cardiac arrests, 202, 228
cardiac output, 139
    dobutamine, 175
    supranormal levels, 151
cardiopulmonary arrest, 140–41
cardiovascular system, 137–40, 148
    blood vessels, 137, 139–40
    heart, 137–39
Carr, Gordon, 202
case fatality rate (CFR), 273n
Casey, Bob, 320
cassette chromosomes, 71, 71n
Celsus, Aulus Cornelius, 8
Centanni, Eugenio, 11–12
Center for Outcomes Research and Evaluation (CORE), 311
Centers for Disease Control and Prevention (CDC), 96, 111, 230, 235
    antibiotic stewardship, 304
    antimicrobial resistance (AMR), 68, 70
    CHIP, 74
    chronic disease, 79

Get Ahead of Sepsis campaign, 319
    hospital-acquired infections, 160
    Hospital Sepsis Program Core Elements, 313
    ICD-9-CM Coordination and Maintenance Committee, 188
    National Healthcare Safety Network, 166, 310
    SENIC, 74
Centers for Medicare and Medicaid Services (CMS), 75, 236, 298
    Deficit Reduction Act, 166, 194
    Hospital Quality Alliance, 194, 195
    Inpatient Quality Reporting program, 194, 195
    implementing antibiotic stewardship programs (ASPs), 75
    NQF and, 166, 195
    pay-for-performance programs, 194–95
    SEP-1 *see* SEP-1
    Sepsis 3 framework, 257
    sepsis mortality measure, 307–8
central venous pressure (CVP), 143
Cerner HealthFacts, 309–10
Chain, Ernst, 48, 69
Charlson, Mary, 129
childbirth and infection, 35, 38–41
Children's Hospital Association, 311–12
children with sepsis, 222–24, 311–12
    fluid boluses, 238
    incidence, 79
    See also Staunton, Rory
cholera, 11, 51
chronic disease, 59, 79–80
citric acid cycle, 146
climate change, 96
clinical trials, 100–102
    animal models, 105, 107–8
    cluster-randomized trial (CRT), 321n
    conundrum, 102, 319
    patient selection, 104–5
    poorly designed, 101
    randomization, 101–2
    septic shock patients, 174–75
    waiver of consent, 215n
    See also specific trials
Clinton, Bill, 164
Clostridioides difficile (C. difficile), 77–78, 78n, 313
Clostridium botulinum, 10
clotting factors, 92

Codman, Ernest, 195n
Collins, Susan, 320
commensalism, 77–78n
community-acquired pneumonia, 61, 322
Comorbidity Points Score (COPS), 284n, 285n, 309
Comprehensive Hospital Infections Project (CHIP), 74
confirmation bias, 128
Consensus Development Process, 236
Consensus Standards Approval Committee (CSAC), 241
Contagiousness of Puerperal Fever, The (Holmes), 38
Core Elements of Hospital Antibiotic Stewardship Programs (CDC), 303–4, 313
corticosteroids, 110n
  bovine adrenal glands and, 103n
  clinical trials, 104, 113–15
cortisol, 103, 104
  methylprednisolone, 114
Corynebacterium diphtheriae, 11
COVID-19 pandemic, 75, 95–96, 271–80, 283–84, 284n
  burnout among medical professionals, 277
  in-hospital mortality, 278
  mRNA vaccines, 275–76, 275n
  platform trials, 278
  preparedness, 281
  public health measures, 276
  sepsis/sepsis-related problems, 272–74
  social isolation, 278
  treatment guidance, 278
  vaccine and vaccination, 275–76, 278
Cowley, R. Adams, 151, 151n, 174
creatinine, 9, 94, 115, 118, 136, 309
critical care. *See* intensive care
Critical Care Medicine, 290
Crossing the Quality Chasm (Institute of Medicine), 165
Crowley, Joe, 230, 235
Cryptococcus neoformans, 76
Cuomo, Andrew, 230
Cyrurgia (Borgognoni), 28
cytokine, 8, 86–87, 89–91, 90n, 105–7, 139, 176, 177, 177n, 178n
  Bayer's inhibitor, 168–69
  drugs blocking, 107n
  and neutrophils, 122–23
  procalcitonin, 323
  release syndrome, 95, 272, 278
  and sepsis-induced myocardial dysfunction (SIMD), 140n
  shock, 109
  suppressing inflammation, 90–91
Cytovale, 323, 325

D
damage-associated molecular patterns (DAMP), 87–88
Dantes, Raymund, 309n, 310
Davaine, Casimir-Joseph, 43
D-dimer, 178n
Declaration of Geneva, 19
Deficit Reduction Act, 166, 194
Dellinger, Phillip, 171–72, 189
Deming, W. Edwards, 167
Denis, Jean-Baptiste, 142
Denny, Melissa, 267
diagnosing sepsis, 7, 16–17, 113, 201–4, 206, 209, 237, 254–58
  overdiagnosis, 265–66
  two-step approach, 131
  See also systemic inflammatory response syndrome (SIRS)
Diagnosis Related Group (DRG), 125–26
Dinarello, Charles, 86
diphtheria, 11, 55
Dobbs v. Jackson Women's Health Organization, 291
dobutamine, 175
Dowling, Michael, 232
Drebbel, Cornelius, 30
drowning, 161–64
Duseja, Reena, 293n
Dwyer, Jim, 217, 230

E
early goal-directed therapy (EGDT), 174–76, 207, 243–47, 259
  ARISE, 198, 244, 244n
  benefits, 190, 197
  central venous catheter placement, 240
  early developments, 151–52
  Edwards catheter, 175, 182n, 186, 240
  in-hospital mortality, 203

as key component of Surviving Sepsis
Strategy, 181–82, 195
multicenter studies, 197–98
NQF#0500, 235–36, 239–40, 241
PRISM, 245, 246
ProCESS study, 197–98, 243, 245–47
ProMISe study, 198, 244
septic shock prevention, 195, 207
skepticism and opposition, 175–76, 197,
197n, 209–10, 237–41
ECMO. *See* extracorporeal membrane
oxygenation
Edwards catheter, 175, 182n, 186, 240
Edwards Lifesciences, 175, 182n, 186, 197n,
240, 240n
Edwin Smith Papyrus, 22–24
Ehrlich, Paul, 51, 55
Eichacker, Peter, 186–87, 19, 340
electronic Clinical Quality Measures
(eCQM), 307–8
electronic sepsis alert (ESA), 223–24
Eli Lilly
eliminating protein C deficiency
status, 178n
PROWESS, 177–80, 186
Prozac, 187
Sepsis Alliance and, 190
SSC and, 182, 186–90, 192
Eichacker report, 186–87
Xigris *see* Xigris (drotrecogin alfa)
EMCrit, 248
Emergency Medical Treatment and Active
Labor Act (EMTALA), 158n
emergency rooms/departments,
158–60, 217–18
alert system, 261–63
interruptions, 266–67
empyema, 136
endocrine system, 103–4
endothelial cells, 92
endothelial-derived relaxation factor
(EDRF), 148
endothelium, 148
endotoxin, 11–13, 85, 86, 105–6
blocking, 106
endotoxic shock, 13, 64, 85, 93, 109,
111, 268
End Sepsis, 232, 319, 320
National Sepsis Forum, 243, 311, 315
epidemiologic transition theory, 77n

epinephrine. *See* adrenaline
equipoise, 215, 215n
errors (medical), 164–65, 166
hectic environment impacting, 266–68
premature closure, 217, 265
See also 100,000 Lives Campaign
Escherichia coli (E. coli), 4–5, 5n, 13, 15, 64,
69, 71, 90, 106, 268, 327, 330. 106
European Medicines Agency (EMA), 198
European Society of Intensive Care
Medicine (ESICM), 170, 172
Evans, Laura, 258, 297, 310, 314, 320, 322
Executive Order 13017, 164
exotoxin, 11, 11n, 78n, 89
extended-spectrum beta-lactamase-
producing *Enterobacteriaceae*
(ESBL), 111
extracorporeal membrane oxygenation
(ECMO), 91, 94

F
Fast Healthcare Interoperability Resources
(FHIR), 310
fever, 8-9, 9n, 22-24, 26, 84, 86-87, 113,119,
120-121, 140, 205, 221, 222, 255
toxin, 12
swamps, 25
fibrin, 92
fibrinogen, 92
Fisher, Ronald Aylmer, 101
Flatley, Carl, 171, 190–91, 230
Flatley, Erin, 170–71, 172
Fleming, Alexander, 48, 68, 71
Florey, Howard, 47, 48, 68–69
fluid boluses, 238–39, 239n, 248,
301–2, 301n
fluid resuscitation, 151, 184, 196–97, 226,
245–46, 300–302, 302n, 324
and COVID patients, 278
incremental, 238–39
six-hour sepsis bundle, 184, **184,** 212,
227, **227**
three-hour sepsis bundle, 227, **227**
folic acid, 62
Fracastoro, Girolamo, 41n
Frank, Edward, 150, 174, 238
Frank, Otto, 138
Frankel, Albert, 54
Frank-Starling Law, 138, *138*

Friedlander, Carl, 54, 54n
Fulton, John, 48
Furchgott, Robert, 148

G
Galen of Pergamon, 8n, 27–28, 100
Galilei, Galileo, 30
gentamicin, 14n, 70n
germ theory of disease, 25–26, 39, 44,
    50, 331
Gesten, Foster, 231–34, 250
Get Ahead of Sepsis campaign, 319
Gilbert, David, 70, 108–9, 109n, 321–22,
    322n, 332
Global Burden of Disease, 79n, 289, 329–30
Global Burden of Sepsis, 79, 289
Global Sepsis Alliance, 232, 241, 319
golden hour, 151, 174, 239
Golden Staph Era, 74, 327
Gordon, Alexander, 37–38, 292
Gordon and Betty Moore Foundation, 191
Gottlieb, Scott, 276, 276n
Grading of Recommendations, Assessment,
    Development, and Evaluation
    (GRADE), 196–97
Gram, Hans Christian, 4, 54
gram-negative bacterial infections, 5, 5n,
    12, 76, 84-85, 89, 107, 110–111
gram-positive bacteria, 4–5n
Gram stain/staining, 4, 4n
gunpowder injuries, 35

H
H1N1 influenza strain, 90, 95
H5N1 avian influenza, 96, 280–81
Halvorson, George, 231–32
Haraden, Carol, 183–84
Harkin, Tom, 241–42
Harvard Pilgrim Health Care
    Institute, 308n
Haynes, Lulu, 320
HCA Healthcare network, 310
health disparities, 79–80, 289–92, 298
    maternal patients, 290–92
    racial biases, 289–90
heart, 137–39
    afterload, 138n
    Frank-Starling Law, 138, *138*
    heart attack, 7, 93, 93n

Heatley, Norman, 48
hemoglobin, 174, 174n
hemorrhagic shock, 143
Henry Ford Hospital, 173, 173n, 194, 197n
Herodotus, 24
Hess, Orvan, 47
Hill, Archibald V., 146
Hill, Bradford, 101
Hill–Burton Act, 58–59
Hillier, Kathryn, 74
Hippocrates, xxii, 24–27
    Book of Prognostics, The, 26
    on fever, 26
    miasma theory, 25
    on pus, 27
    historical evolution of sepsis
        understanding, 20–28
History of Public Health, A (Rosen), 51
HIV/AIDS, 111, 112
Holmes, Oliver Wendell, 38, 292
homeostasis, 103
Homer, 24
Hooke, Robert, 30
hormones, 103–4. *See also* adrenaline
hospital(s), 31–32, 36n, 195n
    best-performing, 128
    code teams, 140–41
    emergency departments *see* emergency
        rooms/departments
    End Result system, 195n
    financial crisis of 2007–2008 impact on,
        195–96n
    hygiene in, 38–41
    infections *see* hospital-acquired infections
    intensive care services, 59, 124–25,
        127, 149
    as laboratories and hubs, 36
    standardization and monitoring, 195n
hospital-acquired infections, 35–41, 74-75,
    77, 80-81, 111, 160, 274, 304, 326. *See
    also* antimicrobial resistance (AMR)
Hospital-Based Emergency Care (Institute of
    Medicine), 159, 328–29
Hospital Inpatient Quality Reporting
    Program, 194
hospital-onset sepsis, 324–25
Hospital Quality Alliance, 194, 195
Hospital Sepsis Program Core Elements
    (CDC), 313
Hospital Standardization Program, 195n

Hôtel-Dieu, Paris, 31–32, 68
humors (vital fluids), 25
hydrocortisone, 110n, 153, 318
hygiene, 38–41, 51

I

Ibn Sina. *See* Avicenna
ICD-9-CM Coordination and Maintenance
    Committee, 188
Imhotep, 22, 24
immunoglobulin therapy, 106
Improving Pediatric Sepsis Outcomes
    Collaborative, 311–12
inequality. *See* health disparities
infection(s), 5
    control, 68n, 74–75, 274, 304, 304n,
        326, 328
    deaths, 112–13, 273n
    dehydration, 9
    opportunistic, 75–78 (*see also*
        antimicrobial resistance (AMR))
    suspected, 261n
    See also hospital-acquired infections
infection fatality rate (IFR), 273n
Infectious Diseases Society of America
    (IDSA), 292, 292n, 302, 303, 306, 321
    on metagenomic sequencing, 70
    on pathogen control, 76–77
    and SIRS concept, 121
    and SSC guidelines, 187, 191, 264–65
inflammation, 7–8
    chemicals, 86
    cytokine suppressing, 90–91
influenza, 90
    H1N1, 90, 95
    H5N1, 96, 280–81
Inpatient Quality Reporting (IQR), 252–53
insects, 25
Institute for Healthcare Improvement (IHI),
    167–68, 183–84, 195–96n, 200, 232,
    299, 312
Institute of Medicine, 183, 194
    Crossing the Quality Chasm, 165
    To Err is Human, 164–66, 168
    Hospital-Based Emergency Care,
        159, 328–29
    National Roundtable on Healthcare
        Quality, 164
IntelliSep (Cytovale), 323

intensive care, 59, 124–31, 127, 149
interleukin-6, 178n, 322
International Classification of Diseases
    (ICD-9), 59
International Pediatric Sepsis Consensus
    Conference (IPSCC), 222, 222n
International Sepsis Forum (ISF),
    168–69, 171–72
International Symposium on Intensive
    Care and Emergency Medicine
    (ISICEM), 168–69
interruptions, 266–67. *See also* errors
    (medical)
intestinal autointoxication theory, 21, 21n
Iwashyna, Theodore, 203

J

Jackson, George Gee, 84–85, 105
JAMA Health Forum, 277
JAMA Network Open, 272–73
Janeway, Charles A., 87
Janssen, Hans, 30
Janssen, Zacharias, 30
Joint Commission on Accreditation, 195n
Journal of the American Medical Association,
    85n, 238
Jukes, Thomas, 73

K

K–12 sepsis curriculum, 319
Kaiser Permanente, 193, 196, 258, 260, 264,
    270, 271, 284, 285n, 301, 307, 324
    emergency room, 217
    lactate levels monitoring, 221
    mortality from sepsis, 201, 214–15, 231
    Northwest Regional Sepsis Initiative,
        200–201, 208–10, 252
    screening tests, 218, 219
Kendall, Edward, 103n
Kerner, Justinus, 10
kidneys, 94
    Gentamicin risk on, 14n, 70
    infections as causes of sepsis, 5
    shut-down as LPS reaction, 13
Kitab al-Hawi (al-Razi), 100
Kitasato, Shibasaburo, 55
Klebs, Edwin, 42
Klebsiella pneumoniae, 54
Kline, Ronald, 299, 305

Knaus, William, 126–28, 130, 130n
Koch, Robert, 11, 43–44, 50
Kolletschka, Jakob, 38–39
Kumar, Anand, 199

L
lactate level
   decrease, 208
   elevation, 147–48, 219, 220
   mortality and, 219–21, *220*
lactic acid, 145–48
Laënnec, Rene, 136
Lancet, 42, 71, 329
Latta, Thomas, 142
Lawler, James, 281
Laws of Medicine, The (Mukherjee),
   16, 293–94
Leapfrog Group, 293
Le Dran, Henri Francois, 4
Leeuwenhoek, Antonie van, 30
leukocytosis, 9, 123
Levy, Mitchell, 169–72, 190, 206, 225, 226,
   237, 321
   and VERICC Task Force, 188
   and sepsis awareness raising, 181–83, 184
lifeguarding, 161–64, 334-335
lipopolysaccharide (LPS), 12–13, 86, 90
Lippershey, Hans, 30
Lister, Joseph, 42, 45, 80
Liu, Vincent, 264
Lower, Richard, 142
lung injury, 61. *See also* acute respiratory
   distress syndrome (ARDS)

M
machine learning systems. *See* artificial
   intelligence (AI) tools
macrophages, 85
Majno, Guido, *35*
malaise, 8
Malcolm, Ian, 68
MALDI-TOF mass spectrometry, 70
Marshall, John, 101, 106–7n, 109n, 116, 119,
   121n, 131n
Martin, Franklin, 195n
mastoiditis, 230
Mate, Kedar, 299
maternal sepsis, 290–92
Maxon, Thelma, 69

McCabe, William, 84–85, 105
McHenry, Justin, 163
mean arterial pressure (MAP), 4, 139
measles, 52n
Measure Applications Partnership, 166
Medicaid/ Medicare, *see* Centers
   for Medicare and Medicaid
   Services (CMS)
medical billing codes, 188
Medicare Modernization Act, 194
Memoires sur les Hopitaux de Paris
   (Tenon), 31
meningitis, 100
Menkin, Valy, 86
metabolism, aerobic, 146–47
metagenomic sequencing, 70
Metchnikoff, Elie, 85–86
methicillin-resistant *S. aureus* (MRSA), 69,
   71n, 111, 133, 145
methylprednisolone, 114
Meyerhof, Otto, 146
miasma, 25–26
Micrographia (Hooke), 30
microscope(s), 29–30
Miller, Anne, 47, 48, 69
Minimum Standards for Hospitals, 195n
Mondeville, Henri de, 28
Moore, Judy Kay, 187n
morbidity, 203–4, 208
Morris, Peter, 188
mortality, 126–31, *130, 131,* 213–14,
   231, 329–31
   clinical trial patients, 116
   intermediate-risk sepsis
     population, 201–2
   lactate level and, 219–21, *220*
   measure, 307–8
   Xigris, 178
Mukherjee, Siddhartha, xii, 16, 55, 293–94
multiple-organ dysfunction syndrome
   (MODS), 132, 312
mummification, 21
Murphy, Edward A., 58
Mycobacterium tuberculosis, 44

N
Naghavi, Mohsen, 79
*National Action Plan for Combating Antibiotic-
   Resistant Bacteria,* 304

National Family Council on Sepsis, 243
National Guidelines Clearinghouse, 181
National Healthcare Safety Network
    (NHSN), 166, 310
National Institute of General Medical
    Sciences, 320
National Institutes of Health (NIH), 59,
    190, 197
National Quality Forum (NQF), 195,
    292–93, 293n
    Consensus Development Process,
      165, 236
    endorsement process, 240–41
    funding sources, 165n
    measure #0500, 195, 235–42, 247–48 (*see
      also* SEP-1)
    as a public–private partnership, 165
    Serious Reportable Events in Healthcare, 166
National Roundtable on Healthcare
    Quality, 164
Nature, 96
necrotizing fasciitis, 26
Neufeld's *Quellung* reaction, 56, 56n
neutrophil extracellular traps (NET), 122
neutrophils, 122–23, 123n, 259, 268
New England Journal of Medicine, The, 67,
    70n, 87, 114, 182n, 186, 189, 249, 275
New York State Sepsis Initiative, 232–34,
    249–50, 260
New York Times, 217, 230
Nightingale, Florence, 124
nitric oxide, 148
noncommunicable diseases, 79
noradrenaline/norepinephrine, 103. *See also*
    adrenaline
Northwell Health, 232

O
Obama, Barack, 242
Ofri, Danielle, 39n, 49
O'Grady, Naomi, 187
Ogston, Alexander, 42–43
Oliver, George, 102
Omnibus Appropriations (2023) bill, 313
Omran, Abdel, 77n
Operation Warp Speed, 280
organ perfusion, 174n
Osborn, Larry, 267–68
Osler, William, 49–50, 54, 84, 86–87

oxygen delivery to organs, 174–75

P
Pacini, Filippo, 11
Pakyz, Amy, 302–3, 304
pandemics (viral), 95–96
    COVID-19 pandemic, 75, 95–96, 271–80,
      283–84, 284n
    H1N1 influenza strain, 90, 95
    H5N1 avian influenza, 96, 280–81
Panthagani, Kristen, 276n, 277
Parran, Thomas, 57
Pasteur, Louis, 41–42, 50, 51
PASTEUR Act, 327
pasteurization, 42
pathogen-associated molecular patterns
    (PAMP), 87–88, 90, 93, 95, 108, 176
patient
    advocacy groups, 298
    characteristics, 78–80
    safety, 166–67
Patient Safety and Quality Improvement
    Act, 166
Pattern Recognition Hypothesis, 87
pattern-recognizing receptors (PRR), 87
pay-for-performance programs,
    194–95, 195n
pediatric sepsis. *See* children with sepsis
penicillin, 47–48, 57, 68–69, 71, 72
    anti-staphylococcal, 69
    attacking bacterial cell, 62
    industrialization, 48
penicillin-resistant *S. aureus* (PRSA), 69
pepsis, 25
peptidoglycan, 4–5n, 48
perforated intestine, 32–33
péripneumonie, 136
Pfeiffer, Richard, 11
phagocytosis, 122
phagolysosomes, 122
Phoenix Sepsis Criteria, 311
Piorry, Pierre Adolphe, 36–37
pirotossina, 12
plasmids, 71
platelets, 92. *See also* blood coagulation
pneumonia, 52–58
    antiserum therapy, 53–57
    causes, 55–56, 62
    community-acquired, 61, 322

public education campaigns, 57
time to first antibiotic dose (TFAD), 265
premature closure, 217, 265. *See also* errors
    (medical)
Prenosis, 323
Prescott, Hallie, 301n
PRISM, 245, 246
procalcitonin, 323, 323n
ProCESS, 197–98, 243, 245–47, 248, 253
ProPublica, 291
PROWESS, 177–80, 186
PROWESS-SHOCK, 225–26, 226n
Prozac, 187
Pseudomonas aeruginosa, 288
puerperal sepsis, 37–39
pulse oximetry, 290
pus, 27–28, 42
    putrefaction, 20, 24–25, 36, 41. *See
    also* historical evolution of sepsis
    understanding
pyrexin, 86
pyruvate, 146

R
racial disparities, 80, 289–90
Rammelkamp, Charles H., 69
Ramsay, Graham, 170
RAND Corporation, 165
randomized clinical trial (RCT), 100, 101
    equipoise, 215, 215n
    procalcitonin-guided sepsis
        protocols, 323
Redi, Francesco, 41
Reichstein, Tadeusz, 103, 103n
relative risk reduction (RRR), 275n
REMAP-CAP trial, 278
resuscitation. *See* fluid resuscitation
ribonucleic acid (RNA), 90
"Riddle of Sepsis, The" (Majno), 35
Rinicker, Elaine, 169
Rivers, Emanuel, 173–76, 194–97, 197n, 235,
    240, 243, 245–46, 292n, 293, 319, 325
    on time zero, 237
Roe v. Wade, 291
Rogers, David E., 67–68, 76, 80
Rory's Regulations, 234, 235, 242
Rosen, George, 51
Rosen, William, 71
Rosenbach, Anton J., 43

Roth, Eric, 221
Roux, Emile, 11, 55
Rubenfeld, Gordon, 205
Rudd, Kristina, 79
Rumpel, Eva, 146

S
Safar, Peter, 125
saline, 13–14, 14n
Salmonella, 73
Salmonella typhi, 12
Sanford, Jay P., 85n
Santy, Paul, 142
sarilumab, 278
SARS-CoV-1, 96, 272
SARS-CoV-2. *See* COVID-19 pandemic
Schafer, Edward, 102
Scheele, Karl Wilhelm, 145
Scherer, Johann Joseph, 146
Schmidt, David, 193, 196, 213, 252, 283
Schottmuller, Hugo, 44–45
Schumer, Charles, 229, 235, 320
selectins, 122
Semmelweis, Ignaz, 38–41, 80, 292, 313
sensitivity of medical tests, 218
SEP-1, 248–50, **249,** 258, 260, 274, 292–93,
    298, 301–3, 305–8, 311–15, 321
    alert system, 284
    as a mandate, 252–53
    non-shock sepsis patients, 285–86
    opposition to, 264–65
    performance analysis, 284–87
    using outdated criteria, 257
sepflation, 254, 308, 309
sepsis, 3–4, 118–22
    causes, 5
    conditions, 330
    as a continuum, 132, *132*
    diagnosing *see* diagnosing sepsis
    as a disease within disease, 20
    end-of-life scenario, 311
    etymology, 20
    funding, 320
    as a heterogeneous disorder, 109–10, 116,
        121, 244
    historical evolution of
        understanding, 20–28
    maternal, 290–92
    misperceptions, 234–35

morbidity, 203–4

mortality *see* mortality

as orphan disease, 319, 320

pediatric *see* children with sepsis.

pepsis *vs.*, 25

prevention, 325–30

puerperal sepsis, 37–39

signs and symptoms, 7

survivors, 202–3

See also specific entries

Sepsis 1, 120–21, 129, 133, 168, 177, 246, 253–54

Sepsis 2, 169–70, 206, 254

Sepsis 3, 253, 254–58, 258n, 318

SEPSIS Act, 320

Sepsis Alliance, 190–91, 208, 232, 293, 319

sepsis-associated encephalopathy (SAE), 269n

sepsis bundles, 167, 300–301

  compliance, 212–13, 313

  dose-response effect, 214

  ethical and logistical difficulties, 215

  implementing, 206–7

  management, 184, **184**

  process-based care, 300–301

  resuscitation, 184, **184**

  sicker patients, 300n

Sepsis ImmunoScore, 323, 324–25

sepsis-induced myocardial dysfunction (SIMD), 140, 140n

Sepsis Scout, 325

Sepsis Transition and Recovery (STAR), 311n

septic shock, 4, 12–13, 57, 142

  blood creatinine level, 115

  blood vessel dysfunction, 139–40

  cryptic patient, 207n

  intermediate-risk patients, 207

  levels, 129n

  management, 150

  prevention, 195, 207

  protocolized shock treatment, 152

  steroids, 114, 129n

  vasopressors, 143

  See also early goal-directed therapy (EGDT)

Sequential Organ Failure Assessment (SOFA), 257, 257n, 323

Serious Reportable Events in Healthcare (NQF), 166

severity-of-illness scoring systems, 126–27

sex (as a contributor to sepsis risk), 79

sex hormones, 104

Shah, Nirav, 231–34, 250, 280, 280n, 296

Shapiro, Nathan, 219

shock, 4, 141–44

  endotoxic, 12–13, 64, 85, 93, 109, 111, 268

  septic *see* septic shock

  traumatic, 137, 150–52, 174

Shoemaker, William, 150–52

Sibbald, William J., 118, 119

Siegel, Jay P., 180, 180n

signal-to-noise ratio, 253, 253n

SIRS. *See* systemic inflammatory response syndrome (SIRS)

Social Security Amendments of 1965, 59

Society for Healthcare Epidemiology of America (SHEA), 74, 292n

Society of Critical Care Medicine, 118, 172, 188

Spallanzani, Lazzaro, 41

Spanish flu. *See* H1N1 influenza strain

Special Study Group on Gram-Negative Bacteremia, 107–8

specificity and sensitivity of medical tests, 218

spontaneous generation theory, 25, 28, 36, 41

Sprung, Charles L., 118

Staphylococci, 43

  Staphylococcus aureus, 43, 49, 68, 74

  Staphylococcus epidermidis, 77n

  Staphylococcus sepsis, 144

Starling, Ernest, 138

Staunton, Rory, 89, 172, 211–12, 216–17, 221, 224, 228–30, 315

  parents of, 216–17, 216n, 229–30, 232, 233n, 235, 242–43, 313, 337

  See also Rory's Regulations

steroids, 116

Stewart, Ian, 311

Stone, Judy, 226

Stop Sepsis, 216, 216n, 217

Streptococcus, 39

  Streptococcus pneumoniae, 55–56, 62

  Streptococcus pyogenes, xvi, 89–90, 228, 317

  Streptomyces griseus, 72

stroke, 3

Study on the Efficacy of Nosocomial
Infection Control Project (SENIC), 74
succus, 33–34
sulfapyridine, 57
superantigens, 89–90
surveillance bias, 111n
Surviving Sepsis Campaign (SSC), 164, 172,
198–99, 298
controversy, 185–92
database, 184–85
Dellinger on, 189
funding, 181–82
GRADE, 196–97
guidelines, 181, 182–84, 196–97
IDSA and, 187, 191
learning and performance improvement
collaboratives, 185
lifesaving therapies, 182
NQF #0500, 195
performance measures, 185
quality improvement program, 182–84
resistance against, 227
self-evident therapies, 196–97
sepsis bundles, 184, **184**, 212–13, 227, **227**
terminating sponsorship and financial
ties, 191
Townsend and, 184, 191, 195, 235–38,
292n, 293, 301
treatment recommendations, 182
Xigris (drotrecogin alfa), 186–90, 197, 198
syphilis, 51
systemic inflammatory response syndrome
(SIRS), 119–21, 170, 253–55
clinical case of Miguel, 117–18,
122–24, 132–34
controversy/skepticism around, 121–22,
130–32, 206, 227–28
epidemiologists on, 214
IDSA on, 121
IPSCC pediatric sepsis definition, 222n
noninfectious conditions, 206
screening process, 207–8, 218–19
systemic vascular resistance (SVR), 139

T
tachycardia, 32
Tenon, Jacques, 31–32, 36
Thomas, Lewis, 87-88
Thomas, Vivien, 137

Thompson, Tommy, 188
thrombus, 92, 93
Tiffany, Sandra, 188, 190
time to first antibiotic dose (TFAD), 265
tissue factor, 92
tocilizumab, 278
To Err is Human (Institute of Medicine),
164–66, 168
Townsend, Sean, 183–84, 191, 195, 235–38,
292n, 293, 301
toxins, 10–13
bacterial, 10n
as biological poisons, 10
botulinum, 10–11
fever, 12
Tracey, Kevin, 232, 315
traumatic shock, 137, 150–52
golden hour, 151, 174
tuberculosis, 43–45, 101, 112
tumor necrosis factor-alpha (TNF-α),
107, 177n
typhoid, 51

U
United Nations Ad Hoc Interagency
Coordination Group on Antimicrobial
Resistance, 71
United States Department of Health and
Human Services, 242
United States Lifesaving Association
(USLA), 163–64
United States Veterans Affairs Medical
Centers, 304n
University of New Mexico Hospital,
218–19, 254
urinary tract infections (UTI), 5–6

V
vaccination, 278
and AMR, 327, 329
mRNA vaccines, 275–76, 275n
historical importance, 51–52
and pneumonia, 57
Value-Based Purchasing Program, 253, 305
Values, Ethics & Rationing in Critical Care
(VERICC) Task Force, 188
van Beneden, Pierre-Joseph, 77–78n
vancomycin-resistant *Enterococcus*
(VRE), 111

van Ermengem, Emile Pierre-Marie, 10
Varro, Marcus Terentius, 26
vasopressors, 143
ventricular fibrillation, 154, 154n
Vibrio cholerae, 11
Vibrio vulnificus, 26–27
Vienna General Hospital, 38–39
Vincent, Jean-Louis, 257
Virchow, Rudolf, 8n, 42
von Willebrand factor (vWF), 92, 93

W
waiver of consent, 215n
Wall Street Journal, 197n
water treatment program, 51
Watts, Amy, 259, 263, 266–69, 283–84,
    295, 334
Weil, Max Henry, 147, 150
Weiss, Scott, 222, 223, 312
When We Do Harm (Ofri), 39n, 49
white blood cells, 105–6, 119, 123, 222n,
    290, 323
  inflammatory cytokines, 87
  macrophages, 85–86
  neutrophils, 122–23, 123n, 259, 268
  non-septic patients, 217
  Rory's blood tests, 216, 217
Will Rogers effect, 214, 254
World Health Organization (WHO), 40, 59,
    80–81, 272, 280, 291, 326
  Global Burden of Disease patient
    database, 289
World Medical Association, 19
World Sepsis Day, 241–42
wound care, 21–24
Wunderlich, Carl Reinhold August, 9n

X
Xigris (drotrecogin alfa), 225–27, 244, 318,
    319, 325
  anticoagulant mechanism, 179
  bleeding complications, 198n
  diagnostic codes and, 188–89
  efficacy, 177–80
  European Medicines Agency (EMA)
    and, 198
  FDA review and approval, 178–80, 186,
    188, 225
  market withdrawal, 225

  mechanism of action, 225
  mortality, 178
  new technology status, 188
  PROWESS, 177–80, 186, 226
  PROWESS-SHOCK, 225–26, 226n
  recombinant DNA technology, 177
  sales, 187
  SSC's recommendation, 186–90, 197, 198

Y
Yersin, Alexandre, 11

Z
zona fasciculata, 104
zona glomerulosa, 104
zona reticularis, 104

About the Author

Dr. Parsa Shahinpoor is a frontline hospitalist, teaching physician, and quality improvement leader at Kaiser Permanente Northwest, where he has spent nearly two decades advancing sepsis care—a role that has connected him with experts around the world. He completed his medical training at the University of New Mexico School of Medicine, where he served as an assistant professor of medicine and director of the internal medicine medical student clerkship. Blending science, history, and narrative, he writes to make one of medicine's most urgent challenges vivid and accessible.